Evaluation of
Health Promotion
and Education Programs

Evaluation of
Health Promotion
and Education Programs

RICHARD A. WINDSOR
University of Alabama, Birmingham
School of Public Health

THOMAS BARANOWSKI
University of Texas Medical Branch
Division of Preventive Medicine and Community Health

NOREEN CLARK
University of Michigan
School of Public Health

GARY CUTTER
University of Alabama, Birmingham
School of Public Health

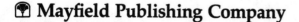 Mayfield Publishing Company

Library of Congress Catalog Card Number: 83-062834
International Standard Book Number: 0-87484-561-0

Manufactured in the United States of America
10 9 8 7 6 5 4 3 2 1

Mayfield Publishing Company
285 Hamilton Avenue
Palo Alto, California 94301

Sponsoring editor: C. Lansing Hays
Manuscript editor: Zipporah W. Collins
Managing editor: Pat Herbst
Art director: Nancy Sears
Designer: Michael Rogondino
Cover designer: Michael Rogondino
Illustrator: Pat Rogondino
Production manager: Cathy Willkie
Compositor: G&S Typesetters, Inc.
Printer and binder: Bookcrafters

Contents

Preface

This book focuses on the technical skills that staff members of health promotion programs can use to evaluate their programs. It has been prepared for several audiences: (1) senior undergraduate and master's level students specializing in health education and related social and behavioral sciences, (2) students in health-related fields enrolled in health education program evaluation courses, and (3) practitioners in the field, including health educators, nurses, physicians, and allied health professionals who are responsible for planning, implementing, and evaluating health education or health promotion programs.

Better documentation and assessment of program impacts and processes will be needed as technology increases and society expects reasonable returns for efforts invested in health education and promotion. Community health programs will be expected to demonstrate effectiveness, and program planners will be held more and more accountable for their efforts, particularly in a period of diminishing resources. The paucity of self-contained literature for practitioners, policymakers, funders, and program planners on achieving more rigorous evaluations of community health promotion and disease prevention programs provided the impetus for this text.

Three major documents were used as guiding sources for the content: "Guidelines for the Preparation and Practice of Professional Health Educators," developed by the Society for Public Health Education (1977); the role specification section for evaluators of the *Initial Role Delineation for Health Education: Final Report*, prepared for the National Center for Health Education under contract with the Department of Health and Human Services (U.S. DHHS, Public Health Service, 1980a), reprinted as appendix B of this book; and *Promoting Health/Preventing Disease: Objectives for the Nation*, by the U.S. DHHS, Public Health Service (1980c), which specifies quantitative objectives in fifteen areas of particular use to community health promotion programs in the 1980s.

We believe that a dramatic improvement in the qualitative, quantitative, and analytical skills of practitioners in health education and health promotion will occur in the 1980s. Those who lack technical competence will not reflect the state of the art in their practice and will not be as competitive in the marketplace. Through analysis of individual program experiences, evaluators will expand the knowledge base in the field; by sharing concepts, such as those discussed in this text, through the professional literature, they can improve the practice of health education and promotion. This may, in turn, improve an individual's or organization's ability to affect policies and resource allocations relating to health promotion.

This book fills an apparent gap in the literature on evaluation of health promotion programs; it is a dissemination document for use in health education training programs and by practitioners in the field. Health education specialists who develop the technical skills to plan, implement, and evaluate programs and to collaborate with other professionals will achieve greater professional success, will enhance the profession, and will play a more significant role in achieving the health objectives of the United States in the 1980s.

Chapter 1, "An Introduction to Evaluation," sets the stage by discussing the evaluation movement, particularly over the last two decades. A common set of evaluation terms and a description of three interrelated levels of evaluation are introduced. The purposes and expectations of program evaluation are considered. Particular attention is given to encouraging program planners to set more realistic program objectives and to appreciate the role of politics in program planning and evaluation. The philosophical and ideological orientations of program directors and planners and their impact on what an evaluator can accomplish are discussed. We examine the continuing issue of underutilization and nonutilization of evaluation reports and studies by policymakers and why this happens. The realization that every program evaluation cannot and should not be conducted as a clinical trial (an experimental study with randomized treatment and control groups) is stressed. Both qualitative and quantitative evaluation methods are important for improving the effectiveness of health education and promotion programs.

Chapter 2, "Conducting Evaluations and Promoting Organizational Change," discusses how to approach an evaluation as a staff member within an organization. Emphasis is given to identifying: (1)

the purposes of the evaluation, (2) the organizational structure and principal decision makers, (3) how major program decisions are made, (4) the role staff persons see the evaluator playing, (5) what is necessary to encourage decision makers to promote and accept change within the organization, (6) who the evaluator's major audiences are, and (7) what behavior changes are possible within the organization and by the social group for whom the program is planned.

Chapter 3, "Health Education Program Planning and Planning for Evaluation," presents the principles of program planning as they relate to evaluation. Of concern here, and in the "real world," is the question: Can the staff of this organization implement a particular program and evaluate it? The "staff" may consist of only one person, for example. The steps used to develop a plan of work are identified, and methods to create a plan are proposed.

Chapter 4, "Conducting Process Evaluations," identifies a number of procedures for conducting a quality assurance review of a program. Periodic audits of the procedures used to implement a program must be performed. We examine the planning and conduct of formative assessments of program content, methods, materials, and media, using qualitative and quantitative approaches.

Chapter 5, "Evaluating Program Effectiveness," discusses the importance of having a preconceived evaluation design and explains how to select an appropriate one. Getting the most out of what is available—which is usually more than the program staff thinks is possible—is a theme of this chapter. Emphasis is placed on examining problems and constraints of the real world. The concepts of internal and external validity, selection of the control or comparison group, and decisions about sample size and statistical power are examined. Methods to adapt the scientific method to a practice setting are explored. We suggest ways to organize a community program to control for common problems that may confound results. Complex concepts and procedures are broken down into their most basic and practical elements for use in meeting day-to-day program issues. Dimensions and issues of design that are often unfamiliar to the practitioner but are directly applicable to practice settings are provided. Case examples illustrate applications of all the principles and methods presented.

Chapter 6, "Issues in Data Collection," deals with another common problem area in program planning and implementation: determining what data to collect and how to collect them. Special attention is given to how to select and develop an instrument or questionnaire and the importance of identifying existing instruments and data collection methods from similar programs. Types of validity and reliability are discussed. Specifying what data are to be collected, collecting data of high quality, and employing sound methods of data collection are the core concepts emphasized in this chapter.

Chapter 7, "Methods of Data Collection," discusses the various methods and identifies the strengths and weaknesses (biases) of each. Consideration is given to other issues in method selection. Several straightforward steps for developing an instrument and implementing the method are outlined. The various methods are considered in two broad categories: obtrusive and unobtrusive data collection.

Chapter 8, "Simple Techniques for Analyzing Program Data," discusses commonly used statistical techniques for analyzing data. The techniques and skills presented represent those within the capabilities of a graduate-trained person. While individuals involved in large-scale evaluation research or clinical trial studies usually employ a variety of complex analytical techniques, most programs are faced with two or three basic questions requiring less statistical sophistication. The determination of program impact, however, requires a comprehension of statistical tests and the ability to apply analytical techniques to interpret data. The issue of statistical significance versus program importance is addressed in this chapter.

Appendix A, "The Health Education Evaluation Report," discusses the basic purposes and elements of an evaluation report. Report writers need to determine in advance who should receive the report and learn the explicit expectations of key personnel (e.g., policymakers, administrators, and contract officers) before preparing interim and final reports. It is advantageous to reach agreement beforehand on the format, length, and depth of the report and its various subsections.

Appendix B, "Specification of the Role of Entry-Level Health Educator, Area of Responsibility V: Evaluating Health Education," describes the minimum functions, skills, and knowledge (i.e., the credentials) necessary to evaluate health education and promotion programs.

Appendix C, "First Principles of Cost-Effectiveness Analysis in Health," is a nontechnical discussion of the principles and procedures used to conduct cost analyses of health promotion and disease prevention programs. Comprehension of and ability to apply the knowledge embodied in this report are essential areas of mastery for the health educator of the 1980s and 1990s.

Acknowledgments

We would like to express our gratitude to our colleagues who read preliminary drafts of the chapters in this book, shared their insights with us, and gave us many valuable suggestions. Our thanks to: Lillian H. Bajda, Edward E. Bartlett, Mary K. Chelton, Myra Crawford, William H. Creswell, Jr., Sigrid G. Deeds, Rosalind J. Dworkin, Michael P. Eriksen, Brian S. Flynn, Teneke Freni, Nell H. Gottlieb, Godfrey M. Hochbaum, James Kouzes, Brick Lancaster, Kevin McCaul, Paul Mico, Joyce Morris, Patricia D. Mullen, Hod D. Ogden, Thomas W. O'Rourke, Marcia G. Ory, Marcia L. Pinkett-Heller, Amelia G. Ramirez, Edward J. Roccella, Karen Rosenberg, Wendy D. Squyres, Frank Willard, Joan Wolle, Rose Yunker, and Jane Zapka.

The text also benefited from the critical reading given by these reviewers: Charles R. Baffi of Virginia Polytechnic Institute and State University, Lorraine G. Davis of the University of Oregon, Robert S. Gold of Southern Illinois University at Carbondale, Don Iverson of Mercy Medical Center in Denver, Jennie J. Kronenfeld of the University of South Carolina, and James H. Price of the University of Toledo.

We would like to thank Marjorie Sorenson for her secretarial assistance. We would like to especially acknowledge the administrative and secretarial assistance of Dorothy Liddell.

1

An Introduction to Evaluation

"We know what needs to be done in health education. The big question is how to evaluate it."

"It was hard to develop conclusions because the program kept changing as we were trying to evaluate it."

"The exciting part was to see our assumptions borne out by the data, both statistically and in the comments of the people surveyed."

"It was rewarding to show our board that our program worked. Knowing about designs really helped."

The purpose of this book is to examine the underlying theories, principles, methods, and procedures used to plan and carry out an evaluation of the educational, informational, and behavioral components of a health promotion program.

As noted in *Promoting Health/Preventing Disease: Objectives for the Nation* (U.S. DHHS, Public Health Service, 1980b), consensus exists on broad national goals for improving the health of Americans for the remainder of the decade. Based on the efforts of over 500 individuals and numerous organizations, this federal document established objectives for 15 priority areas: (1) high blood pressure control, (2) family planning, (3) pregnancy and infant health, (4) immunization, (5) sexually transmitted diseases, (6) toxic agent control, (7) occupational safety and health, (8) accident prevention and injury control, (9) fluoridation and dental health, (10) surveillance and control of infectious diseases, (11) smoking and health, (12) misuse of alcohol and drugs, (13) physical fitness and exercise, (14) control of stress, and (15) violent behavior.

Objectives for the Nation offers the planner and evaluator a thorough discussion of prevention and promotion measures and their relative effectiveness. Education and information, service, technological, legislative and regulatory, and economic measures are specified for each of the 15 priority areas. Program evaluation and evaluation research are identified as essential requirements in the 1980s to advance knowledge of the most effective and efficient means of achieving these objectives. This text discusses salient issues common to evaluating each of the identified health promotion/disease prevention areas and others that an organization or individuals may select.

In this chapter we introduce a number of basic concepts. A set of common definitions used in discussing evaluation are presented. To give you an idea of what is happening in the field of program evaluation and health education, we examine discussions in the past literature and review the history of the evaluation movement during the last two decades. The more recent gestational period of the 1970s is briefly examined to give you an idea of where evaluation is now and where it needs to go. The level of professional competence in evaluation now required by health specialists is explored. Over the years evaluation skills have been considered essential for a master's degree in health education. We present the various levels of evaluation organized into a hierarchy: process evaluation, program evaluation, and evaluation research. Finally, the purposes of program evaluation, the role of evaluation in an organization, the uses of program evaluation reports, and the importance of setting realistic goals and developing feasible program plans are examined.

EVALUATION TERMINOLOGY

In evaluation, as in most specialty fields, a set of common terms has developed. An understanding of each is essential to comprehend the evaluation literature. The following terms are frequently used in this text with the meanings specified here:

> *Formative evaluation*: An evaluation that produces information used during the developmental stages of a health education program, to improve it. A common procedure in a formative evaluation is conducting a pilot study, using alternative methods of assessing the immediate or short-term cognitive, affective, or psychomotor (skill) effects of elements of the program.
>
> *Process evaluation*: An evaluation that provides documentation on what is going on in a program and confirms the existence and availability of physical and structural elements of the program. It is part of a formative evaluation and assesses whether specific elements, such as facilities, staff, space, or services, are being provided or being established according to the given program plan. In the clinical vernacular, a process evaluation might be referred to as a *quality assurance review* or study (QAR). Process evaluation involves documentation and description of specific program activities—how much of what, for whom, when, and by whom. It includes monitoring the frequency of participation by the target population and is used to confirm the frequency and extent of implementation of selected programs or program elements. Process evaluation derives evidence from staff, consumers, or outside evaluators on the quality of the implementation plan and on the appropriateness of content, methods, materials, media, and instruments. Some reports refer to this type of evaluation as *efficiency evaluation* or *quality monitoring*.
>
> *Summative evaluation*: An evaluation that provides a summary statement of a health promotion program's effectiveness over a specified period of time. It enables decision makers to plan and allocate resources.
>
> *Program impact evaluation*: An evaluation that assesses the overall effectiveness of a program in producing favorable cognitive, belief, and behavioral effects in the target population. It measures the relative effectiveness of different types of programs in meeting selected objectives—for example, decreases in smoking by adolescents, or increases in use of maternity health services by pregnant women. Its principal purpose is to determine whether

changes have occurred over time in the dependent variable and if the changes can be attributed to program efforts.

Health outcome evaluation: An evaluation that assesses changes or improvement in morbidity, mortality, or other health status indicators for a specified group of people. Because of the natural history of most contemporary chronic diseases, health status indicators may not be the end point of a health promotion program unless the program has sufficient resources and continues for several years.

Effectiveness: A measure of the extent to which the program achieves its preestablished, measurable objectives; i.e., did it work?

Efficiency: A measure of the cost in resources to accomplish program objectives; i.e., how much did it cost to achieve what? This may be expressed in a number of ways, such as a ratio between input and output or cost per unit.

Cost-effectiveness analysis: Determination of the relationship between observed outcomes and program cost, expressed as cost per unit of impact achieved.

Intervention: A planned and systematically applied combination of program elements designed to produce cognitive, affective, skill, behavior, or health status changes among individuals exposed at a specified site and during a specified period.

Internal validity: The degree to which an observed effect can be attributed to an intervention.

External validity: The degree to which an observed effect that is attributable to an intervention can be generalized to similar populations and settings.

THE EVALUATION MOVEMENT

The interest, energy, and resources spent on evaluating health programs have been considerable, particularly in the last two decades. The interest in evaluating health education and promotion programs has paralleled the interest in public health and in health care. At present, almost without exception, programs are expected to include some type of evaluation plan.

Awareness of the importance of evaluating health education and promotion programs is not a contemporary phenomenon; leaders in the field have been saying for a full generation that evaluation is needed. Several early comprehensive statements about evaluating programs designed to produce changes in health behavior were presented by Rosenstock (1960), Roberts (1962), and Young (1968). The need to perceive evaluation as a diagnostic process and the need to improve both the quality and the quantity of empirical work were put forth throughout the 1960s by Hochbaum (1962, 1965), Campbell and Stanley (1966), Campbell (1969), Steuart (1965, 1969), Suchman (1967), Deniston and Rosenstock (1968a, 1968b), Schulberg, Sheldon, and Baker (1969), and Cochran (1969). Throughout that decade, program evaluation and evaluation research were perceived by many in the health field as areas of considerable interest and future growth in the United States.

The close relationship between program planning and program evaluation and the salience of making educational diagnoses as part of the planning and evaluation process have received consistent emphasis. Yet the health education literature of the 1950s and 1960s has only a few empirical examples of rigorous evaluation studies. Early reports noted this conspicuous absence. A recurring concern has been that the health education profession has in the past relied principally on evaluations that measured how much effort or how many resources were put into a program or described how the program was conducted—structure and process efforts. Behavioral results were seldom evident, and changes attributable to program inputs, if evident, were seldom unequivocal.

The gap between scientific theory and professional practice is another issue frequently expressed in literature on program evaluation and in social and behavioral science research. Sophisticated and rigorous quantitative methods, well described in research texts, often fall short in examining dimensions of programs whose focus is not a planned behavior change. The problems of adapting a broad range of social and behavioral science methods to evaluate health programs and the influence of values on evaluation are as apparent today as they were up to 25 years ago (Knutson, 1959; Young, 1968; Campbell, 1969; Baric, 1972, 1980; Green, 1977; Mullen and Iverson, 1980; and Windsor et al., 1980).

The *Report of the President's Committee on Health Education* (Larry, 1973) provided documentation of the paucity of evaluation literature in health education and promotion. This state-of-the-art report identified the need for the profession to emphasize determining the effectiveness and efficiency of health education programs in a variety of settings, including schools, hospitals, community health clinics, and industries. National interest in evaluation was also stimulated by reports such as *Promoting Health: Consumer Education and National Policy* (Somers, 1976), from the Task Force on Consumer Health Education. The need for far greater precision in furthering the state of the art was the basis for recommendation 6 of the task force report: "Provide federal support for research and development in consumer health education techniques, methodologies, and programs, and their evaluation." Although much discussion of the importance of evaluation took place from 1955 to 1975, few reports of rigorous health education evaluations appeared in the United States until the early 1970s. The literature suggested that the dissemination and application of evaluation principles, concepts, and methods in planning health education programs lagged behind the underlying disciplines of communication, sociology, psychology, and epidemiology.

EVALUATION ON THE CUSP

The 1970s represented a gestational period for evaluation research and program evaluation in health education and health promotion. Federal and private agencies began to include evaluation as part of practically all demonstration projects. Seminal works by Rossi and Williams (1972), Weiss (1972, 1973a, 1973b), Arnold (1973), Deniston and Rosenstock (1973), Green et al. (1975), Rosenstock (1975), Cook and Campbell (1983), Shortell and Richardson (1978), Schulberg and Baker (1979), and Rossi et al. (1979) reflect the degree of interest in evaluation during the past decade. The current interest in evaluation of components of health promotion programs is largely a reflection of a broader national interest in the topic. Formal evaluation is increasingly perceived by administrators as the principal method for program accountability and decision making (Michnich et al., 1981).

A survey of 23 consumer health programs by Arthur D. Little, Inc., in 1976, indicated that the field had witnessed a surge of evaluation studies. Program evaluation was identified as an essential element by the National Health Planning and Resources Act of 1975 (Public Law 93–641) and the National Consumer Health Information and Health Promotion Act of 1976 (Public Law 94–317). As a follow-up to Public Law 94–317, procedures for evaluating community health education programs were recommended for health planning groups (Sullivan, 1977). Almost without exception, presentations at national health education meetings during the middle and late 1970s suggested that the methodology of program evaluation had moved beyond the rudimentary stage and was improving in quality. Reports from the International Union of Health Education (IUHE) meetings in Paris (1973), Ottawa (1976), London (1979), and Hobart, Australia (1982), also highlighted evaluation and the pervasive interest in the subject internationally.

The need to develop a literature base through the standardization of procedures, strengthening of designs, and replication of studies in a variety of settings was a consistent theme in the literature of the last decade. To expand on the existing knowledge base in research and evaluation in health education, Zapka (1982) has suggested the following: (1) continued commitment to rigorously controlled experimental and quasi-experimental designs in evaluative research studies; (2) increased attention to and application of qualitative research strategies; (3) increased attention to integration of formative and summative approaches to evaluation design; (4) diversification of the settings in which evaluative research studies are conducted and of the focuses of investigation; (5) increased case studies by field practitioners, to demonstrate modest evaluation strategies applied to well-planned programs; (6) evaluation studies placed in a larger, health education, quality assurance framework; and (7) rigorous analysis of critical broad issues related to research and evaluation.

Several evaluation studies that have been reported in recent years represent successful models of large-scale community health education programs: the North Karelia Cardiovascular Risk Reduction Projects of 1972–78 in Finland (Puska et al., 1979), the Stanford Heart Disease Prevention Study of 1973–76 in California (Farquhar et al., 1977), and the Multiple Risk Factor Intervention Trial (MRFIT) of 1974–82 (Neaton et al., 1981). Selected aspects of these and recent smaller scale health education evaluations by Baranowski et al. (1980), Windsor et al. (1980), Windsor (1981), Clark et al., (1981), and Windsor and Cutter (1981) are presented in later chapter discussions. These studies point to the value and feasibility of planned designs and methods in evaluating health promotion programs and education efforts.

PROFESSIONAL COMPETENCE

Professionals and training institutions have consistently perceived competence in evaluation methods as a major skill of graduate-trained, health education specialists. The function of evaluation was first identified by the American Public Health Association Committee on Professional Education (1957). Evaluation techniques have long been identified as critically important and an integral component of health and community service programs by standard-setting organizations such as the World Health Organization (1954, 1969), the American Public Health Association (1957), the Association of Schools of Public Health (Boatman et al., 1966), the International Union for Health Education (Kaplun-le Meitour, 1973), and the Society for Public Health Education (1968, 1977a).

The need for health education specialists with master's degrees to know and use research and evaluation skills was reaffirmed in 1976

Table 1.1 Guidelines for the Preparation and Practice of
Professional Health Educators

Area Four: Research and Evaluation

Skill Area	Master's Level Function
1. Statistical methods	Collect and use quantitative data and perform standard statistical tests to understand and analyze the relationships between variables and draw inferences for work activities
2. Research design and research methods	Design and conduct studies on health-related behavior, health education methods, and behavior-change problems
3. Design methods of evaluative research	Design health education programs so that evaluative measures are incorporated, with provision for continuing process evaluation
4. Methods of data collection and analysis	Determine which data are needed to analyze a health problem and where they can be obtained Use standardized measurement instruments Analyze research findings relevant to health-related behavior change and draw implications for application Design action research and demonstration projects
5. Computer science; technologies for storage and retrieval of data	Understand appropriate applications of computer technology for planning, conducting, and evaluating educational activities
6. Knowledge and skills possessed by other professions and disciplines in research and evaluation, and how these resources can be utilized for health education	Use expert help as needed for design and conduct of research

---

Source: Society for Public Health Education, Ad Hoc Task Force on Professional Preparation and Practice of Health Education, "Guidelines for the Preparation and Practice of Professional Health Educators," *Health Education Monographs* 5(1) (1977): 75–89.

by approval of the "Guidelines for the Preparation and Practice of Professional Health Educators" by the National Board of Trustees of the Society for Public Health Education (SOPHE) (1977a) (see table 1.1). These guidelines set forth the minimum competencies for graduate-level training in research and program evaluation. The importance of having baccalaureate-trained health educators assist in program evaluation was confirmed by "Criteria and Guidelines for Baccalaureate Programs in Community Health Education" (SOPHE, 1977b) and *Initial Role Delineation for Health Education: Final Report* (U.S. DHHS, Public Health Service, 1980a). The section of the latter entitled "Area of Responsibility V: Evaluation Health Education" is reprinted as appendix A of this text.

CLASSIFICATION OF LEVELS OF EVALUATIONS

Three interrelated general levels of evaluation can be used to organize an approach to evaluation of health education efforts. Level 1 is process evaluation; level 2 is program evaluation; and level 3 is evaluation research. Level 3 subsumes all the characteristics of levels 1 and 2.

Level 1 typically employs nonexperimental or preexperimental evaluation designs; level 2, quasi-experimental designs; and level 3, experimental designs. This book focuses mainly on levels 1 and 2: process and program evaluation.

To delineate what is and what is not a program evaluation, we can compare it to other common evaluation activities performed as part of a process evaluation. Examples of these activities include assessing employee performance, periodic review of departmental functions, a budget review, and evaluation of the performance of a new system for monitoring participants. In these process evaluations, standards and criteria for determining acceptable performance are derived from independent professional judgment, experience, or available guidelines from accrediting agencies, procedure manuals, consultants, and professional associations.

Program evaluation can be distinguished from process evaluation activities by its use of the scientific method to complement professional judgment. Program evaluation attempts to determine the congruence between performance (i.e., what occurred) and objectives (i.e., what was supposed to occur) and to isolate the cause(s) of a specific outcome. Formal program evaluation and evaluation research are different in that the former is designed to supplement "real world" decision making; the latter is designed to add to the knowledge base of health education.

An increasing degree of sophistication is needed to perform evaluations of each higher level. Levels also rise in their demands for time, training, skill, and resources. Purposes, methods, and characteristics of adjacent levels overlap, however. General characteristics of levels 1, 2, and 3 are presented in table 1.2 and the next three sections of this chapter, while a fuller discussion of each level is provided in chapters 4 and 5.

Table 1.2   General Characteristics of Levels of Evaluation

Level	Selected General Characteristics
1. Process evaluation	Applies nonexperimental designs Assesses operating procedures Examines structure and process Conducts observational analyses Performs qualitative observations Monitors effort–activity Reviews–audits data and records Employs formative evaluation methods
2. Program evaluation	Applies quasi-experimental and experimental designs Assesses behavioral impact Uses nonrandom or random assignment Emphasizes internal validity Uses simple analysis and comparisons Applies tested interventions Employs formative and summative evaluations
3. Evaluation research	Applies experimental designs Uses randomization and controls Tests hypothesis on behavior change Uses multivariate analyses Improves knowledge base Is grounded in theory Emphasizes internal and external validity

Level 1—Process Evaluation: Program Quality Assurance Review

Ongoing programs need to conduct process assessments. Part of a program quality assurance review (QAR) consists of observing and assessing the quality of procedures performed by program staff. This involves examining the situation, events, problems, people, and interactions as a program unfolds, e.g., during program development, program implementation, and data collection. QARs assess structure and process variables in the delivery of services. Elements of an ongoing program are assessed for staff adherence and participants' responses to a plan and the quality of the procedures being used. This review should suggest ways to improve the design and operation of the program. A quality review also examines program activity data, monitors data collection and recordkeeping procedures, and examines the completeness and quality of the recordkeeping system.

The review of interactions between program staff and client should be part of a QAR. It may be a written consumer appraisal or participant observation of staff performance in providing the educational service. Using standard procedures, a review of interaction patterns provides feedback and is useful to identify problems being encountered by staff. Qualitative techniques should be used to define the content, methods, materials, and elements of a program (Mullen and Iverson, 1980). Detailed discussions that elicit insights from both the consumer and the provider on how they feel a program is operating and progressing are a basic feature of the quality assessment process (Cook and Reichardt, 1979; Patton, 1980).

QARs of selected elements should be planned, occur routinely, take a short period of time, and expend modest resources. In general, a QAR should be conducted as unobtrusively as possible. It should be performed in a timely manner, particularly in the early stages of implementation of a project, and at least once a year thereafter. Data from routine records, monthly activity reports, quarterly program reports, participant observations, discussions with staff, and discussions with consumers of the service are examined. These sources should provide valuable insights about revising program structure and process.

Evaluators conducting QARs should stress simple and direct observations that can be used as a basis for improving efficiency and effectiveness. Lists or rating systems and open-ended questionnaires and forms can be used. A detailed study of various program inputs and elements may then be made. The QAR should be planned with full staff input into its objectives, process, and scope. In chapter 4 we provide a more extensive discussion of standards and quality control procedures for conducting process evaluations.

Level 2—Program Evaluation: Effectiveness Assessment

The objective of most program evaluations is to determine the impact of an intervention applied at a given location to a specified population. Because of time and resource limitations, and since programs are (and should be) concerned about what works in their setting for their people, a greater emphasis is usually placed on internal validity than on external validity. One assumption in a program evaluation is that the model or theoretical basis of the intervention has been confirmed by previous evaluation research. In other words, health education and promotion programs rarely break new theoretical ground. Yet this assumption is infrequently demonstrated. A common problem that may contribute to a program failure is not looking at the programs previously conducted in an area to learn what level of skill or behavioral impact it is possible to achieve. Program evaluation is in a class of programs often referred to as service or demonstration projects. Evaluations of health promotion programs seldom include the testing of formal hypotheses. Implicit, however, in conducting any evaluation is the belief that certain educational methods will produce certain outcomes. Health promotion programs need to be more concerned about accounting for hypothesized effects and relationships when they occur.

In varying degrees, most programs use information, methods, and materials that have been established in the literature. Yet only a limited review of the supportive materials may be made when choosing an intervention method. The program may then attempt to determine whether that intervention is generalizable to several different settings. Program evaluators need training and skill in sophisticated measurement and design, although not as extensive grounding as evaluation researchers.

While program evaluation designs should be as rigorous as possible, they tend, in practice, to be less rigorous than evaluation research designs. One principal difference is that a program evaluation usually deals with a fluid program and has to adapt to organizational and situational changes, while evaluation research tends to be more rigid in its inputs and methods, attempting not to deviate from a protocol and research design. Although control for bias of program results is an important issue in conducting a program evaluation, a control or comparison group may be difficult to establish. Program evaluations tend to be multifaceted. Since randomization may not be feasible in a program evaluation, various quasi-experimental research methods are usually employed. Capabilities are usually more limited within a program than with a research design, e.g., less extensive and frequent data may be collected.

Program evaluation focuses principally, although not exclusively, on the internal validity of program results—did this program work in this setting, and did it produce the observed change? In contrast, evaluation research is concerned with both internal and external validity—did this program produce an observed change, and would the program produce a comparable impact at other sites with a comparable population? Elements of formative and summative evaluation usually represent the principal parts of the evaluation plan in a program evaluation. The need to produce well-grounded conclusions imposes demands on program evaluations (and on evaluation research) that are often difficult to meet in practice. A convincing argument of a cause-and-effect relationship between exposure to a program and cognitive, affective, skill, or behavior changes is necessary; it needs to be confirmed and supported by ruling out alternative explanations.

Level 3—Evaluation Research

Because of its nature and complexity, evaluation research (ER) almost always demands extensive resources, often beyond what a community, school, business, or hospital program in health education has available. Evaluation research is most often conducted in specialized centers for research as a collaborative effort between health education research scientists and other investigators with training in the psychosocial, quantitative, and health sciences. Extensive training in measurement, design, statistical analysis, and analytical skills is essential to an investigator in ER. The major concern of an ER study is appraisal of the impact of an innovation on groups of individuals. It is the principal method of testing a theoretical model. The model may have single or multiple components and may entail mass, group, or individual methods of communication. Evaluation research attempts to produce evidence in support of a research hypothesis and to demonstrate a cause-effect relationship between the educational intervention and the outcome. The objective is to obtain knowledge that is generalizable to similar groups in other settings. Therefore, the researcher is concerned with both internal and external validity, and ER must necessarily be designed to yield conclusions that are convincing. Alternative explanations for an observed, significant impact have to be ruled out (Cook and Campbell, 1983). From a practical perspective, ER represents the best mechanism to examine "age-old truths" and "new fads."

A number of elements of evaluation research further distinguish it from program evaluation. First, ER uses operationally defined and empirically testable hypotheses. The importance of hypothesis testing is paramount and is characteristic of all ER. While program evaluation tends to be multifaceted, ER by definition is more narrowly focused.

Another prerequisite in conducting ER is a thorough review and synthesis of primary source material. This gives the evaluator and staff an understanding of the state of the art in a particular area of health behavior change. The ER team can then develop interventions that are built on accumulated knowledge, e.g., what factors influence smoking cessation among pregnant adolescents. The interventions thus have a sound theoretical grounding. Other characteristics of ER include use of an equivalent control group, the attempt to reduce sources of error and bias by controlling for extraneous variables through standardization of program procedures, and the selection of an appropriate experimental design. The principal ingredient in ER is the application of scientific methodologies to test hypotheses concerning the impact of one or more interventions.

ER examines the effectiveness of different types of interventions, most often using at least two treatment groups and one control group. It generally involves a standard set of procedures: (1) specification of research questions or hypotheses, (2) selection of an appropriate population to test the hypotheses, (3) selection of a site and maintenance of subjects in treatment categories, (4) designation of a data system that produces early estimates of immediate and short-term program effects and estimates of long-range effects, (5) selection of data sources of high quality, and (6) selection of an evaluation design that maximizes internal and external validity.

Ultimately, evaluation research attempts to add to the state of the art by empirically testing hypotheses that can be used in theory building. In addition it should provide information to policymakers who allocate resources, provide support to the field of practice and study, and provide insight to the public health profession on how to have the most favorable impact in a specific area of health education practice.

PURPOSES OF PROGRAM EVALUATION

On a conceptual level, program evaluation is seen by different people in different ways. To some it is a means to ascertain the extent to which a program has succeeded or failed. To others it is a management tool, a means to improve the planning and implementation process or to have an impact on policymaking. Many see it as collecting data from participants to determine their degree of satisfaction with or acceptance of the program's process and content. Irrespective of the evaluator's viewpoint, pragmatically, most program evaluations have to be concerned with five broad questions (Rossi et al., 1979, 20):

1. Is the intervention reaching the appropriate target population?
2. Is it being implemented in the ways specified?
3. Is it effective?
4. How much does it cost?
5. What are its costs relative to its effectiveness?

Most people expect a well-designed evaluation to confirm, with varying degrees of certainty, what parts of the program contributed to the overall success and what parts impeded the achievement of program objectives. Identifying reasons for lack of success may prove as fruitful for program development as a success, although obviously failures or partial successes are not as well received as successes. From the perspective of program effectiveness, the sine qua non of evaluation is determination of the degree to which observed behavior changes can be attributed to the program. The ability of a program to demonstrate behavioral effects, however, is always related to the problem, characteristics of the setting and target audience, and available resources (time, personnel, and money).

Ten major purposes often cited for an evaluation are:

1. Determining the rate and level of attainment of program objectives

2. Ascertaining strengths and weaknesses of program elements for making decisions and program planning

3. Monitoring standards of performance and establishing quality assurance and control mechanisms

4. Determining the generalizability of an overall program or program elements to other populations

5. Contributing to the base of scientific knowledge

6. Identifying hypotheses for future study

7. Meeting the demand for public or fiscal accountability

8. Improving the professional staff's skill in the performance of program planning, implementation, and evaluation activities

9. Promoting positive public relations and community awareness

10. Fulfilling grant or contract requirements

It is probably unrealistic to expect any one evaluation to achieve all the listed purposes, but an evaluator needs to consider the relevance of each to a given program or setting. The imaginative and skilled practitioner can accomplish a number of purposes at once.

ROLE OF EVALUATION IN AN ORGANIZATION

In an organization, the interest in, expectations of, and funding for an evaluation tend to have a tidal quality, ebbing and flowing. Some participants see evaluation as a necessary but meaningless exercise, while others believe it is a way to gain insight into what happened and why. Whatever the evaluator's position is, however, he or she must deal with political realities. The evaluator who fails to recognize the political dimension of resource allocation is in for a rude awakening. Although, theoretically, an evaluation's objective evidence on the outcomes of a program is used in future allocation of resources, in practice economic, philosophical, and political orientations play an equal (perhaps greater) role in how policy is made and resources allocated. Chapter 2 discusses this issue at greater length.

Program staff members and evaluators need to recognize that the principal reasons for conducting a program evaluation differ from situation to situation and site to site. The expectations and demands of the audience for the evaluation will influence its purposes. The purposes, organizational and programmatic, will help to define the following: (1) the objectives to be evaluated; (2) the type(s) of evaluation to be performed; (3) the evaluation design to be used; (4) the measures appropriate to program input, process, outcome, and impact; (5) the types and amount of data collected; (6) the analytical demands of the program; and (7) the time, staff, and resources needed to accomplish the evaluation. The evaluation process is enhanced when particular emphasis is placed on having program staff members perceive evaluation as an opportunity for professional growth.

UTILIZATION OF PROGRAM EVALUATIONS

A legitimate question commonly asked about an evaluation is, "Is anyone going to pay attention to it?" Literature on the history of the use of evaluations reveals a mixed but generally pessimistic picture. Reasons suggested for the seeming indifference to evaluation reports are varied. Wholey et al. (1970, 23) describe four basic reasons for low utilization of many evaluation reports by organizations:

1. Organizational inertia. Organizations tend to maintain the status quo and to resist change. Evaluation usually implies that changes are needed.
2. Methodological weakness. Poorly conducted studies produce poorly respected conclusions. Decision makers tend to trust their own instincts or experiences rather than the results of poorly done studies.
3. Design irrelevance. Critical programs and vital policy issues often are unrelated to the evaluation undertaken.
4. Lack of dissemination. Concerned policy and decision makers might never see or hear about the conclusions of the evaluations. Sometimes the evaluation is deliberately buried to keep the information from being communicated to relevant individuals and organizations.

Formal evaluation reports may not play a substantial role in organizational policymaking and programming for two reasons: they do not support the reason for existence of an organization or a bureaucracy, and they frequently communicate equivocal results. A related and continuing problem is staff turnover in an organization, which impairs program and evaluation continuity. In addition, organizational goals, organizational constraints, and the role played by the health education practitioner in the planning and allocation of finite resources affect the valuing, conduct, and use of an evaluation. Evaluations, program design, policy development, and the allocation of resources are all based on value choices. Persons who direct or assist in program evaluation need to become adept at influencing the un-written agenda of an organization that determines what will actually get done. As Weiss (1973b, 50) has noted:

> Only when the evaluator has insight into the interests and moti-vations of other actors in the system, into the roles that he him-self is consciously or inadvertently playing, the obstacles and opportunities that impinge upon the evaluative effort, and the limitations and possibilities for putting the results of evaluation to work—only with sensitivity to the politics of evaluation re-search—can the evaluator be as creative and strategically useful as he should be.

An examination of the use of federal health evaluations suggests that reported results have often exerted little or no influence on pro-gram and policy decisions. This situation is paralleled in the broad field of evaluation research and program evaluation. Revealing dis-cussions by Suchman (1967), Weiss (1972, 1973b), Patton et al. (1977), and Zweig and Marvin (1981), encompassing areas of discussion sel-dom examined in the literature on health education/health promo-tion, confirm the nonutilization or underutilization of evaluation research by management and policymakers and examine the reasons. Although it is easy to blame methodological defects when an evalua-tion's conclusions are not heeded, correcting these is only part of the answer. Many factors impinge on a program, and evaluators need to understand them fully. Lamenting health education specialists must realize that improvements in the methodological quality and analyti-cal sophistication of a study may not improve its impact. In fact, the quality of methodology may receive little consideration. While these improvements are important and necessary, they may not persuade a superintendent, health officer, or chief executive officer to apply the evaluation's conclusions.

Part of the lack of attention given by decision makers to evalua-tion reports is explained by inadequate definitions of program im-pacts. Current thinking suggests that evaluators need to assess more elements than impact-outcome variables. Both qualitative and quan-titative assessments need to be performed to characterize a program's evolution and effect more fully—not just the presentation of a statis-tically significant increase at the 0.05 level. While impact evaluation can help to decide if a program should be continued or repeated, it does not help to judge the quality or how it might be improved.

At least *one* principal purpose of evaluation reports must be to assist decision makers in an organization to make program and policy decisions. If program staff get too wrapped up in their own objectives and activities, they may lose sight of or become insensitive to what they are doing, why, and for whom.

Increased use of evaluation research and program evaluation results will come about only by broadening the utility of results to those who fund evaluation studies. As discussed in appendix B, one of the functions of an evaluation report is the translation of findings into recommendations. The report should also attempt to persuade the reader, within the constraints of reality, of course. Prudence suggests that the results of an evaluation report should be translated into alternative recommendations, identifying program strengths and weaknesses, for administrative and policymaking use. Evaluators in both practice and academic settings need to become more adept at relating relevant information to principal decision makers to answer their questions and respond to their agendas. This need for improved translation must be given much greater emphasis by the profession. Increased concern about the effective dissemination of methods and results should increase the utilization of evaluation research and program evaluations in health education and health promotion.

SETTING REALISTIC GOALS AND PROGRAM PLANS

As noted in chapter 3, the first dimension of evaluation planning is goal setting. The program staff needs to determine what is possible for a program to achieve and what is not. A comprehensive program evaluation is seldom possible, given the resources and circumstances of most ongoing programs. Therefore, one of the first steps taken by program staff should be to specify reasonable expectations. In general, program staff should set more modest expectations for their programs than they do (Ogden, 1978, 1980). Trying to evaluate what cannot be evaluated given resources and expertise, attempting to evaluate a program before it has had a chance to be established in a setting, or evaluating inappropriate outcomes represent common problems faced by health program staffs. They also need to remember the law of common sense. Every aspect of a community program usually cannot, and in most cases should not, be evaluated.

Individuals who are planning health education and promotion programs should recognize that there may not be a "good" evaluation design, or definitive method, to apply to their situation. The best evaluation outcomes will be produced when methods and designs are matched to the program questions being asked. Designs are better or worse, or more or less appropriate, for particular situations. Data are of better or poorer quality or can be collected more or less easily or expensively in different situations. Proof derived from a sophisticated design, e.g., a randomized clinical trial with treatment and control groups with extensive resources, still may not provide a definitive answer to the given research questions. Part of the problem is that practically all programs and studies are plagued by implementation problems. Another part is that unequivocal proof of intervention effectiveness is a very evasive phenomenon. In general, the best an ongoing program evaluation may be able to do is to rule out several less plausible reasons for an observed change and support one or two reasons why the program worked. The serendipity of program outcomes also needs to be acknowledged.

In conducting evaluations, program managers and staffs need to reach a consensus on the criteria of success; compromise is almost always evident. Plans must include both qualitative and quantitative criteria. While criteria obviously vary from organization to organization, the bottom line in the 1980s and 1990s will increasingly be the effectiveness and efficiency of services rendered, often measured in economic terms.

Program evaluators need to approach the creation and revision of an evaluation plan with an insight into how different parts, methods, and designs relate to each other conceptually and operationally. Adjustments in one dimension almost always affect another dimension. Attention to detail at the outset will, in general, improve the ability to revise and adapt the plan as it unfolds. Weiss (1973a, 51) cogently argues that evaluations can be made more responsive and suggests how this can be accomplished:

> for the evaluation to be relevant, agreement on several prior issues is essential: (1) the goals of the program, (2) the nature of program service (and any variants thereof), (3) measures that indicate the effectiveness of the program in meeting its goals, (4) methods of selection of participants and controls, (5) allocation of responsibilities for participant selection, data collection, descriptions of program input, etc., (6) procedures for resolving disagreements between program and evaluation personnel, and above all, (7) the decisional purposes that evaluation is expected to serve.

An evaluation plan is a guide that (1) defines program objectives, outcomes, and impacts; (2) specifies tasks, methods, and procedures to be employed by whom, for whom, over what period of time, and (3) describes what resources will be allocated to achieve the objectives. The plan should assist the program and the evaluator in resetting objectives. Failure to specify and operationalize the objectives and outcomes is a common omission in a program plan. It almost always prevents the assessment of process and outcome. When the evaluation plan is designed, however, a number of decisions and assumptions are made. Moreover, not all aspects of a program evaluation are evident during the program planning and early initiation stages. Opportunities to examine selected dimensions of a program may exist prior to program initiation or in the early stages of implementation and may not exist at a later time. One of the purposes of this book is to improve an evaluator's ability to participate with confidence in preparing or revising a program plan, realizing as fully as possible the alternatives and consequences of each part and its alteration.

CONCLUSION

Contemporary thinking in professional preparation, practice, and policy dictates that the practice of health education and promotion be perceived in a more experimental and qualitative fashion. Evaluation should serve as a mechanism not only to assess and improve programs but also to test innovations. It represents one of the most important channels for improvement of the health education profession and should become one of the major sources of personal and professional growth. Program evaluation and health education practice need to be perceived as the spawning ground for collaboration between trainers, persons in training, and practitioners within the profession. Of the three levels of evaluation, program evaluation seems to have the most potential for bridging the existing gap between academically oriented and practice oriented health professionals. The work of people of both orientations improves or diminishes the state of the art. While both groups experience frustration at the energy and sophistication needed to plan, implement, and evaluate a program with limited resources, individuals in practice and academic settings need to strive to work well with what they have and to get more of what they need. This book is intended to assist in that process.

The development, implementation, and adaptation of an evaluation plan to unanticipated situations can be one of the most creative exercises in which a health professional participates. If health education and promotion are to prosper as part of the public health, health care, and educational systems in the United States, professionals need greater technical skill and sophistication. Responsibility for the extra effort it takes to master the technical skills to conduct health program evaluations rests with you, the health education specialist. With improved skills, you will perceive what is possible, probable, or impossible, given available resources and time.

2

Conducting Evaluations and Promoting Organizational Change

"I worked for two years on that evaluation, and no one even read the report."

"We were the first to employ an elegant factorial design in evaluating this program, and the administrative decision ignored our findings."

"The only reason the agency hired me is that the feds require an evaluator on staff. These people don't even know what an evaluator does."

"I really threaten our program people. They keep me at arm's length. I can't even get a meeting with them."

Professional Competencies Emphasized in This Chapter:

- ability to analyze political processes related to health and health education

- ability to identify social, cultural, environmental, organizational, and growth and development factors that affect health behavior, needs, and interests

- ability to acquire ideas and opinions from persons who may affect or be affected by the educational program

- ability to secure administrative support for the program

- ability to secure the cooperation of those affecting and affected by the program

- ability to incorporate results into planning and implementation processes

- ability to contribute to cooperation and feedback among personnel related to the program

- ability to reconcile differences in approach, timing, and effort among individuals

The concept of evaluation has been defined to mean the act of placing a value, positive or negative, on something. Negative value implies something is wrong and should be changed or improved. Anything less than full positive value implies that the object of evaluation can be improved through some change. Since program evaluations are often conducted by comparing a program's performance against a standard, some negative value is implied by almost all evaluation results. From this perspective, one part of the job of the evaluator is that of an agent of change: working to improve a program in the many ways identified by evaluation results.

The comments at the beginning of this chapter reveal the frustrations experienced by many evaluators in getting the results of their evaluations implemented within an agency. Program evaluators spend many hours specifying their evaluation objectives, laboring over their instruments, collecting and analyzing the many facets of their data, and communicating their results to a variety of audiences. Despite all this effort, their reports are rarely used in an obvious and straightforward way. Ineffective programs are rarely dropped. Obvious improvements are only infrequently made. Effective programs are allocated little, if any, additional money. While people in evaluation might wish that an agency's operation were governed by a rational decision equation into which evaluative data could be plugged and appropriate decisions would then be derived, unfortunately no such equation exists. Evaluators may become exasperated at the lack of immediate rewards for their extensive technical effort.

This state of affairs highlights the political nature of evaluation. Evaluations are conducted by people, for other people, about other people. That is, evaluation is conducted within a "social context" (Levine and Levine, 1977). The evaluator becomes a part of the struggles, conflicts, and movements in the agency. To be effective in this context, an evaluator needs a variety of skills related to the politics, or interpersonal relationships, of health education and its evaluation. These proposed skills were identified in the report of the Role Delineation Project (National Center for Health Education, 1980):

> *I. E. 6. The health educator must be able to analyze political processes related to health and health education.*

As human activities, health education and the evaluation of health education programs occur between and among people. Conflicts necessarily occur between individuals and the institution those individuals create. Concepts are needed to understand these conflicts, and methods are needed to minimize the disruption, and maximize the benefits, brought about by each conflict.

> *II. A. 2. The health educator must be able to identify social, cultural, environmental, organizational, and growth and development factors that affect health behavior, needs, and interests.*

Of particular note for this chapter, evaluation is most often conducted in an organizational context. While this text cannot provide a complete analysis of organizational dynamics, some organizational theory and strategies can be related to the conduct of evaluation.

> *III. A. 1. The health educator must be able to acquire ideas and opinions from persons who may affect or be affected by the educational program.*

Involvement by the participants in program planning and evaluation may ensure their continued satisfaction with and participation in the program. Involving the participants is an important strategy in improving program evaluation and promoting program change, as well.

III. A. 5. The health educator must be able to secure administrative support for the program.

Without administrative support, a program is doomed to failure.

V. B. 3. The health educator must be able to secure the cooperation of those affecting and affected by the program.

Administrative support alone is not enough. The evaluator needs skill to facilitate the participation of both administrators and others in the agency in planning and evaluation, particularly the consumer.

V. D. 3. The health educator must be able to incorporate results into planning and implementation processes.

This statement is the first to recognize that planning and evaluation are processes, and by implication a system and strategy must be developed to help these processes meet the needs of the participants and the agency. As part of this system, mechanisms must be created to enable participants to review evaluation methods and results.

VI. A. 1. The health educator must be able to contribute to cooperation and feedback among personnel related to the program.

Within the system that is developed, the health educator must become proficient at providing feedback to all the participants, as part of an effort to promote cooperation.

VI. A. 2. The health educator must be able to reconcile differences in approach, timing, and effort among individuals.

Each staff member, manager, and participant has a personal way of doing things and a personal schedule. The system must reflect the differing preferences of all the participants.

Along these same lines, the Joint Committee on Standards for Educational Evaluation (1981, 56) proposed a standard for ensuring the political viability of evaluations: "The evaluation should be planned and conducted with anticipation of the different positions of various interest groups, so that their cooperation may be obtained, and so that possible attempts by any of these groups to curtail evaluation operations or to bias or misapply the results can be averted or counteracted."

To promote these skills, we will introduce several ideas on the organization of human services and a problem-solving strategy for reconciling differences among participants in a program planning and evaluation process. These ideas and this strategy provide the foundation for the health educator to develop the listed skills. Practice in real world settings is necessary to develop these ideas and methods into personal abilities that can be employed successfully in conducting agency evaluations.

In particular, we cover the following issues: What are the major components of an organization in conducting an evaluation? How do these components usually function? What are the sources of conflict among the components? How might the evaluator relate to these agency components? What strategy might the evaluator use to minimize the conflicts and move the components to some consensus about agency change? Practical examples are provided at many points in the chapter.

DOMAINS AND INTEREST GROUPS

Services are provided by agencies or organizations. Agencies may be very simple with one service provider and a limited clientele (e.g., a private health education consultant and clients), or they may be large and complex with many clients (e.g., the American Heart Association or the National Foundation March of Dimes). There are many models for agencies and many characteristics in which an evaluator might be interested.

The agency decides which services to provide and what essential ingredients to include. Agency decisions and actions can be complex. To understand how agencies function, Kouzes and Mico (1979, 1980) found it useful to identify three "domains" of decision making and action in human services organizations: policy, management, and service. The *policy domain* consists of a board of directors; the *management domain* usually consists of agency administrators; and the *service domain* consists of agency staff members who render the services (see figure 2.1). For example, a state affiliate of the American Cancer Society (ACS) will have at a minimum a board of directors responsible for deciding in which activities the statewide organization becomes involved (*policy*); a state vice-president responsible for raising funds and managing staff to achieve the board's objectives (*management*);

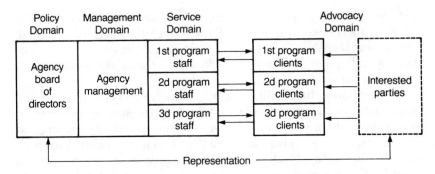

Figure 2.1 A Model of Agency Domains

and a statewide activity coordinator (staff) who motivates and organizes volunteers to conduct ACS activities (*service*).

Although a particular person in an organization may perform activities that fall within all these domains (e.g., the manager who makes some policy decisions, manages, and also provides services), it is useful to talk about the functions characteristic of each domain. The function of the policy domain is to set direction and overall guidelines for the agency. Questions addressed by the policy domain include: What services will this agency provide? With what other agencies should it collaborate? How and where should it seek funding?

The function of the management domain is to run the agency within the direction and guidelines set by the policymakers. Questions considered by management include: Given the funds available, how many and what kinds of staff members will the agency hire? Where should the staff be located? How can the staff be organized to provide quality service?

The function of the service domain is to provide the specific services selected by the policymakers and organized by management. Questions relating to service include: What should each service include? How should various services available from this agency be employed to meet the needs of a particular client best? How does this agency define *quality* for the services provided?

The agency functions by providing service units to a clientele. The clients in turn justify the agency. A dramatic example of the importance of this relationship occurred when the March of Dimes Foundation participated in successfully eliminating polio as a national scourge. The foundation had to find another target group to justify continuation of its extensive and powerful fund-raising organization. It did so by emphasizing birth defects and problems of pregnancy, delivery, and infancy. This new set of problems justified the effective fund-raising and service delivery activities of the March of Dimes.

The clientele in turn has various interested parties, i.e., groups interested in the welfare of the agency's clientele. For example, the Juvenile Diabetes Foundation is interested in young diabetics; the Citizens Council for Hypertension Control is interested in hypertensive patients; the National Welfare Rights Organization is interested in welfare clients.

In a sense, clients constitute a domain: the *self-advocacy domain*. If organized, clients can exert significant influence on agency activities. To be "organized" means that a clientele has some political or self-help group that works for the perceived interests of the clients. An unorganized client group may exert influences on an agency as well. Lack of organization, however, tends to reduce the direct influence clients exert on the decisions and actions of the other domains.

It is important to note that each domain addresses a different set of questions, and all the sets are important to the agency's effectiveness. The concerns of one domain are no more important than those of another for the viable functioning of the agency.

Some examples will give a clearer picture of how the domain ideas apply in specific situations. Three types of agencies are discussed: (1) health education staff in local clinics or community hospitals; (2) divisions of state health departments engaged in risk-reduction programs; and (3) state affiliates of voluntary health agencies.

Example: Local Clinic

A locally run primary-care clinic will often have a board of directors, a central management unit, and a variety of service providers to meet local needs. The board of directors constitutes the policy domain. Boards are usually composed of individuals and representatives of groups who are interested in health issues and influential in the local community, e.g., representatives of local industry, labor unions, churches, potential health care consumers, and individual benefactors. Three reasons for inviting people to be on a board of directors are that they represent groups that can provide financial or professional resources, they are sources of clients, or they represent influential opinions in the community. Having these people on the board gives the agency more direct access to the resources represented and feedback on how the agency is perceived in the community.

Central management is usually composed of a director and other staff members, who manage the books, collect and pay bills, obtain funding and materials, maintain the buildings and facilities, hire personnel, and plan services and facilities to meet the needs of the local community.

The services staff includes doctors, nurses, dietitians, health educators, technicians, and various other professionals who provide health services. These service providers are usually organized into divisions, e.g., pediatrics, radiology, and pharmacy. The directors of these divisions often experience role conflict because they operate in both the management and the service domains and experience the demands of both.

Clients in this system are patients who come for acute or chronic disease care and people who benefit from clinic outreach programs, e.g., weight-reduction programs and hypertension screening.

Example: State Health Department

Divisions that operate risk-reduction programs within state health departments present a more complex domain structure. The policy domain has several components with separate responsibilities. High-level policy for risk-reduction programs is formulated to one degree or another by Congress, the federal executive branch (the U.S. Department of Health and Human Services), the state legislature, and the governor's office. Policy guidelines from these sources tend to be broad enough so that local programs have latitude for action on specific needs. The state-level policy function is most often provided by the director of the state health department, and a statewide risk-reduction advisory board. Advisory boards are usually composed of representatives of organizations that can contribute to a statewide risk-reduction program, e.g., voluntary health agencies, university departments, other divisions of the state health department, and individuals who have been particularly active in risk reduction.

Management is also complex. State health departments often have a variety of divisions that are concerned with management functions, e.g., finance and personnel. In addition, the risk-reduction program director is in a position analogous to the service division director in a clinic, with both management and service responsibilities.

Service staff in a statewide risk-reduction program includes the director of the risk-reduction program and all paid staff members promoting risk-reduction programs throughout the state. From the evaluator's point of view, the service domain also includes all people who volunteer their time to help achieve objectives of these programs.

In a statewide risk-reduction program, all the residents of the state are potential clients. Primary clients, however, are the groups that have been targeted by specific risk-reduction projects, e.g., people with a high risk of cardiovascular disease, or smokers, or alcoholics.

Example: Voluntary Health Agency

In a state affiliate of a voluntary health agency, the policy domain includes groups that provide direction to the affiliate, most often the national (parent) organization, its representatives and staff, and the affiliate's own board of directors or board of professional members (e.g., physicians). These boards usually have committees to govern policy formation and implementation in many facets of the agency's activities.

The management domain consists of the director, staff, and volunteers assigned to management tasks, e.g., fund raising and personnel. The service domain in a voluntary health agency usually is comprised of a director and volunteers engaged in program activities. The clientele is all residents of the state with the particular afflictions targeted by the agency. A more specific client domain consists of afflicted individuals for whom the agency has developed specific service programs.

In some cases, the board is also drawn from the volunteers; the manager may also be a major service provider. In these cases, the same person may function in several domains. The rest of this chapter must be understood by considering one function at a time. Conditions in agencies vary so greatly that it would serve no purpose to detail the many possible functions and interrelationships. The "domain" is a useful concept for understanding the interests that intersect in agency operations and for dealing with them effectively.

OPERATING CHARACTERISTICS OF AGENCY DOMAINS

Why is it important to know about an agency's domains? Kouzes and Mico (1979) proposed that the agency domains differ in their operating characteristics: governing principles, success measures, organizational structure, and working modes. The differences are summarized in table 2.1, where they are overstated to clarify the ideal. Although no agency functions in exactly this manner, a clearer understanding of the ideal operating characteristics may help the evaluator work better with these domains in a particular agency.

Kouzes and Mico described the policy domain as using the "consent of the governed" as their governing principle. This means that policymakers usually employ a parliamentary form of governing in which all members are considered equal. In theory, the consumer representative is the equal of the physician in the policy domain. Policymakers often assess the success of their activities by whether there is some equitable (right, just) distribution of resources among interests

Table 2.1   Operating Characteristics of the Domains in Human Services Organizations

Domain	Governing Principles	Success Measures	Organizational Structures	Work Modes
Policy	Consent of the governed	Equity	Representative Participative	Voting Bargaining Negotiating
Management	Hierarchical control Coordination	Cost efficiency Effectiveness	Bureaucratic	Use of linear process tools
Service	Autonomy Self-regulation	Quality of service Good standards of practice	Collegial	Client-specific problem solving
Self-advocacy	Client advocacy Agency oversight	Increased or improved services for clients	Varied, depending on history of development	Protest Conflict Participation

and concerns. Thus, members of the Heart Association board might be satisfied if the agency's resources were equitably distributed among hypertension, heart disease prevention, and heart disease rehabilitation programs. The structure for their meetings is representative (each member representing a particular interest) and participative (each member participating in policy deliberation). Setting policy is most often accomplished by voting, bargaining, and negotiating. Different interests may have different weights in setting policy due to personality, political, or economic influences. In some agencies, policy may be set by a "dictator," malevolent or benevolent.

The management domain typically employs a hierarchical mode of organization: relationships among nonequals. People at the higher levels are considered to have more responsibility and skill and, therefore, coordinate the activities of people at the lower levels. This has been described as a bureaucratic organizational structure. The clinic director may employ directors of finance, personnel, and purchasing, who in turn employ staffs, including support personnel. The people in management usually use a variety of analytic tools, e.g., budgeting systems and cost-effectiveness analysis, which have as their criterion of success some aspect of effectiveness or efficiency. This focus on efficiency and effectiveness naturally follows from the constraint that management provide services within the limits of available resources. Thus, a risk-reduction program can work with only as many communities as its staff, printing, telephone, and travel budget will permit.

The service domain most frequently is comprised of human services professionals, people who are as responsive to and interested in the values and activities of their colleagues at other agencies as they are in the mandates and directives of their own agency. These service renderers belong to professional organizations at which standards are propounded and discussed. The way professionals typically relate to one another is as colleagues: peers with similar skills and responsibilities providing complementary services with a common purpose. This is certainly true *within* classes of professionals (e.g., physicians, nurses) but not necessarily *between* classes of professionals, a potential source of conflict. Service staff members tend to protect the professional autonomy of their own domain and class of colleagues, and thus they prefer to control their practices through professional self-regulation. Peer review committees for professional self-regulation are common in a wide variety of disciplines. The work mode of professionals is characterized as client-specific problem solving; techniques for this are developed and defined by consensus among professionals.

Outlining the four organizational characteristics of the advocacy domain is a bit more difficult. The measure of success is clearly increased and improved services for the agency's clients. Hypertensive patients want more and better hypertension control services from the Heart Association. The organizational structure, however, may be representative and participative, autocratic rule by a charismatic leader, bureaucratic, or even anarchistic, depending on the circumstances and leadership at the inception of the organization. The advocacy domain can provide a crucial impetus for improved agency performance at least from the perspective of the client (Dinkel et al., 1981). To implement the governing principles of client advocacy and agency oversight, clients may alternatively use protest, conflict, and participatory work modes, as appropriate. Conflict and protest were common work modes among client groups in the 1960s and early 1970s. In the mid-1970s many agencies formulated rules (Windle and Paschall, 1981) and developed mechanisms (Zinober et al., 1980) for promoting the participation of clients and client groups.

COOPERATION AND CONFLICT AMONG DOMAINS

A health education program can most easily be evaluated in agencies where (1) domains are cooperating to achieve the agency's ends; (2) there is mutual respect for each domain's operating characteristics; and (3) each domain is open to the possibilities for growth and change. This state rarely exists, because conflict is more common than cooperation. The evaluator must understand the tensions and conflicts within agencies to deal with them effectively.

The pattern of conflict and cooperation among domains can be complex. For example, disagreement may exist on the long-term goals of an agency, but agreement and cooperative behaviors may exist on short-term goals. Domains may cooperate in some areas of activity, but be in conflict in others. Coalitions may form to cooperate on certain issues but not on others. Coalitions may be in conflict with other coalitions. A variety of factors may lead to conflict or cooperation, including salary level, prestige, fringe benefits, perquisites, and control over resources (power). Resources are always in short supply. For example, only limited funding is available to any agency; no agency has all the funds it would like. If one division or domain gets increased funding, that may mean less funding for the others. Colleagues do not shower prestige on everyone (or else it would not be considered prestige). Resources and incentives go to some people in preference to others, to reward their effort and skill, to keep them working at a high level, and to demonstrate to others that increased skill and effort will be similarly rewarded.

A certain amount of conflict in an agency must be understood as a natural and healthy outcome of the competition for scarce resources. The desire for more salary, more benefits, more recognition from superiors and colleagues or more resources is universal. At times, however, conflict can go beyond some poorly defined acceptable bound.

Conflict may also stem from the structural differences among domains. People in one domain tend to relate to individuals in other domains by using operating principles that have worked in their own domain. Imposing one domain's operating characteristics on another can have disastrous effects. For example, although it is possible to conceive of a clinic manager employing a completely representative, participative management structure there would be little specialization of activity under such a structure. Thus, secretaries may do accounting; accountants may do janitorial work; and janitors may make program management decisions. This implies a violation of the "efficiency" measure of success, a strong component of management's operating characteristics. Similarly, it is difficult to conceive of physicians using voting as their work mode for deciding on the best therapy for a patient.

Different operating characteristics lead to conflicts among domains. For example, improving the quality of health education programs often requires increasing the expenditure of resources (more staff, more money, more educational materials, etc.); the expenditure of resources may violate the cost-efficiency measure of success held by management. An extra expenditure of resources per unit of service may incur the wrath of managers who have to take the resources from other activities to meet the demands of the new activity. For example, health educators have been told by third party payers that patient education programs can be implemented only if the costs of their programs reduce the cost of medical care by at least an equal amount (a cost-effectiveness criterion) (Baranowski and Fuller, 1981).

THE EVALUATION DOMAIN

The domain concept is also useful in demonstrating the conflicts between health program evaluators and people in each of the domains—conflicts that lead to the types of comments at the beginning of this chapter. Although evaluation is usually located in the management or policy domain, the common conflict between evaluation and management (Connolly and Porter, 1980) indicates that evaluation has a unique set of operating characteristics and thereby justifies consideration as a separate domain. We will describe the operating characteristics of the evaluation domain in terms of dominant "ideal types"; few organizations manifest these characteristics precisely as characterized.

The evaluation domain can be structured in two ways. If the evaluator is based in a university, the organizational structure is often collegial. If the evaluator works in a contract research organization, or for the agency itself, the structure is likely to be bureaucratic, with some attempt to create a collegial atmosphere. The governing principles are autonomy and self-regulation among university-based evaluators but hierarchical control and coordination among others. The primary work mode is the use of social science (linear technique) methods within a client-specific problem-solving framework (rather than a hypothesis-testing framework). That is, the evaluator attempts to address particular problems, case by case, using one or more social science tools. The measures of success often include: direct use of the results in agency decision making, more effective agency performance (as a result of evaluative efforts), and production of a respectable report.

Conflicts with Other Domains

The identification of these evaluation operating characteristics points up differences from the other domains and highlights the conflicts that face an evaluator working within an agency. Conflicts have been recognized in the literature at the interface of the evaluation and management domains (Connolly and Porter, 1980). For example, Cox (1977) reviewed the management literature and identified aspects of "managerial style" that sharply conflicted with evaluative style. First, he noted that managers must deal with tremendous amounts of information and make many different types of decisions within very short periods of time. In contrast, evaluators intensively focus on a limited set of issues over a long period of time. The speedy managerial pace implies that the manager must deal with many and varied issues in a brief and fragmented manner, while the evaluator is usually attempting to achieve some integrated conceptual whole. Managers are more interested in action, the evaluator in contemplation. Verbal communication fits more easily into the manager's style, while written communications are more useful to evaluators attempting to provide a comprehensive picture. The manager prefers faster (less well formulated) information to the slower, better formulated information preferred by the evaluator. Hawkins et al. (1978) empirically validated Cox's contention about the manager's preference for informal verbal information. Managerial style, therefore, comes into direct conflict with the more reflective, intensive, written, and documented style of the evaluator.

Gurel (1975) identified related conflicts encountered by evaluators. He noted that agencies are often caught in a dilemma: The organizational need for stability is in conflict with the need for change or adaptation to new problems and new understandings of problems. Managers and staff are often on the side of maintaining stability, while the evaluator is often working for organizational change. Gurel also noted that, despite the popular perception of science (particularly the physical sciences but also the social sciences) as omnipotent, the social sciences have not even established the technology for promoting change. Agency people at all levels may thus have unrealistic expectations of how an evaluator can help them accomplish their goals. In addition, most people believe that effort expended in the service of a worthwhile end will produce positive results. Agency people find it hard to accept evaluation findings that are predominately negative. Such findings threaten the self-esteem of all agency domains and may in fact threaten the financial security of particular projects. Finally, Gurel noted that evaluations are frequently conducted on programs in serious trouble. Given the lack of effective technologies for change, evaluators and their methods can hardly assist such programs. From Gurel's perspective, the social setting in which evaluation is usually conducted generates tensions and conflicts before the evaluator has begun the task.

Weiss (1972) and Conner (1979) classified conflicts between the evaluative and management domains into major categories: personality differences; differences in roles (management of and commitment to the project as is, versus assessment and change of the project); lack of clear role definition (the activities and responsibilities of evaluators have never been clearly spelled out); conflicting goals, values, interests, and frames of reference; institutional characteristics (primarily the conflict between the organizational structures and working modes of the two domains); and aspects of evaluation methods and techniques (the obtrusiveness of questionnaires, random assignment, etc., into agency operations).

No one has reported on relationships between the evaluative and the policy, service, and advocacy domains. Undoubtedly similar categories of conflict exist where these domains interface, as well.

This brief overview of agency structure and interrelationships raises a series of questions about evaluation. Is an objective evaluation always possible? Which domain's or faction's interests does a particular evaluation serve? What are the roles an evaluator can play in relation to other domains? How does an evaluator deal with all domains and factions in an agency?

Effects of Domain Conflicts on Evaluations

Clearly, evaluations employing objective techniques are not always possible. For example, a clinic manager may want to reduce the number of health educators employed by the clinic. The manager may direct an evaluator to assess the demand for and effectiveness of health education services per unit of medical service. Money is not available for an observation study, however, so the evaluator must depend on specially designed forms completed by the health educators themselves. The manager and the health educators have a severe conflict of interest. The tensions and conflicts between these two domains may be so high that the health educators will actively subvert the evaluation. They may falsify records to improve their own performance image or devalue the manager's. Domains and factions tend to focus on a limited number of performance indicators to the detriment of overall performance (Campbell, 1975). The evaluator is, thus, always at the mercy of the people who complete the records to be used in evaluative assessment. Unless a large evaluation budget is available, these record completers are always agency staff who are members of the various domains and factions, with their vested interests.

Within a cauldron of conflicts and competitiveness, the perception of interest may be crucial. An evaluation introduced by one domain in conflict with another will be greeted with suspicion, fear, and defensiveness. In the above example, a full-blown evaluation focusing on health educators' achievements may not be the best approach. A variety of other evaluation options (reviewed in chapter 1) are available that the health educators would find programmatically useful and not threatening.

Possible Roles of the Evaluation Domain

Uzzel (1978) recently noted that the community researcher (this would include the program evaluator) can play four roles in relation to an agency and/or a research audience. Traditionally, the evaluator has played the role of "dispassionate outside observer or chronicler of social activity." An evaluator, however, might also play the roles of educator, broker of conflicts, or advocate of change. When each role is most appropriate will vary with circumstances. The evaluator may be in a position to remedy a knowledge deficit in the agency. When conflict exists between two domains, the evaluator may attempt to get each side to understand the other's positions and may negotiate differences. Finally, an evaluator may be an advocate of his or her self-perceived need for change, or may work with the self-advocacy domain to help its members achieve their perceived need for change.

This last role identified by Uzzel, advocate of change, points up another sticky situation in which many evaluators find themselves. The common concept of the evaluator as an objective observer conflicts with the concept of an evaluator as an agent of change. This conflict reinforces the notion of evaluation as a separate domain. Evaluators, too, have vested interests in a variety of agency activities and actively pursue those interests. The interests include not only pay and fringe benefits but also influence in the agency, i.e., utilization of evaluative reports in policy formulation, agency management, and delivery of services. Maintaining the distinctness of the evaluation domain from the policy, management, and service domains simultaneously may assist evaluation in being more "objective" in its findings and recommendations.

The rest of this chapter discusses how an evaluator might conduct an evaluation that is likely to be effective in promoting the changes identified in the final report, while negotiating the conflicting interests of the various domains and other vested interests in the agency.

UNDERSTANDING CHANGES THAT OCCUR NATURALLY

Change can be brought about in an agency despite conflict and the potential opposition of vested interests. Some change, after all, is a normal part of human experience. A change may be small and relatively insignificant—for example, new typewriters, new time schedules for a service, or new recordkeeping forms. Other changes, such as a new activity or procedure (e.g., contracting) introduced in connection with a service (e.g., smoking cessation), have major impact. Some of these changes may occur naturally as a result of changing circumstances, the decisions of leaders, or decisions made by other agencies. Other changes may be managed by individuals to achieve their own ends.

One approach to studying change that occurs naturally is associated with the theory of *diffusion of innovations*. This literature, reviewed by Greer (1977) in the area of health care organizations, has been primarily concerned with patterns in the introduction of a change to a set of organizations over time, rather than with the change process within a particular organization. Several authors have mapped the rate of change in introducing a new practice, i.e., the number of agencies adopting a new idea or practice over sequential units of time. This rate of change has been labeled the *diffusion cycle*.

Diffusion theorists have studied differences between those who adopt new ideas or practices early in a diffusion cycle (early innovators) and those who adopt them later. They have also studied differences in the characteristics of innovative ideas or practices that may result in quicker or slower change. These studies suggest that, within each organization, change occurs in three stages. According to Greer, they are: (1) idea entry and consideration, (2) change decisions, and (3) change implementation. She described these stages as follows (Greer, 1977, 519):

> In the idea stage, information and creativity are very important. This stage requires flexibility, circulation of ideas, a variety of perspectives, and freedom from threat of excessive discipline. At the adoption (decision) stage, other factors become important: motivation, resources, and the ability to reach a consensus. In the final implementing stage, such factors as perceived legitimacy, disruptiveness, displacement, and trust become important.

This concept of stages or phases in organizational change is useful for evaluators.

Another approach to understanding change that occurs naturally derives from analysis of the conflict among domains and factions (vested interests). Greer (1977, 525–26) reported on the principles of intraorganizational change propounded by Roos (1974) from a political analysis of organizational decision making:

> Changes occur:
> (1) when there are changes in the goals of powerful groups . . . ;
> (2) when the power of opposition groups is decreased . . . ;
> (3) when the power of proponent groups increases . . . ;
> (4) when the old structure becomes obsolete for achieving goals . . . ;
> (5) when performance gaps provide impetus for change.

These general rules about relationships among domains or factions in promoting change should apply to any agency. The health program evaluator should, therefore, know the goals of powerful groups in the agency, the relative power of these groups, how aspects of the organizational structure are used to achieve each group's ends, and differences between expected and actual performance for each group. The evaluator might be particularly valuable in designing alternative structures and might play an influential role by maintaining records of performance.

In addition to the important rules gleaned from studies of change that occurs naturally, evaluators need models for how to promote needed change.

PROMOTING ORGANIZATIONAL CHANGE

Three models for the management of agency change have been identified: the management consultant, the evaluator-managed, and the open system problem-solving models.

Management Consultant Model

The management consultant model for promoting change through evaluation has been most clearly described by Ziegenfuss and Lasky (1975a, 1975b, 1980). They proposed that the evaluator develop a relationship with the management domain and focus primarily on management concerns in five areas: administration, agency services, fiscal management, legal matters, and service system. Their focus was not service outcomes but primarily organizational structure. Two examples of evaluative questions raised within this model are: Is there a statement of board roles and responsibilities? Are there procedures to protect the civil rights of clients, e.g., protecting the privacy of people who attend health education programs?

Ziegenfuss and Lasky saw this type of evaluation as useful early in the development of a program, to ensure that the program was developing along rational lines. For example, failure to protect privacy could result in the client's embarrassment or worse. In a sense this method takes the easiest approach to evaluation: dealing primarily with one domain, management. Although all domains (except the clients') participate in self-assessment precipitated by evaluator questions, the report is made primarily to the management. This can be an effective model early in an organization's development, when there is little conflict among domains, and in cases in which the primary concerns of all domains are expressed in the report. There is no provision in this model for the resolution of conflicts among domains, but an evaluation of this type may result in clarification of potential problems.

Evaluator-managed Model

Several authors (Schulberg and Jerrel, 1979) have suggested that the evaluator align with management. This course is recommended because the manager is usually in the pivotal situation, relating to all other domains and dispensing resources. While attractive, this approach fails to recognize that management is not the sole domain to make decisions. Each domain, in its own area, makes decisions crucial to achieving agency goals: the board makes policy decisions; management makes management decisions; service renderers make service decisions; clients make advocacy decisions. A balanced evaluation should reflect the interests and perspectives of each domain; this will improve the evaluation, prevent one domain from foisting an evaluation on the others, and prevent one domain from subverting the evaluation.

Polivka and Steg (1978) have provided examples of evaluator-managed change. They report on an overhaul of the organizational structure of the Florida Department of Health and Rehabilitative Services placing the evaluation unit in a position to approve the continued funding—and structure—of all agency units and programs. An evaluation analysis and policy development process was established in which management and service domains of all programs periodically participated in evaluations to reach a consensus on recommendations for continuity and change. Many evaluators would find this an exciting model, since they have "clout" in the agency's decision making. However, the authors reported that, after six months, the evaluation unit was given more and more administrative responsibilities, becoming in effect part of the management domain. The danger of this approach is that evaluators may assume the conceptual styles, concerns, working modes, etc., of management and lose their perspective and objectivity on the needs and operating modes of other domains.

Open System Problem-solving Model

French and Becker (1975) saw particular promise for an open system problem-solving approach to managing change. In this model, the evaluator is no longer the font of truth for other participants but instead uses data collection and analysis, among other techniques, to clarify problems and promote compromise, cooperation, and coordination among the competing domains and vested interests. Many authors have contributed to and commented on this approach (Argyris, 1970; Delbecq, 1978; Dickey and Hampton, 1981; Glaser and Taylor, 1973; Reppucci, 1973; Van de Ven and Koenig, 1976). The approach of Van de Ven (1980a, 1980b) is presented here in greater detail, because it encompasses the major ideas of the other authors and has been shown by experimental study to be superior to a method in which no systematic planning is conducted.

The basic problem-solving model was first presented by Van de Ven and Koenig (1976), who proposed a seven-phase model for program planning and evaluation: phase 1, prerequisites to planning; phase 2, problem exploration; phase 3, knowledge exploration; phase 4, program design; phase 5, program activation; phase 6, program operation and diffusion; and phase 7, program evaluation. In later publications (Van de Ven, 1980a, 1980b), phases 5–7 were condensed into a single phase. The primary characteristics of each phase as applied to the concern of conducting an evaluation are described in table 2.2.

The phases may best be explained by means of an example. At a rural primary care clinic in a coal mining area, the board of directors insisted that a smoking-cessation program be developed because of evidence that black lung disease (coal miner's pneumoconiosis) develops primarily among coal miners who smoke. The health educator on staff developed a program to be used by the nurses in the clinic with all coal miner patients. Since implementation required considerable nursing time and other clinic resources, the board wanted to make sure that the benefits justified the effort.

In response, the health educator developed a program evaluation. As a first step, the health educator arranged with the chairperson of the board and the clinic administrator to establish a committee to consider evaluation (phase 1). The committee included the board member who was most vocal in instigating the smoking-cessation program, the director of clinic finances (the person who raised the issue about the project's costs), the nurse who was most interested in implementing the program, a patient (client) with whom the program seemed to have been successful, and one with whom the program had failed.

The first meeting was spent primarily in having committee members get to know one another. At the second meeting (phase 2), the committee agreed that smoking cessation is a true need of coal miners. They also agreed that there were enough nurses to implement the program, but they were concerned that the nurses did not have adequate interest in and skills for the project. Several of the nurses had said that they were already overworked and didn't need additional responsibilities.

Two specialists from the local state university were invited to attend the third meeting (phase 3). The smoking-cessation specialist indicated that the methods employed in the program were standard and seemed to work well with volunteer smokers. The nursing educator specialist noted that nurses in high-volume rural primary care clinics were prone to "burnout" because of extensive responsibilities, seemingly endless demands on their time, and their perceived lack of control over specific tasks, a lack that deprived them of the satisfaction of achievement.

The fourth meeting had to be cancelled because the two coal miners on the committee had to attend a union meeting. At the fifth meeting (phase 4), the evaluation committee decided that three questions had to be answered in evaluating the project: (1) whether the

Table 2.2 Characteristics of the Problem-solving Approach to Program Evaluation

Phase	Conceptual Set	Task	Primary Participants	Strategy	Function
1. Evaluation prerequisites	Problem mindedness	Establish an evaluation committee representative of all domains and interests Identify the evaluation unit Agree to an evaluation activity sequence	Leaders of all domains		Involvement of all domains in the process
2. Problem exploration	Problem mindedness	Conduct an assessment of agency and program strengths and weaknesses, as perceived by all domains	People selected from all domains	Inspiration	Problem appreciation
3. Knowledge exploration	Problem and solution mindedness	Bring the best available expertise to bear on conceptualizing program functions, nature of deficiencies, and potential solutions to the problems	Experts	Judgment	Raising the program staff's ideas above the level of public consciousness
4. Evaluation design	Research design mindedness	Reach agreement on the major issues facing the agency program Design a method of evaluation that further clarifies the problems and assists in selecting from among potential solutions	Leaders of all domains	Negotiation and compromise	Debate of ideas Negotiation of each leader's vested interest in dominance
5. Evaluation implementation	Research conduct mindedness	Conduct the evaluation and produce a detailed report	Evaluators	Computation	
6. Evaluation dissemination		Work with all domains in reviewing evaluation findings and in drawing implications for program and agency structure and process	Leaders of all domains	Negotiation and compromise	Institutionalization of selected ideas

program was reaching miners; (2) whether the miners were stopping smoking at least as frequently as reported in the literature on smoking cessation in the general population; and (3) how the staff nurses felt about the program.

Before the sixth meeting the health educator designed a survey of nurses' attitudes toward the project, and a survey of miners who had been in the clinic's care for the duration of the project. The miner survey aimed to determine if miners had been contacted by a nurse about smoking cessation and if they had given up smoking during this period. At the sixth meeting, the committee accepted the design of the evaluator's study and decided to expand the second survey to include a random sample of all adult patients (18 years or older) registered with the clinic. Data collection (phase 5) started following the sixth meeting.

At the seventh meeting, the evaluator reported on the progress of data collection. As a result, the nursing representative spoke to several nurses to speed up their return of nursing questionnaires. The board and client representatives were asked to contact several noncooperating clinic patients to get them to agree to an interview.

At the eighth meeting the committee learned that all the nurses but two were antagonistic to the new smoking-cessation program; the program was reaching more nonminer patients (mostly women) than miners; and approximately 50 percent of all patients reached by the program had given up smoking for up to two months. The data indicated, however, that about 50 percent of people not reached by the program had also given up smoking in the last six months. In addition, 50 percent of the miners expressed interest in quitting smoking; of these, 75 percent preferred self-learning materials to an intensive clinic-based program.

Before the ninth meeting, the committee members discussed the evaluation results with members of their respective domains. The board member still felt that a smoking-cessation program was important for reaching miners and preventing black lung. The nurse was still excited about the program but was receiving very negative comments from her colleagues. The finance director was concerned about costs. Both patient representatives appreciated the attention given to all health care consumers at the clinic.

At the ninth and tenth meetings (phase 6), a compromise was reached. All but two nurses were relieved of responsibility for the program. These two, who had been most supportive, were assigned primarily to implementation of this project. The two nurses and the health educator were also asked to develop a smoking-cessation self-instruction package for miners. Once these materials were developed, the clinic clerical staff were to contact all miners in the clinic, find out which ones smoked, and discover which of those were interested in a self-instruction package for stopping smoking and which would participate in a smoking-cessation clinic. To avoid overburdening the staff, miner patients were to be contacted over the next two years. Other clinic patients were offered places in the intensive smoking-cessation group sessions, filling slots left empty by miners (thereby reducing costs).

The committee decided that some collaborative planning process should have been used in designing the original smoking-cessation program to avoid some of the problems that surfaced. The committee also agreed on an evaluation procedure that could be implemented with the start of the new smoking-cessation program.

This approach resulted in a smoking-cessation program for coal miners with greater chance for success, reflecting the interests and concerns of each domain. The committee was able to facilitate various stages of the evaluation process.

Why did French and Becker (1975) suggest that this open system model was such a valuable approach? Van de Ven (1980a) presented data showing how it was used in 11 experimental and control group communities. The experimental communities performed better on several outcome indicators. The open system procedure effectively dealt with social change by enabling conflicting interests to focus on only a limited set of issues at one time and by negotiating and resolving the conflicts step by step (Van de Ven, 1980b). Dickey and Hampton (1981) have argued that such a problem-solving evaluation model will promote intraagency (interdomain) communication patterns that identify and solve problems more effectively.

Other studies support various aspects of the open system problem-solving model. Weeks (1979) found, to his surprise, that the greater the number of people participating in an evaluation decision (especially early in the evaluation design process), the more likely it was that the evaluation information would be used. Dunn (1980, 530) assessed five different models from a review of over 100 case studies of evaluation utilization. He found moderate to strong support for the following hypothesis: "The greater the overall influence of social scientists, policy makers and other *stake-holders* in each phase of the policy-making process, the greater the knowledge utilization."

Windle and his colleagues (Dinkle et al., 1981; Windle and Cibulka, 1981; Windle and Paschall, 1981; Zinober et al., 1980) have argued that clients and interested citizens have a right to participate in an agency's evaluation. They further hold that the evaluation results will more likely be used as a result of client's participation.

Under the open system model, maintaining evaluation as a separate domain has important advantages. Evaluators will not be perceived as foisting one domain's set of operating characteristics or interests on other domains. Working separately enables the evaluator to facilitate resolution of the conflicts among other domains. What is most important, evaluators can define and maintain the operating characteristics appropriate to their own activities, which differ from those of the other domains. In this way, the evaluation domain can become a creative force within an agency, attempting to promote change that makes the agency's programs more responsive to internally and externally perceived needs.

Working as a separate domain also involves certain risks, especially the isolation of evaluators from other domains. Conner (1979) emphasized the importance of evaluators maintaining a cooperative and collegial attitude to all evaluation participants and showing up at service delivery sites to demonstrate a shared commitment to the project. Conner argued that these activities assisted in the development of trust between evaluators and the other domains, which led to mutual respect and a minimum of conflict. In other words, evaluators must appreciate the interdependence of all domains and work to promote trust, respect, and cooperation in the evaluative task.

SUMMARY

This chapter has emphasized one of the evaluator's many roles: as an agent of change. To promote change effectively, the evaluator must be aware of the domains and interest groups in an agency, their self-interests, and their operating modes. In working with domains and interest groups, the evaluator must promote a problem-solving orientation in which evaluative techniques are used to solve jointly defined problems. This problem-solving process requires the competing interests within an agency to collaborate in a phased sequence of steps in which problems are clearly defined, the greatest number of alternatives are clearly specified, and data are used to make selections from among alternatives. The project design must incorporate the most appropriate scientific approaches and data collection methods for answering questions about the program under evaluation. The evaluator must be aware of the forces that tend to perpetuate the status quo and have the ability to control them. These propositions, if followed, are likely to result in evaluations that are on target, have the support of all concerned, and result in improvements to the benefit of all concerned.

3

Health Education Program Planning and Planning for Evaluation

"Why didn't we think of this before the program began?"

"Good grief, you mean we've been teaching breathing exercises, and they have no relationship to improving a person's asthma?"

"I thought this program would lead to fewer hospitalizations, but that outcome was never logically possible."

"I don't understand why the medical department won't cooperate in this program."

Professional Competencies Emphasized in This Chapter:

- description of the influence of the sponsoring organization on a health education program

- description of the membership and usefulness of a health education planning network

- definition of needs assessment

- analysis of a health problem and the logical connections between the problem, an educational program to address it, the impact of the program on learners, and related outcomes

- enumeration of the steps of health education program planning

- development of a health education program plan

Chapter 2 focused on the role of the evaluator and the potential for evaluation to bring change within an organization and community. In this chapter, we discuss development of the educational program to be evaluated. In many, if not most cases, the health educator oversees the planning, implementation, *and* evaluation of an educational program. The program plan is the health educator's road map—the blueprint that ensures that the program is logical, addresses learning needs, and can be evaluated. The plan consolidates the thinking of the health educator and other collaborators. Among the collaborators in health education planning, of course, are the learners. Frequently, it is possible to involve potential learners directly in planning. At a minimum, individuals who represent the learners' interests must be among the planners.

In addition to ensuring that the program is well conceived, good planning also enables the health educator to mobilize beforehand the information, people, and resources critical to program success. Often the plan is necessary for securing funds. The plan, then, is the comprehensive document that ensures that a program is sound and engenders the support needed for implementing it.

This chapter focuses on the steps for developing a program plan and emphasizes planning for the program evaluation. Initially we discuss some basic concepts of particular importance to the program developer: the organizational context for planning, the planning network, needs assessment, and the links from a program to new behavior and related outcomes. Later in this chapter we discuss step by step the process of developing the program plan.

THE ORGANIZATIONAL CONTEXT FOR HEALTH EDUCATION

When researchers and academicians set about to plan health education, they try as best they can to manipulate the environment so that theories can be applied and hypotheses carefully tested. In the day-to-day practice of health education, however, practitioners must accept realities and try to build into their plan ways to manage existing situations. Often health educators have limited control over the conditions in which programs are developed and delivered. Nonetheless, a standard of practice is that programs are based on excellent principles and theories. Achieving this end can be difficult. For example, existing theory suggests that developing ongoing peer support groups with the same members meeting over time may enable people with a chronic disease to acquire the social support needed to manage their illness (Yalom, 1970, 317). But, given the work schedules of potential learners, available meeting places, a limited budget, or other factors, it may be impossible to apply this principle fully.

In actual practice, educators try to come as close as they can to the theoretical conditions that enable positive change to occur in learners. As discussed in chapter 2, they continually try to bring about needed changes in employing organizations and communities, changes that will enable them to come even closer to creating optimum learning conditions (Clark, 1978). Evaluation research, or level 3 evaluation as discussed in chapter 1, generally manipulates the environment to test hypotheses, to test the application of knowledge. Program evaluations, or level 2 evaluations, contribute to the knowledge base of health education by assessing and describing the application of knowledge in similar settings and situations (Suchman, 1967). Ultimately, the program evaluations you will conduct as part of your daily health education work are the basis on which a theory comes to be accepted as generally workable and therefore good. The challenge for the field of health education is to develop programs and conduct evaluations that successfully bridge the theory-and-practice gap.

Philosophy of the Organization

In the main, health educators are employed by health-related agencies and organizations to develop programs, and it is primarily to these health educators that this book is addressed. Working with an organization means that you, as a health educator, must represent in programming not only your own view, objectives, and philosophy of health education but also those of your employing organization. Sometimes there is conflict between what an individual health educator believes and the goals of the organization. If you find yourself in such a quandary and no reconciliation of ideas can be achieved, you will need to make a personal and professional decision about whether to work with organizational goals unlike your own. This is difficult to do and would probably preclude effective work. You may, instead, find another organization and setting where the philosophy and views are more in line with yours. Some health educators volunteer their assistance to individuals and groups to develop programs that espouse particular political and philosophical views. The health educators can then emphasize views they believe are particularly important, unencumbered by the need to represent an employer. In presenting the steps of program development in these pages, we have assumed that the health educator must pay attention to the interests of an employing organization with specified health goals. We also assume that the health educator has chosen employment with an agency whose goals, in the main, are consistent with the educator's own values.

Impetus for the Program

In the field of practice, there are three basic ways in which health education programs come into being. The health educator sees the need to design a program: "Boss, we really need to develop a hypertension education program for the elderly. We've got to improve the quality and the cost-effectiveness of our service. Shall I develop something for you and the budget people?" Or the health educator is asked to design a program that, according to someone else, the agency's clients need: "Larry, the board of directors feels we should get a hypertension education program for the elderly off the ground. Please develop something that we might get the budget to support." Or the health educator is asked to design a program on the basis of what clients want: "Joan, what kind of health education do our elderly clients need and want? Find out and put together something. Then let's see what kind of budget we'd need."

Orientation and Goals of the Organization

Regardless of who initiates the program, it is likely to be organized in one of two ways: (1) as part of ongoing activities providing related health services directly to clients; (2) as a project by groups that provide no direct medical or nursing service. For example, hypertension education may be part of the senior citizen program of a local health department. Health department physicians or nurses may be on staff and available to treat program participants diagnosed as hypertensive. Similarly, the program may be part of the services of a general medical clinic that has a large elderly population and where physicians routinely see hypertensives. In other words, health education is developed to be integrated into ongoing work of an organization with a wider set of health service activities.

On the other hand, the hypertension education might be developed as an activity of a senior citizen center where the aim is to assist the elderly with many concerns, including health. In this case, participants will be referred elsewhere if they need medical or nursing services. Similarly, the education may be developed by a private voluntary agency, say Citizens for a Better Community, and directed to all the elderly in an area. Such a program might recruit medical and nursing staff members to cooperate in the program if they are needed or might refer people to available services when necessary. The important aspect to note about these latter two examples is that the health education is part of a broader community effort and not of medical or nursing services.

It is also likely that, in organizations where health education is part of a larger set of medical and nursing activities, health may be narrowly defined to mean primarily those conditions that signal absence or reduction of the diseases in which the organization is interested. Health related to hypertension, for example, may mean having a sufficiently low blood pressure. In organizations where health education is not tied to medical and nursing services, health may have a much broader definition. Health for the senior citizens, for example, may include such things as practicing a range of good personal health habits (Meals for Millions Foundation, 1981) or being socially integrated with other people (Pratt, 1976; Pilisuk and Minkler, 1980). In medical settings, health is frequently defined in light of medical or nursing objectives. In community settings, health is frequently defined more holistically.

The emphases of evaluations conducted by an organization will depend on how health is defined within that setting. In other words, both the goals of health education and the goals of evaluations are greatly influenced by the orientation of the organization that sponsors the program.

Table 3.1 categorizes organizations that sponsor health education by their orientations and health goals. The classification is not meant to be absolute or comprehensive. Few organizations fit exclusively into one cell. The table illustrates, however, that every organization has a basic goal and orientation. Organizations give priority to programs that further their primary goals. Health organizations tend to be oriented primarily toward communities or individuals and toward disease management or prevention.

Table 3.1 Basic Orientations and Goals of Organizations Sponsoring Health Education

Goal	Orientation	
	Community	Individual
Disease management or cure	Voluntary agencies: arthritis, epilepsy, muscular dystrophy, etc.	Hospital in-patient services Specialty clinics Chronic care agencies: home health care, nursing home health-related facilities
Disease prevention and health promotion	Health departments Voluntary associations Community centers Community action agencies Government and quasi-governmental agencies Church-related groups	Schools and universities Well-baby clinics Group practices Wellness centers Insurance agencies Business Industry Unions

If an organization has an individual orientation it will tend to focus on what people as individuals can do to improve their health. Such an organization—a hospital, for example—might develop health education that assists diabetic patients to administer medications themselves. The focus is on the individual and an individual solution to the health problem. If an organization has a community orientation it tends to focus more on a broader kind of change. It looks for communitywide solutions.

As a case in point, assume a health problem exists in an area because health services are inadequate or because people cannot afford to engage in healthful behavior such as eating nutritious food or securing adequate housing. An organization with a community orientation might organize and educate people to work collectively to bring about changes in health care delivery or might develop cooperatives to cut costs of buying food or better housing. In other words, health education favored by a community organization might focus on assisting groups of people to change conditions that have a negative impact on their health.

A cardinal rule for the program planner, then, is to know the organizational context *well* before starting a program. You must understand the goals and orientation of your organization as they relate to the health problem in question.

As you review table 3.1 and consider health education in light of the variety of organizations that sponsor it, you may ask a question frequently posed: Is the objective of education always behavior change? We would answer yes and point out that behavior change is always sought within the context of social change. Rarely is an individual's behavior under that person's total control. Virtually always, health education tries to stimulate organizational and community changes that will enable people to acquire the resources and services necessary for healthful living (Clark and Wolderufael, 1977). This is particularly apparent when education has a community action orientation; but it is also the case, as discussed in chapter 2, when the program is oriented toward individual change.

Educational programs operate on the assumption that people will be different as a result of their participation. This assumption is easy to understand when a program focuses on individuals and disease management. Hypertension education for an elderly woman, for example, should enable her to reduce her sodium intake—that is, to behave in a new way. It is more difficult to see behavior change as the goal if the program focuses on communities and prevention. Assume, for the sake of discussion, that education is to assist people to improve inadequate housing in a community. A goal may be to organize groups to demand service from the city housing authority or to bring suit against recalcitrant landlords. While housing may improve because the housing department or landlords send workers to make repairs, the behavior of participants in the program has presumably led to this outcome. Even when the goal is to change the conditions that obstruct good health, it is people who bring about the change by behaving in a different way. These behaviors may include such things as being more assertive, being more vocal, exercising more community leadership, and participating more in cooperative activities (Clark and Pinkett-Heller, 1977; Clark, 1978). An important part of planning a program evaluation, therefore, is to anticipate what changes in behavior and what other changes might occur and to determine if and how such changes might be measured. We will discuss this further in a later section.

THE HEALTH EDUCATION PLANNING NETWORK

Regardless of the type of organization sponsoring the education, program planning is never a unilateral activity. The design, implementation, and evaluation of a program almost always involve a network of people: representatives of the learners, you (the program planner), others in your organization, and representatives of outside organizations that can provide needed services and resources. Another cardinal rule of program development is that effective health education is planned with the participation of major interest groups.

If a program fails to account for the learner's perspective, it cannot possibly appeal to potential learners' motives or enable them to see the relevance of the learning to their situation. Without the participation of potential learners, it is entirely possible to plan a program that misses the vital ingredient that will enable learners to behave in a new way or will change conditions that inhibit healthful behavior (Bruner, 1973). Without the views of those who provide needed related services, it is very difficult to mobilize the resources and cooperation to carry out a comprehensive program. Without a clear understanding of the interests of your own organization, it is impossible to determine in what ways your organization can best serve learners and in what ways it cannot address their needs. In other words, it will be difficult to find fit between what you and your organization are able to do and what the learners want and need to bring about change.

Good health seems to be everyone's goal, but views on what it is and how to get it differ enormously. Therefore, part of program planning is to reach some agreements with those who will collaborate with you in the program. Figure 3.1 illustrates the network of contacts

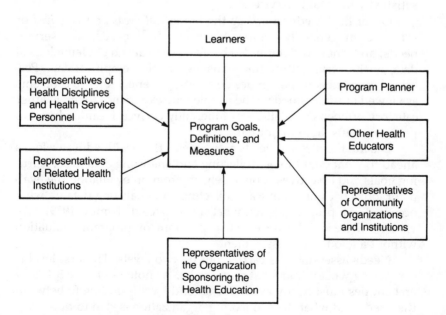

Figure 3.1 The Program Planning Network

health educators generally establish when planning a program. You will want to involve representatives from some or all of these entities in decisions about learning needs, program objectives, learning activities, and evaluation procedures.

NEEDS ASSESSMENT

The health education program planner, in one sense, is seeking to match learners' needs and wants, the sponsoring organization's needs and wants, and the community's needs and wants. Needs assessment, therefore, comprises a large part of program planning. Needs assessment is generally defined as the process by which the program planner identifies and measures gaps between what is and what ought to be.

Some health educators borrow from marketing terminology and refer to *service needs* and *service demands* or *wants* (Luck et al., 1978; Kurtz and Boone, 1981). As they relate to health education, generally service needs are those things health professionals believe a given population must have or be able to do in order to resolve a health problem, while service demands are those things learners say they must have or be able to do in order to resolve a health problem. Service demands also include things a learner wants in order to be more satisfied with health services.

Other health educators use the terms *real needs* and *perceived* or *felt needs* in generally comparable ways. Real needs, like service needs, are generally determined by using clinical and epidemiological data, health service utilization statistics, or other empirical data. Perceived or felt needs, like service demands, generally refer to problems as viewed or understood by the people who experience them. Neither category of needs is infallible or inherently correct. Health education programs must account for both.

During the steps of needs assessment, the health educator looks ahead to what ought to be, collecting and analyzing data to set learning goals and objectives. Conversely, in program evaluation the evaluator looks back on what was, collecting and analyzing data on what occurred in a program, given what was expected (Trimby, 1979). Obviously, there can be no effective program or program evaluation without a good needs assessment.

Needs assessment is carried out on two levels. The first level is comparing what is and what ought to be. As noted in figure 3.1, several entities must be involved. The second level is finding fit between the needs and what the sponsoring organization is able to do.

Keep in mind, as you develop a program, that it must provide some benefit to your employing organization, or the organization will have no reason to continue sponsorship. A program that benefits the organization at the expense of the patient, however, rarely will succeed. For example, a program goal to educate clients to keep clinic appointments is at best of dubious value. Keeping appointments may or may not be related to improved health status. If clinic hours are scheduled not to the advantage of clients but to the advantage of health service personnel, the goal is even more suspect. Achievement of program goals must yield rewards primarily for the learner.

Needs assessment can provide data on how collaborators in the program will benefit if goals are met. To illustrate, consider the conclusions drawn by planners of two actual programs after they analyzed their needs assessment data. First, in a project sponsored by a large metropolitan hospital to help families with a child who has asthma learn to manage the illness better, planners asked: What do families need and want in regard to this problem? What does the hospital need and want? Existing and newly collected data provided the following picture: Asthma is the leading chronic illness of childhood in terms of the numbers it strikes and the days of absenteeism from school that it causes (U.S. DHEW, NIH, National Institute of Allergy and Infectious Disease Task Force, 1979). Fear associated with asthma is the source of much disruption and stress within a family (Creer et al., 1976). It leads to excessive emergency room visits. It detracts from a child's positive self-image and self-esteem (Pless and Pinkerton, 1975; Freudenberg et al., 1980). From this picture, the planners could postulate the following benefits: If a family were assisted to develop confidence and expand its range of asthma management skills, the family might well experience less stress and a normalization of activities, i.e., an improvement in the quality of life. The hospital might benefit by reducing the number of inappropriate and expensive emergency room visits. The community might benefit by cutting down the costs to the school system of chronic absenteeism. Medical and nursing personnel might benefit from patients who are more involved in their own care and who "do better" in their treatment plans.

The second example is an employee diet and exercise program for cardiovascular risk reduction, sponsored by a large insurance company. Again the planners asked: What do employees want and need? How would the company benefit from such a program? Employees, they determined, might benefit more by simply feeling and looking better than from the knowledge that they theoretically would reduce their chances of heart attacks (Morris, 1980). Families might benefit by having a happier, healthier member. Employers might benefit because the employees' satisfaction with their work might increase and worker illness and absenteeism might be reduced (Corroll, 1980).

In short, it is reasonable to believe that participating groups in a health education program will find rewards for participating and that a program will answer needs, real and perceived. It is also reasonable for evaluators to measure the extent to which a program met the needs of participating groups that it was expected to meet.

THE CONNECTION BETWEEN PROGRAM, IMPACT, AND RELATED OUTCOMES

The purpose of needs assessment is to look forward, to determine what ought to be, and to set learning objectives. The primary purpose of evaluation is to measure, as much as possible, the subsequent impact of the program on the learners. Impact is the extent to which learners behave differently as a result of their participation in a program. Generally, when you are evaluating a program, you also want to know if new behavior is associated with improved physiological and psychological health in the learners. In addition, you want to know if changes in behavior and health status led to other outcomes. In an asthma education program, for example, these may include a reduced number of hospitalizations, fewer emergencies, and lower medical costs. If the education is for community action to improve housing and nutrition, outcomes may include an increased number of repairs to correct housing violations, increased membership in food buying cooperatives, and a permanent positive change in the services of local health facilities. Presumably your program will change behavior, and the new behavior will stimulate other changes. There is a logical sequence that underlies program development, from the problem to the broadest goal, as illustrated in figure 3.2.

As an example of how the logical connections are made, consider again the case of asthma education. Following a needs assessment, planners may decide that intended new behaviors should include using breathing exercises and postural drainage at the sign of an asthma attack. Improved health status will be defined as improved pulmonary functioning and fewer severe wheezing episodes. Parents who learn breathing exercises and postural drainage and who learn to distinguish minor from serious symptoms may be less fearful during a child's wheezing episode and may be better able to calm the child. As a result of less fear and improved ability to distinguish symptoms, families may seek emergency services less often. Consequently, the hospital may save money or spend less on emergency services for children with asthma. In other words, the program and program evaluations must be planned in a logical sequence making links from the problem to learning activities to new behavior to improved health status and to related outcomes.

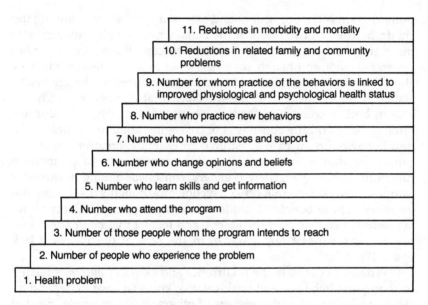

11. Reductions in morbidity and mortality

10. Reductions in related family and community problems

9. Number for whom practice of the behaviors is linked to improved physiological and psychological health status

8. Number who practice new behaviors

7. Number who have resources and support

6. Number who change opinions and beliefs

5. Number who learn skills and get information

4. Number who attend the program

3. Number of those people whom the program intends to reach

2. Number of people who experience the problem

1. Health problem

Figure 3.2 Logical Relationship of a Health Problem, a Program, and Anticipated Outcomes

You can see immediately from this example that, when programs are planned to bring people to new behavior and to realize related outcomes, the health educator must depend to a greater or lesser degree on the knowledge and actions of professionals in different fields. As a health educator, you must determine what encourages or hinders a family in adopting new behavior. You must know, for example, what conditions, factors, information, and skills will enable the family with asthma to practice breathing exercises. Similarly, you must know how to organize and deliver a program that will assist a family to increase its information, develop skills, change conditions, and behave differently. However, you will often count on colleagues in other fields. In the asthma example, the health educator must turn to medical colleagues for knowledge of the factors linked to improved pulmonary functioning and the symptoms of severe wheezing. These are medical issues that the health educator should comprehend.

Suppose basic epidemiological research and clinical trials do not illustrate a connection between breathing exercises and pulmonary functioning or that the association is dubious. When you wear your evaluator's hat, you may not see an improvement in the pulmonary health status of children in the program even if the children loyally practiced the breathing exercises.

The measure of the success or failure of the asthma health education program is the occurrence and extent of new behavior among the children. The positive effect of the behavior on the physiological status of the child is a measure of medical success. If the connection between behavior and health status does not exist, the health educator should not include the behavior in a program aimed to change health status. If the connection is questionable (that is, basic research has shown both a connection and no connection), the health educator often depends on the consensus of colleagues about the efficacy of a new behavior. In the case of asthma, for example, breathing exercises cannot be shown to have a definitive connection with pulmonary functioning. However, there is general consensus among health educators and physicians that other psychological benefits result from the exercises. These benefits include increasing a person's ability to relax, sense of control over the illness, and feeling that he or she is taking an action (not being passive) in the face of the illness (Clark et al., 1980).

When you evaluate the occurrence and extent of *outcomes* related to changes in behavior and health status, you also have to depend on the good judgment and decisions of others. If, for example, needed health services are not available, or are too costly, or are inappropriately organized, it may take much more than an asthma education program to realize desired outcomes. Assume, for the sake of illustration, that the optimum management of asthma (management that is least disruptive and time consuming for families) entails periodic preventive visits to a clinic. Assume also that health services in the community are financed in such a way that it is cheaper for a family to visit the hospital emergency room in a time of crisis than it is to visit the clinic on a regular basis. An asthma education program may provide valid information that preventive visits are best. However, the structure of services at the hospital may not make such behavior beneficial to families. If this is the case, it is likely that frequency of emergency visits and related costs to the hospital will not decrease as a result of the program. Planners might then decide that a more appropriate health education program would inform and organize families to push for changes in the structure and financing of community health services.

The efficacy and effectiveness of a health education program, then, is affected by the knowledge and actions of people in other disciplines. By involving professionals from relevant disciplines in the planning process, you obtain the expertise needed to forge clear links between the program, new behavior, and related outcomes. In planning the program evaluation, the knowledge of professionals in relevant fields can help you determine which changes can and should be measured. Since new behavior is the objective of education, it has priority for program evaluation. Once you have planned how to document the occurrence and extent of new behavior, you can move to deciding which related outcomes can and should be evaluated.

THE BASIC PROGRAM PLANNING QUESTIONS

In order to design a program that will ultimately meet the needs of a group of learners, a sponsoring organization, and a community, you must find answers to several questions, posed below. The first six concern existing needs. In securing the answers to them, you are doing a needs assessment. In answering questions 7 and 8, you are planning the program evaluation. Answers to question 9 will give you a good idea of what educational methods and materials will be effective. Questions 10 and 11 deal with administrative aspects of a program. Answers to them will enable you to plan for training, logistics, and finances.

The basic planning questions are:

1. What are the dimensions of the health problem? There are at least two ways to analyze this: Condition-specific and people-specific.

   a. *Condition-specific*: How does the health problem you are interested in (e.g., cardiovascular disease, asthma, unhealthy lifestyle, or mismanagement of minor illnesses) specifically occur in the group of learners in question (say, middle-class senior citizens or low-income mothers or blue-collar employees)? What is the incidence, rate, and prevalence of the problem in the group? What aspects of the problem are unique to the group? What would you expect the situation to be if the problem were addressed through education? How would people behave? What would their lives be like regarding the health problem?

   b. *People-specific*: What is the health problem of greatest priority for the group of people you want to assist? How does that health problem occur in that group? What would you expect the situation to be if the problem were addressed through education? How would people behave? What would their lives be like regarding the problem? How would conditions be different?

2. What specific behaviors must learners acquire or strengthen to reduce the effect of the problem?

3. What information and skills must a person have to be able to behave in the new way?

4. What resources, personal and material, must a person have to behave in the new way? (For example, a child rarely learns to brush teeth well and regularly without encouragement and a toothbrush.) Are these resources available, or can they be obtained?

5. What kind of related health services, community services, or other conditions are needed to enable people to change to the desired behaviors? Are these available or can they be arranged?

6. Which behaviors can be addressed in an education program? What learning objectives would be consistent with your organization's capabilities, orientation, and goals?

7. Which behavior changes can and should you try to measure? What specific measures will you use? When will measurements be taken?

8. What wider changes in conditions and situations would you expect to see if learners adopt the new behavior? What changes would you see in individuals, families, and communities? How can these outcomes be measured? Which ones will you try to measure? When will you take measurements?

9. What educational technique will best present information, develop skills, provide support, and create an appropriate learning environment, given your particular learners and the desired behaviors? How can you monitor the quality and efficacy of the educational activities?

10. What organizational and logistical arrangements are needed to support the program? What kind of orientation or training is needed for program personnel?

11. What budget do you need? Can you mount the program within your given budget or at a cost your organization is willing to bear?

THE STEPS OF PROGRAM PLANNING

Finding the answers to these 11 questions constitutes the 11 steps in program planning. We consider each step in greater detail next.

Step 1: Analyzing the Health Problem and the Learning Group

In evaluation research, which is designed to develop a profession's knowledge base, there is often a high degree of freedom to select problems and define them as hypotheses to be tested. In the usual practice of health education, however, the educator generally selects or is given problems based on the interests and immediate goals of the employing organization. These problems tend to be people-specific or condition-specific. The more narrowly defined the problem is and the more narrow the focus on a specific group of learners, the higher the chance of successfully documenting change. Although some health educators continue to mount general information programs for a general audience, the relative value of these efforts in achieving behavior change is difficult to ascertain. The relationship between general information programs and broader community change is virtually impossible to document.

A goal in the first step of program planning is to specify the health problem in narrow enough terms so that you begin to understand how education may help to resolve it. Similarly, you must understand enough about the potential learners to be sure you see the problem the way they see it. You must be sure that the education will be relevant and appropriate.

Assume, for example, that the health problem is lack of exercise. Obviously, this problem and education addressing it are quite different for senior citizens than for schoolchildren. They would be different for residents of a middle-class suburban community than for those of a poor, urban one; for fully healthy people than for those with health problems; for families than for individual learners; or for new mothers than for women with grown children. The information, skills, resources, and support needed to change behavior vary from group to group. This is not to say that there are no differences within groups; there certainly are. The first step, however, is to describe the group of people with whom you will work, in terms of some pervasive similarities and common experiences with the problem: demographic, geographical, psychological, physiological, or historical. Similarities may also relate to the way people use health services, what they expect about health, or similar factors that give rise to common experience.

As discussed earlier, you may decide to begin with condition-specific planning. In that case, you start with the health condition, e.g., lack of adequate exercise, and determine, given the range of clients you serve, for which group it is a priority problem. Alternatively, you may decide on people-specific planning, and select a condition only after you analyze a particular group and determine what is the highest priority for them. You might find, as a result of step 1, that exercise is not an important concern to your particular group, but diet, or increasing social contacts, or safety, or some other issue is.

Step 1 is the first step of needs assessment. Through the needs assessment process (steps 1–5), you will come to see a problem comprehensively. You will learn, for example, that controlling asthma is not just a matter of having a patient take medicines as prescribed by medical personnel, but rather that there is a complex interplay of factors and conditons that the family must control and that is not within the domain of physicians and nurses. You will begin to understand that controlling asthma is largely a matter of self-management, which is influenced by a person's beliefs and values and by certain skills. You will develop an idea of what self-management entails and of how difficult or easy it is for a particular group, e.g., low-income families.

Through initial analysis of the problem and the learning group, you are doing your homework, becoming versed in theoretical and empirical explanations of the problem and the kind of learning that may best address it. At the end of step 1, you should be able to describe the health problem in detail, describe in general terms the behavior associated with resolving it, describe in some detail the learners you are interested in, describe the relative importance of the problem to the learners and their perspective of it, describe the kind of program learners will be motivated to take part in to address the problem, describe what the relevant professions say about the problem, identify colleagues in related fields who might collaborate with you in a program addressing the problem, determine how they see the problem, have some idea of how willing they are to work with you, and enumerate the benefits of a health education program to the learners, your colleagues, and your own organization. What is most important, you should be able to describe in some detail the logical chain connecting a problem to a health education program to expected change in behavior to expected related outcomes.

Whether you begin with a particular group of people or a particular health condition, there are basically two kinds of data to use to understand the people and the problem: secondary data, those that are already available from other sources; and primary data, those you collect yourself.

Secondary Data. Epidemiological data are frequently used to determine the importance of particular health conditions, the kinds of problems arising in given segments of the population, the factors associated with health conditions, and characteristics of people who experience them. Often these statistics are made available by government agencies, research institutes, or academic centers. Currently, for example, the diseases causing the greatest number of deaths among United States citizens are heart disease, cancer, and stroke (U.S. DHEW, 1979). These are accepted as major national health problems precisely because many people experience them. The toll taken by heart disease is particularly high among middle-aged men and, as a result, you may decide to focus health education about heart disease on that group. Frequently, money is made available by government only for programs on problems that have a wide impact.

Epidemiological data, however, need not be national in scope to signal a problem for particular groups. Spiegel and Lindaman (1977) reviewed New York City Health Department records and documented falls by children from windows as an important source of morbidity and death. Dr. Stephen Rosenberg, Associate Professor, Division of Health Administration, Columbia University School of Public Health, reviewed hospital medical records and noted a high incidence of morbidity caused by lead paint poisoning among low-income children seen in the emergency room (personal communication, 1979). Each of these findings led to the development, implementation, and evaluation of successful health education programs.

Other secondary data from surveys, systematic observations, and experimental studies are available for defining problems. Findings from research appear regularly in professional journals and are presented at conferences. With increasing frequency, they are also reported on television. What does the literature say about the problem? What do the experts say? Such data are widely available and call attention to the existence of important health problems, the groups of people in jeopardy, and potential solutions.

Primary Data. Despite the range of secondary data, frequently you will find you must collect data yourself to understand a problem fully. You may know, from secondary data, which problems are widespread and which group of people in general is most affected by a particular health problem. However, you may not know how the problem is viewed by those people, how they specifically behave in relation to the problem, or what specific factors enable or inhibit desired behaviors. Sometimes you will be interested in problems for which few data exist at all. Even if much information is available, you may want to collect additional data from a specific group of clients so you can be sure the problem is acknowledged by them as important. You might want to begin with a recognized problem and show the association of another one, e.g., one found to be important in the epidemiological data. Motivation to learn is obviously much higher when the subject interests the learners. Primary data are those collected by going directly to the potential learners to discover their perceptions of, priorities about, and experience with a particular health problem.

The intention of data collection in the needs assessment steps of program development is to look forward, to ensure that the intervention designed fits the problem and population for which it is intended. The intention of data collection for evaluation is to look back, to see what occurred. The process of data collection for needs assessment, however, can often be used to create a baseline against which to measure change during evaluation.

The range of methods available for collecting needs assessment data is not different from that available for evaluation. Quantitative and qualitative methods can be used for both. Qualitative approaches are discussed at length in chapter 4 and quantitative ones in chapter 5, so they will be mentioned here only briefly and in light of their usefulness for program planning.

Discussion Groups. If your aim is to discover how problems are perceived or which problem is most important to a group, you can form a discussion group. The group should be comprised of representatives of the learners in which you are interested. Group members are volunteers who agree to discuss the issues they find most pressing or aspects of a health problem that concern them most. Members might be people who hold a position with community health groups or other organizations, or they may simply be interested individuals who experience the problem and are likely to know the viewpoint of their peers. Such a discussion group has the advantage of allowing people to discuss and even vote on something of immediate interest.

When conducting group discussions for needs assessment, you must make clear what actions your sponsoring organization is prepared to take in light of the perceptions and concerns of the group. Sometimes when your organization has little or no assistance to bring to problems directly uncovered by discussion, you can help group members to locate appropriate assistance. Indeed, the whole domain of community organization and action within the field of health education is based on this role and function. McKnight (1978) has used a very effective approach combining discussion groups, analysis of secondary data, and action. He assists members of community organizations to translate statistics from their local hospital or health department or some other source into a picture of the actual problems experienced in the neighborhood. By examining available data, community representatives explore how the particular problem occurs in their area and then can select one aspect of the problem to address in action.

Sometimes health educators convene meetings specifically to discover the priorities of individuals or community groups. In such a meeting, group members, led by the educator, determine which problem or aspects of the problem are most important. The Nominal Group Process, Delphi Technique (Delbecq, 1974), or a similar approach is frequently used by health educators in situations where varying points of view must be reconciled. These techniques enable group members to select problems and reach consensus on aspects of problems without letting individual views dominate.

A disadvantage of discussions by volunteers is that you never know exactly whose views the group members represent. Some representatives of organizations may have clear-cut constituencies, and statements by them may accurately present the case for their constituents; but this is not always the case. Similarly, concerns expressed by unaffiliated individuals may be uniquely felt. The views and attitudes of one suburban mother of young children do not necessarily reflect those of similar women. It is difficult to know, in other words, how far to generalize the opinions and experiences of these volunteers. If a disparity eventually emerges between the views of the representatives and the learners you aim to reach, fundamental problems can plague your program. Nonetheless, discussion groups can generally shed much light on the problems potential learners confront, can help establish priorities among these problems, and can provide rich insights on dimensions of the problems.

Surveys. The purpose of a survey, whether a mailed or telephoned questionnaire or a face-to-face interview, is to elicit specific information from a specific group of people. Like information collected from discussion groups, survey data are used to delineate the problem and describe the population of learners. If the survey is of the exact people who will eventually be in the program, the answers can also be used as baseline data for measuring change.

In conducting a survey, the health educator generally samples a population. Sampling has been defined simply as the selection of a few observations that will serve as the basis for general conclusions (Babbie, 1979). Sampling is used to overcome the problem of representativeness (remember the disadvantage of discussions by groups of volunteers). By selecting people (e.g., women who come to the organization for counseling) at random, using a systematic procedure (e.g., every third woman who visits), you have a basis for expecting the data to be representative; in other words, the sampled women's views are likely to be similar to those of people not surveyed, whereas volunteers might be different in some respect from the larger population you hope to reach. Sampling and techniques for conducting surveys are discussed in detail in chapter 5.

Fieldwork and Observation. Other ways to assess needs from primary data include fieldwork and observation. These have the advantage of not interrupting the normal events surrounding the target audience and the problem you are interested in understanding. Simply, doing fieldwork means becoming part of the natural events where the problem occurs. Fieldwork tends to be rather costly in terms of time and generally is manageable only for reaching relatively small numbers of potential learners. Nonetheless, fieldwork can generate rich data for planning. For example, you might decide to observe in the clinic or participate in the activities of a family with the health problem in question. Using checklists, protocols, or a log, you might systematically record your observations and experiences. Being systematic in the way you collect and compile data is crucial. Often, if the people observed are the same ones who will take part in the education, data from checklists and observation schedules can be used as baseline measurements.

The fieldwork approach can yield data of a depth and richness not available in other approaches. Most health educators believe that, regardless of what other means are used in program planning, a period of fieldwork is mandatory and will lead to better program development.

Analyzing Secondary and Primary Data. Through analysis of the data collected in step 1, you should begin to see whether there are connections that link certain information, skills, and conditions on the part of particular groups to certain behaviors, and whether those behaviors are linked to certain outcomes. During this initial step, you also identify the theories that describe why people behave as they do in relation to the particular problem. That is, you must locate and analyze the theories that predict the kind of behavior you are interested in. Often, available theories also explain how people change their behavior, and these, too, must be examined. Every health education program is based on theoretical assumptions about behavior and learning. A critical part of step 1 is locating useful theories and making them explicit in your program plan.

Steps 2 and 3: Delineating Behaviors to Resolve the Health Problem; and Delineating Needed Information and Skills

In these steps of needs assessment, you must zero in on specific behaviors that will aid learners to manage or resolve the health problem and the information and skills that the learners will need.

A set of circumstances is briefly described below to illustrate how a health educator delineates needed behaviors and identifies information and skills. Assume that you have been hired to develop an employee education program. Data show that middle-class men, 45–60 years of age, who are employed in sedentary office jobs, who smoke, are overweight, have high blood pressure, and do not get adequate exercise, are at high risk of cardiovascular problems. Your employer, a large insurance firm, wants to develop a cardiovascular risk-reduction program for its male employees in an urban community. You expect that the target population will benefit from such a program by looking and feeling better, more "healthy," and more active. The company is expected to benefit by increasing the satisfaction of these employees with their employer and the benefits it offers. In the long run, the company also expects some benefit from reduced costs of cardiovascular-related illness among its employees.

The physicians and nurses of the employee health service are willing to cooperate. In general, employees express interest in such a program. Most who do not engage in "good health practices" readily admit that they don't and feel as if they should. You have carried out step 1. You have read the available literature on risk reduction, including critical factors predicting behavior and describing the kind of learning that has been shown to bring about change. You have convened representative middle-aged, middle-class men from each department of the company to discuss issues of risk reduction. You have also drawn a random sample from the employee roster and surveyed 200 of the 2,000 men employed by the company who fit the description "middle-aged, with a sedentary job." You used a questionnaire partially developed from data collected from the employee representatives in the group discussions. These data reflect employee concerns. The questionnaire also included questions addressing concerns of the medical professionals in the employee health service. You led the group discussions and constructed the questionnaire using principles discussed in chapter 5 and based on factors discussed earlier in this chapter. The return rate from the survey was 84 percent, and you calculate that about 40 percent of the male employee population is at risk, that is, engages in one or more negative health practices.

Now what? You begin to sift the primary and secondary data for the *specific* factors associated with changing behavior. You have four separate but interrelated risk-reduction behaviors to consider: smoking, lack of exercise, overweight, and high blood pressure. Here we will select overweight as the risk to follow through to illustrate how to find the behavioral dimensions to include in a program.

Assume that 20 percent of the population you surveyed weigh at least 20 pounds more than desired for their age and height. No man in the group has associated physiological problems to account for the weight. A good emphasis in the program, therefore, would be to help this number of men to drop the extra pounds. What do all your data reveal about losing weight? Assume that the data show the following:

1. The knowledge level of the group is low regarding the kinds of foods that are low in fat.

2. Most of the men eat breakfast and dinner at home and eat whatever their spouses prepare for them.

3. Most have many business lunches and must travel for business, often eating in restaurants.

4. Most believe that "healthy food" refers to something flower children and hippies eat.

5. Many claim to have little time or inclination to seek out exercise during the business day and say they are too tired on weekends.

6. A majority describe an interest in exercise but say it is hard to fit into a busy schedule. Some claim not to be the exercise type.

7. Most believe that middle-aged men are susceptible to cardiovascular problems but believe they themselves are not at much risk.

8. The men report that the most important things to them are their families and getting ahead in the company.

9. Many, but not all, say they believe that being healthy benefits their families and improves their work.

10. Most do not consider being overweight much of a deterrent to "getting ahead."

By slowly and carefully culling your data, you begin to get a behavioral picture of the people you intend to assist, of how they behave, how they perceive the problem, and the priority of the problem to them. The accuracy and specificity of this picture, of course, depends on the relevance and completeness of the initial data you acquired and collected.

Assume that you know, from the literature and from discussions with your nutrition colleagues, that the desired health status (lower weight) is, except for those with psychological or physiological problems, a function of eating the right combination of foods, eating the right amount of food, and getting adequate exercise (Glanz, 1980). What new behaviors, given your population and the context in which it must function, do these men need to acquire? You can diagram the problem as shown in table 3.2. You begin with current behavior and move to behavior to be learned that is instrumental to ideal behavior. What are some behaviors to be learned by the overweight men you aim to help? You know from the literature review that nutrition knowledge is associated with receiving clear, accurate information (McNutt, 1980). The target men must learn which foods and how much food to eat. They must, for example, (1) be able to select from a restaurant menu foods that will be beneficial to their diet; (2) be able to recognize "fat" foods from "skinny" foods; (3) be able to distinguish too big a portion from an adequate portion and choose the latter; and (4) be able to substitute foods they like or at least favor for

Table 3.2   Three Types of Behavior Included in Program Planning

Current Behavior	Instrumental Behavior (Behavior to Be Learned)	Ideal Behavior (Outcome Behavior)
Eating "wrong" foods	Selecting correct foods, combinations, amounts	Eating "right" foods
Getting little exercise	Finding and practicing exercise that fits one's temperament and schedule	Getting adequate exercise

foods they love that are too fattening. In addition, the men must rethink their behavioral patterns regarding exercise. For example, they must (5) be able to find time and fit exercise into their busy schedules; and (6) choose, and even rehearse, a type of exercise suitable to their temperament and personality and determine an appropriate routine for its use.

At this stage, the educator must review the behavioral picture the data provide and ask: What must the men be able to do, given their situation, in order to eat "right" and get exercise? This process enumerates the behaviors that must be learned and simultaneously suggests the needed information and skills.

Initial data have also made clear that the men hold values and beliefs about health and nutrition. Most men, for example, highly value family and job. There are some theoretical connections between maintaining weight, maintaining health, and benefits to a man's family and work. It is likely that men who accept the connections would also value losing weight. The men who will take part in the program may come to accept the connections, or they may reject them. In either case, the program should provide the opportunity for them to analyze the relationships and understand their own views (Simon et al., 1972). Many men in the group do not consider themselves susceptible to cardiovascular accidents. You know, as a result of your literature review, that people who believe themselves susceptible are predisposed to new health actions (Becker, 1976). The program, then, should enable the men to recognize overweight as a risk factor and recognize that overweight coupled with additional negative practices places a man at high risk.

In these examples of steps 2 and 3 of planning, we have used only a fragmented behavioral picture of the men. When you, as the health educator, review all the data collected in step 1 in the way recommended, you are likely to find an even wider range of information and skills that the potential learners need. This is especially so in a risk-reduction program that also addresses other problems, e.g., smoking and blood pressure control. In step 2 you must try to be comprehensive about the problem and its associated behaviors. Carrying out this process enables you to see the people, the problems, and the needed information and skills in a larger context. When the time comes to select a smaller number of behaviors as the target of the program, you will understand clearly how one behavior or set of behaviors relates to another.

Steps 4 and 5: Identifying Needed Resources and Related Services

If your learning program is to enable people to change behavior, you need to recognize the kind and extent of resources, both personal and material, that are available to the learners. For example, again consider the weight-loss component of the employee risk-reduction program. The literature review shows that a primary influence on the way a man eats is his wife (Becker and Green, 1975). Without the agreement and support of the spouse, a person is less likely to change eating behavior (Witschi et al., 1978; Schafer, 1978; and Saccone and Israel, 1978). Further, the potential learners have reported that at home they eat mainly what their wives prepare. Clearly, the educational program will have to find a way to reach these spouses. The literature review also shows that peer support is important to people who change behavior (Levin et al., 1976). Eating, for these potential learners, is significantly associated with business. The men will therefore have a more difficult time if their colleagues and bosses do not acknowledge the value of their efforts to lose weight. The men also might not stick to their diets if they continue to equate eating healthful foods with "health nuts and hippies." The behavior of the learners will be influenced by others in the work setting who might give or withhold support, and the education must accommodate to this fact.

It is likely that the potential learners have access to healthful food. Assume that they earn enough money to afford balanced meals, and they live in an area where fresh fruits and vegetables and a range of other foods are readily available. The men probably have other needed material resources. Most have a bathroom scale to monitor their weight. Most reside in communities where recreation facilities and parks exist, where they can exercise. These material resources could not be assumed in a poorer population, however, and would need to be accounted for somehow.

Assume, as well, that needed health and community resources are available to the group. For example, the physicians on your planning committee are likely to recommend a physical exam for each man before beginning a weight-loss program. Assume your group can be examined by the employee health service at no extra cost to the men. Should physical problems be detected, they will be referred for service, and the costs will be covered by their employee health plan. Let's say, then, that your group is a lucky one with services organized and financed in a way appropriate to their needs. Often a program to help people learn to behave differently entails an initial phase of securing needed related services and, especially with low-income populations, this can be the most inhibiting factor of all.

In steps 4 and 5, you review each ideal and instrumental behavior, while asking: What personal and material resources must potential learners have in order to change? What services must they have? This process enables you to see outside factors that will enable or inhibit the change. A goal at this stage is to identify ways to obtain needed social support, resources, and services. In the hypothesized case, it is evident that most resources are plentiful, but somehow your program will need to engender support from the spouses and colleagues of the men to foster change.

As a result of steps 1–5 of the planning process, you will have amassed considerable information:

A comprehensive picture of the people and the problem

A comprehensive list of outcome behaviors—that is, the "ideal behavior" to resolve or manage the problem

A corresponding list of instrumental behaviors—what people must learn to do to behave in a new way

A compilation of the information and skills that are entailed— the content of what must be learned

A compilation of the factors outside the individual that will most inhibit or enable learning—personal and material resources and needed health or community services

Step 6: Enumerating Expected Changes and How to Measure Them

In step 6, you begin to lay the groundwork for evaluation. This is the time to identify which changes might occur and how they might be measured. Continuing with the weight-loss example, previous steps identified the kind of behavior that resolves or reduces the problem of being overweight. Next, the measurable outcomes related to new behavior must be identified.

The first changes to be evaluated concern the impact of learning on the men. You will want to know if participants changed their eating and exercise patterns. The *impact of education* on the patient (remember our earlier discussion) is what they do differently. You will also want to know if they lost weight and if they kept it off. A *change in physical health status* is whether the participants lose weight. Related *changes in psychological health status* might also result, e.g., whether the men feel better, think they look better, think better of themselves—increase their self-esteem (Weller et al., 1977). Both physiological and psychological changes are likely.

Now envision a number of these newly thin, happy, healthy employees. What related changes might be expected? Over time, the men may reduce their risk of cardiovascular-related illnesses, i.e., they might get lower scores on risk-assessment tests. There may also be a reduced number of cardiovascular illnesses in the group, but that outcome would be measurable only quite a while down the line. Some men may feel a higher degree of job satisfaction, due in part to their increased self-esteem and in part to receiving health education as an employee benefit (Stoner and Fioullo, 1976). There may be fewer days of absence from work due to illness (Employee Health Fitness editors, 1980). In other words, this phase of planning involves outlining the anticipated results of successful education of the men to eat "right," get exercise, and consequently lose weight.

At this point, you must think carefully about how each of these changes might be measured. While many changes might occur theoretically, only some can be easily measured empirically. For example, it should be easy to measure whether eating patterns change. As an evaluator, you might ask participants to keep dietary diaries or recalls, to record their eating habits. Or you might ask them to describe their typical meals for a period of time, e.g., a month preceding and following the program. You might telephone spouses on a few random occasions before and after the program and ask for a description of the meal the participant ate that night.

You might measure the outcome of weight loss by having the men weigh in and weigh out before and after the learning program. You might measure cardiovascular risk reduction by asking the men to complete an assessment before and after the program. You might measure job satisfaction or self-esteem before and after by developing an index or using a standardized one. Measuring actual reductions in cardiovascular disease might be more difficult. Such a measurement might be taken at some future time, by reviewing personnel files or employee insurance claims.

The focus, depth, and extent of evaluation of related outcomes is a function of how much time and how many resources are available to you. Following step 6, however, you will have a very good idea of which outcomes seem most likely, which can be measured empirically, and how difficult and expensive evaluation will be.

Step 7: Selecting Behaviors to Address and Outcomes to Measure

Step 7 in the planning process might be called a "reality test." This is the time when you and your colleagues in planning must agree (get out the consensus exercises) on the specific things that your program can indeed achieve. While it is desirable during the initial steps to touch on all aspects of behavior related to the problem, and while those planning steps may have revealed the complexity of the problem, paradoxically, now is the time to narrow the problem and to arrive at a feasible, manageable, affordable set of behaviors and outcomes to address and measure in the program.

The importance of taking a detached look at the emerging program cannot be overstressed. You must ascertain the appropriate scope for your program, given all you know about the problem and what is needed to resolve or reduce it. You must reassess whether the direction in which you are moving is appropriate for your organization.

Assume, for example, that you are quite sure by this stage that one set of instrumental behaviors to bring change has to do with a wider kind of action, i.e., something more than just personal health behavior of the learners. In the asthma example used earlier, suppose that analysis has brought you to conclude that several equally important factors are involved in better management of childhood asthma: taking medicine in correct doses at correct times, practicing relaxation exercises, using prearranged and rehearsed strategies in the face of an attack, and maintaining a favorable living environment. These practices, in large part, involve personal instrumental behaviors; however, analysis may reveal that maintaining a suitable environment is exceedingly difficult for the particular targeted learners, because they are poor, urban residents of substandard housing. They cannot afford to rebuild their living quarters to eliminate falling plaster. They cannot afford to move to other apartments to get away from the broken down elevators, dampness, and lack of heat that contribute to the onset of infections and wheezing.

Based on analysis of the data, you may feel that reaching desired outcomes depends on the ability of families to change these conditions. This, however, takes much more than one parent's effort; it takes collective action. The learners might, for example, collectively sue the landlords who are failing to keep buildings in good repair. They might contribute time and materials and help each other repair their apartments. They might organize into a tenants' association and demand services from the city housing department. In other words, people might learn about and be assisted to take legal, cooperative, and political actions that would better enable them to maintain a favorable living environment for their children. Somehow this need for wider action must be addressed if significant change is to be realized.

There are several options for accommodating this kind of learning need. Your organization may see health education for community action as part of its regular health education responsibility, and you can develop the appropriate activities as an integral part of the program. Your organization may not engage in community action and outreach of this type, but one of your collaborating organizations may; you might develop an action component with them. If no collaborating organization is willing, you may be able to refer learners to groups in the area who handle legal and political action. On the other hand, the objectives of your organization might be more in line with fostering collective action than with developing the personal, individual behaviors that are needed. In such a case, at this point, you would need to explore the possibility for addressing the latter dimensions. In some way or another, however, the major needs must be addressed, and you must form your expectations of change according to how well they are addressed.

There are several criteria to use in determining which behaviors to include and measure in the program. They have to do with what is relevant, appropriate, and feasible for the learners, for you as the health educator, and for your organization. A behavior is a priority if the answer to most of the following questions is yes:

1. Is the behavior free from outside factors that would inhibit its development, or can you accommodate the important outside factors in your program? (For example, if you include eating correct foods at home as a behavior in a risk-reduction program, can you involve participants' spouses, who control at-home meals?)

2. Is the behavior a critical one in achieving the desired outcomes?

3. Do you know what kind of learning activities will develop the behavior? (Here you may want to review theories related to health behavior and learning and the lists of needed information and skills that emerged in steps 2 and 3.)

4. Is the behavior deemed important, or could it come to be recognized as important by the learners?

5. Do the collaborators (members of your planning network) agree that the behavior is important?

6. Is the lack of this behavior pervasive among potential learners? (If only one or two people are not already doing the behavior, individualized learning may be more effective than making the behavior a focus of the program.)

7. Is educational, medical, or other expertise available to design the needed learning activities?

8. Are needed related services available to support the change?

9. Is the cost of implementing education to change the behavior a reasonable one? How about the cost to measure the impact on the learners (the change in behavior that might occur)? How about the cost of means to measure related outcomes?

By completing this step in the process, you have not only winnowed the list of behaviors to address, using criteria of feasibility, appropriateness, and relevance, but also specified which changes to *assess*. At this point, you also begin to explore the appropriate evaluation design, if you feel a controlled evaluation is possible. These designs are discussed in detail in chapter 6.

Step 8: Designing Learning Experiences

By the time you are ready to plan the interventions, you have collected and analyzed enough data so that many aspects of needed learning materials and methods are very clear. In designing learning experiences, you again rely on data from steps 1 and 2. You review the theories and descriptions of previous educational programs and studies describing the factors that enable people to change behavior. You cull your lists of information and skills needed to behave in a new way. You use these data to design learning activities that, given theory, the experience of others, and the particular problems confronting the learners, hold the highest promise of success and address the behaviors most critical to the desired outcome (as determined in step 7).

For example, the data from the potential participants in the cardiovascular risk-reduction program revealed that they held values that discounted the importance of certain healthful foods. Assume one instrumental behavior you want to address is selecting healthful foods from a typical restaurant menu, and you plan to include learning activities to develop this skill as part of the program. You also know that participants will be unlikely to select foods they view as "health foods" or "hippie foods." Another needed learning activity, then, may be a values clarification exercise that enables participants to explore how they react to certain foods and why they feel as they do (Clark, 1981). Such an exploration may help to "unfreeze" their values and, if so, make a wider range of foods available to them.

You also know that the support of spouses who prepare at-home meals will be needed for behavior change, so you may want to organize discussion groups, or information sessions, or demonstrations of food selection and preparation that include the spouses and that introduce new ways to improve family eating patterns (Mojonnier et al., 1980). You may want to establish a mass information campaign at work, focused on the colleagues and supervisors of the participants, to enlist their support of the men's efforts to change. In other words, for each behavior that you want to help the men develop, you select the learning approach best suited to its development and support.

You need to satisfy two levels of concern when designing educational interventions: the *content* of the material (in the above example, health promotion, diet, and exercise) and the *processes* by which people learn to behave differently (consciousness raising, problem solving, rehearsal and practice of skills, values clarification, acquisition of new information, receiving support, and so on). Process and content are interrelated, of course. A group discussion to provide social support among participants, if led by a trained facilitator, may also be the best means to present one or two nutrition messages, to do some values clarification, and even to rehearse skills such as selecting low-fat foods from a list.

When evaluating programs, evaluation researchers feel that it is "cleaner" to assess different interventions separately (Becker and Maiman, 1975)—that is, to discern whether values clarification is a more effective intervention than rehearsal of skills, or problem-solving groups, or counseling. In the daily practice of health education, this separation of approaches makes sense only if previous studies and your own experience say it is the most effective way to proceed. Answering the effectiveness question is currently an important area for evaluation research. Theoretically, combined approaches should be better (Green, 1979). In designing learning events, however, the behavior to be learned dictates the approach and determines the resources and materials needed to support the approach.

It is important to remember that materials in health education (slides, films, tapes, written documents) in and of themselves are not learning methods. Learning is a process often supported by materials. Materials can provide information, stimulate discussion, and reinforce information provided. You can choose the kinds of materials needed only after you have decided on the learning objectives and approaches.

For each learning event, you must determine how participants will demonstrate that they have learned the instrumental behavior.

Often, this is simple. Participants in the diet and exercise program might, for example, complete a checklist of preferred foods at the end of their session on menu selection. Sometimes, monitoring learning activities is more difficult. For example, some men in the program may be unwilling to express how they feel about some aspect of nutrition at the end of a values exercise. For each learning event for which there is a specific objective, however, you must decide how to determine if the objective has been achieved to a satisfactory degree. Monitoring provides important benchmarks for both learners and program personnel (Mezirow et al., 1975). There must be signs that the program has momentum and is moving the participants along.

The duration and frequency of learning sessions and of the program itself are of great concern to program developers in terms of both learning and cost. Some studies have shown that important behavior change has been realized in a single learning session (Green, 1977; Weingarten et al., 1976). At least one study has found that attending more sessions was associated with more change (Clark et al., 1981). One researcher has postulated that extended health education reaches a point of diminishing returns (Green, 1974). Another found this to be the case with nutrition counseling and education delivered at home (Wang et al., 1975). Current data suggest that programs of more than one session that do not drag on over a long time may yield the greatest degree of change. Unless specific data are available from evaluation research to suggest a particular time frame for the type of education you are planning, this determination should be based on the following criteria:

1. What is best for the participants in their view?
2. What have previous studies and programs of a similar type shown to be effective?
3. What is manageable, given the context in which the program must operate?
4. What in your previous experience has been effective?
5. How much material must be covered?
6. What is the location of the program in relation to the participants?

The location of learning is an important consideration. If people are to be convened for learning away from the places where they spend the bulk of their time (that is, school, home, and work), then you must consider a practical question: How often and for how long can people be expected to travel to and from a learning site? If learning is attached to other health services, then the location and frequency of learning sessions may be geared to them, e.g., the sessions will coincide with monthly clinic visits. If school or work or home is the site, more frequent learning sessions for shorter durations may be the best.

You need to base decisions on available data and what makes most sense for the learners. It is standard practice, during step 1 of program planning, to ask potential learners what configuration of time and what location are best for them.

Similarly, the number of learners to include in a program is based on three criteria:

1. The number best suited to the educational approaches selected

2. The number of the population to be reached

3. The practicalities of cost and manageability

Assume that you have decided on group discussion as a format for the employee program on diet and exercise. From the review of the literature in step 1, you know that six to eight members in a group is optimum to ensure full participation in discussion. However, there are almost 1,000 men to be reached eventually. You may decide, therefore, to hold information sessions for large groups with numerous visual aids, self-tests, and a lecturer. These will alternate with discussion and support groups of small numbers of men. In this way, you hope both to reach a big audience with information and to meet the necessary conditions of the more intensive learning approaches within a reasonable cost.

One of the most enjoyable steps in program development is designing the actual learning events. There is a rich and growing literature on both learning and health behavior. Your knowledge of theories and studies, coupled with creativity, can produce excellent learning activities and effective deployment of materials.

Table 3.3 presents a sample summary of goals, objectives, and anticipated outcomes for the asthma education program used as an example in this chapter. The table illustrates planning steps 1–8, the logical progression from a problem to a program to outcomes. From analysis of the problem, the people, and their behavior, the health educator identifies the kind of learning needed to enable learners to behave in a new way.

Step 9: Developing Organizational Arrangements, Logistics, and Personnel Training

If the health educator has faithfully involved members of the program planning network in the planning process, by step 9 the resources and support needed to mount the program should be both evident and available. If, early on, for example, the employee health service has agreed to give medical checkups to employees enrolling in the weight-loss program, now is the time to work out the details of referral, recordkeeping, and so on. If you have developed a program alone, without bringing along those vital to its success, you can expect trouble at this point in trying to secure assistance.

This is when you determine what is entailed administratively and logistically, from recruiting learners through evaluation of the program. What departments, people, and resources are needed and available? Which people must give their approval before the program proceeds? Which facilities are needed for learning events? Have all the parties needed to implement the program committed themselves and where necessary put the extent of their participation in writing? Have all organizational and legal constraints been considered?

Take, again, the asthma education example. Assume you have decided to evaluate reduced school absences as a related outcome of better management. Will the local school let you use its records? Will parents need to sign a release? Assume you have decided to invite tenant organizers to the clinic to talk with parents about improvements in housing. Will the organizers need passes to visit the clinic? Must these visits be noted as referrals in clinic records? Each step of the program you have designed must be reviewed while you ask: Have we accounted for the administrative, legal, and logistical aspects of this element? You should undertake step 9 with the confidence that, because the planning network has been used, major aspects were considered and adequately addressed in earlier steps.

At this juncture, you must also determine what kind of training of personnel is necessary to implement the program. Each type of worker who will have an influence on the learning must be oriented, and some may need special training. Some must be trained to implement education, others to collect data, others to keep records, and so on. Certainly, those who will facilitate discussion groups must be trained. At the very least, the immediate group of health educators must be trained and oriented. Every program is different, because every group of learners is different. At a minimum, the educators must be prepared to work with the particular group of people in the specific context.

The design of personnel training, like the education program, operates on two levels: those who must be briefed and oriented regarding the content or health condition, and those who must be trained in the learning process. Physicians who play a role as counselors in an asthma education program may be very well versed in clinical aspects of asthma but need training in counseling. Health

Table 3.3 Synthesis of Planning Steps: A Program for Managing Childhood Asthma among Low-Income Families

Problem	Determinants of Family Behavior	Learning Objectives (Instrumental Behavior)
Disruption, stress, and high cost to families and communities resulting from childhood asthma	Knowledge of potential management behaviors	Learners will be able to:
	Level of skill in managing	Demonstrate relaxation exercises
Goal	Belief in one's ability to control the illness	Identify signs and symptoms of asthma
Increased ability of parents and children to manage asthma and reduce its negative effects on family life	Belief in one's ability to make judgments	Describe signs of a severe attack
	Perception of effective management measures	Describe strategies for managing a severe attack
	Availability of personal support to self-manage	Identify basic ways to prevent infection
	Availability of material resources	Use guidelines for negotiating with the child to set limits
		Demonstrate ways to question the physician
		Complete an information sheet for the school
		Express confidence in their own ability to manage
		Express belief in their own judgments
		Describe criteria for seeking medical assistance
		Identify allergens
		Seek assistance from relevant community services·

Program	Impact on Learners (Ideal Behavior)	Related Outcomes
Content Taking medicine Setting realistic guidelines for the child Getting information from the physician Keeping the child healthy Helping the child to do well in school Managing an attack *Process* Group problem solving Peer discussion Presentation of accurate information Rehearsal and practice of skills Peer support Counseling Parent and child discussion Parent and child practice of skills together	Increased self-management— learners will: Practice relaxation exercises Accurately assess wheezing severity Take actions appropriate to wheezing severity Use criteria for seeking medical assistance Take actions to promote health and prevent infections Seek information and assistance Remove allergens Set realistic limits for the child Communicate with the physician Establish relations with the school	Reduced stress and fear in the child and the parents Reduced school absences Increased adjustment of the child in school Reduced emergency visits Reduced hospitalizations

educators may be highly skilled in facilitating discussion groups but need a background in the clinical dimensions of asthma.

A rule of thumb is *not* to assume that health personnel already possess the requisite information and skills. In most situations, personnel have uneven levels of skills and information, and orientation and training help to fill the deficits. If different groups of personnel will undertake different tasks, then it is reasonable to train them separately. On at least a few occasions, it is necessary to bring all program personnel together for combined sessions or orientation. If tasks will cut across types of personnel (e.g., physicians, nurses, schoolteachers, and health educators, who must all provide the same basic messages when counseling), then it is reasonable to train them all together. The extent of training is determined by the tasks to be performed, the information to be provided, and the existing skill level of the personnel. In few cases would we recommend mounting a health education program without preparatory training for program personnel.

Step 10: Developing a Budget and Administrative Scheme

When a program is developed, certain costs and administrative needs result simply because the program is new. Costs of planning and development of methods, materials, and evaluation tools are in large part one-time expenses. The configuration of personnel needed to carry out initial planning and development may be different from the pattern needed when the program becomes institutionalized or part of an organization's routine.

The effectiveness of health education is likely to be proportional to the resources made available to a program. Failure to allocate sufficient money to programs has been cited as a reason for the limited success of some health education (Haggerty, 1977). A budget should include a rationale for each person or set of tasks to be undertaken during program development and once the program is going. The budget with its rationale should convince the sponsoring organization or funder that initial investments are warranted and that the program will be affordable over time.

The first concern in step 10, then, is to think through carefully what people will be needed to develop the program and to carry it out initially. Next, job descriptions must be written and personnel costs figured. The following kinds of personnel may be needed: a program director to assume overall responsibility; program coordinators to manage logistics; consultants in particular areas (content specialists, educational methods specialists, materials specialists, data collection and analysis specialists, etc.); educators to carry out the learning program; evaluators to conduct data collection and data analysis; and a secretarial and clerical staff.

Many of these people may already be available in the organization or members of the planning network. Individuals from other organizations may participate, and their services will show on the budget as contributions. To determine the cost of personnel, the simplest method is to estimate the number of hours per week, month, or year a person will need to devote to program activities, and compute the amount that person will be paid per week, month, or year. The proportion of full-time employment the person will give to the program is called the *percentage of effort*.

A budget must show not only the direct cost of personnel, that is, the money they will actually receive, but also the cost of fringe benefits provided them by the sponsoring organization. What will be the cost of vacation, insurance, workers' compensation, etc.? Most organizations have established rates for figuring these costs. Similarly, there are other unseen costs in a program. What is the cost of housing the program? What about services provided by other divisions or departments of the organization, such as the financial office and the personnel office, to support program personnel? The indirect cost of these services must be computed; again, the organization is likely to have an established rate for doing this. It is also likely that one person (you, for example) will have several program responsibilities. A health educator might serve as both program coordinator and teacher. If so, this fact must be spelled out in the budget rationale.

Items other than personal services will be needed to develop the program. Some of these will be ongoing expenses but some will be required only during program development. Expenses likely to be incurred initially include: space, if program housing is not available; equipment—typewriters, desks, and so on; supplies—paper, pencils, and other office needs; telephone service and postage; photocopying; acquisition of studies, articles, and books (that is, secondary data); printing costs for primary data collection and evaluation materials; printing costs for educational materials; computer costs for data analysis (if a computer is available); travel costs to and from learning sites; and training costs.

Once you have determined who and what are needed to carry out the program, the budget must be developed. Table 3.4 illustrates how you might show program costs for the first development year and the following two years. Figure 3.3 presents the rationale that might accompany the budget to explain why the amounts are requested.

Table 3.4 shows that the formula this sponsoring organization uses to compute fringe benefits is 20 percent of a person's salary. In this example, indirect costs are determined to be 20 percent of total

Table 3.4 Budget for Program Development and Implementation

		Year One					
Personnel	Estimated Hours per Week	Estimated Percentage of Effort	Salary per Annum	Fringe Benefits[a]	Total	Amount Available in Current Budget	Amount Requested
Program director Sidney Greenstreet	40	100%	$22,000	$4,400	$26,400	$26,400	—
Program coordinator/educator (To be named)	40	100	18,000	3,600	21,600	—	$21,600
Program evaluator Jamie Stewart	10	25	5,800	1,160	6,960	—	6,960
Secretary Leslie Lawrence	20	50	5,000	1,000	6,000	6,000	—
Consultants							
C. Velez (educational materials)	2	5	—	—	—	Contributed by Heart Association	—
R. Polanski (data analysis)	2	5	—	—	—	Contributed by University	—
Total personnel costs							$28,560
Costs other than personal services							
Books, materials, and acquisition of background data							$ 500
Printing of questionnaires and evaluation materials							350
Telephone, postage							150
Total direct costs							$29,560
Indirect costs[b]							$ 7,390
Total year one request							$36,950
Total year two request							$40,645
Total year three request							$44,710

Personal Services

Program Director   Sidney Greenstreet will devote 100 percent time during year one of program development. He will assume overall responsibility for the program, maintain links with all cooperating agencies, and oversee day-to-day program activities. The cost of the program director is provided for in the yearly departmental budget. In years two and three, it is estimated that Sidney Greenstreet will spend approximately 10 percent time supervising ongoing program implementation.

Program Coordinator/Educator   A person will be hired at 100 percent time to coordinate all day-to-day aspects of program development and to carry out the actual teaching in the program. The cost of the coordinator/educator is requested at 100 percent for all years of the program. After the first year of program development and evaluation, the program coordinator/educator will devote 100 percent time to the ongoing program and to its expansion to four sites by the third year of program implementation.

Program Evaluator   James Stewart will spend 25 percent time in all years of the program and will handle all major evaluation tasks.

Secretary   Leslie Lawrence, a half-time secretary, will handle secretarial tasks of correspondence and recordkeeping. The cost of this position is provided for in the departmental budget.

Consultants   Cosponsors of the program, Local Heart Association and Local University, each will contribute the equivalent of 5 percent consultation time by C. Velez and R. Polanski for development of educational materials and for analysis of initial survey data, respectively. In years two and three, consultation will be provided regarding program expansion and evaluation.

Other Than Personal Services

Books, Materials, Background Data   Although many resources are available in our own resource center and in the library of the nearby university, we will need to acquire some specialized materials from outside sources. This collection of materials will need to be updated yearly.

Printing of Questionnaires and Evaluation Materials   Most of the materials that will be needed for the program are available through existing sources, such as the Heart Association and other cooperating agencies. However, some costs will be incurred in the printing of specialized questionnaires to be used for needs assessment and for evaluation. These costs are likely to be incurred yearly.

Years Two and Three

To compute costs for years two and three, the year one budget has been increased each year by 10 percent to cover inflation and salary increases.

Figure 3.3 Budget Rationale

direct costs. Outside contributions are included in the budget with an indication that no funds are requested from the department for these services. Showing contributed time in the budget more accurately reflects the percentage of effort that will be expended. The bottom of the budget notes that requests will be made in years two and three.

The budget rationale, figure 3.3, explains that, after the first year, the program director will spend only 10 percent time administering program activities. This is likely to be considered a reasonable ongoing program expense. The rationale also states that, in the next two years, the program will be expanded to four sites with no addition of

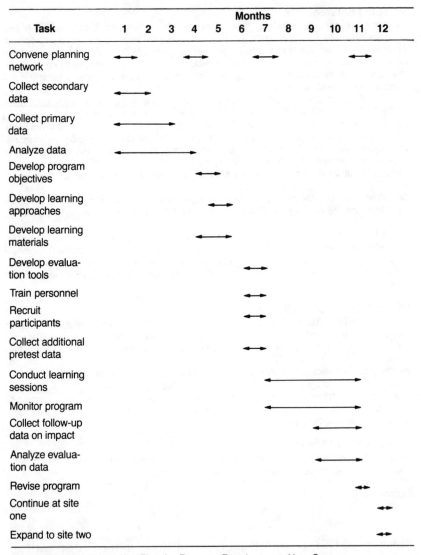

Task	Months											
	1	2	3	4	5	6	7	8	9	10	11	12
Convene planning network	←→			←→		←→				←→		
Collect secondary data	←—→											
Collect primary data	←——→											
Analyze data	←———→											
Develop program objectives					←→							
Develop learning approaches					←→							
Develop learning materials					←→							
Develop evaluation tools						←→						
Train personnel						←→						
Recruit participants						←→						
Collect additional pretest data						←→						
Conduct learning sessions							←————→					
Monitor program							←————→					
Collect follow-up data on impact										←→		
Analyze evaluation data										←→		
Revise program												↔
Continue at site one												↔
Expand to site two												↔

Figure 3.4 Implementation Plan for Program Development, Year One

staff. Each year the budget has been increased by 10 percent to cover changes in salaries and prices of materials.

Once you have developed the budget and budget rationale, you need to outline the time frame for carrying out major tasks. Figure 3.4 gives an example of how the first year of tasks might be presented. Note that representatives of organizations and groups from the planning network will meet regularly over the first year of development. The program will also be monitored continuously during the three months it is operating and will only be expanded to the second site after evaluation and revision.

With a program description, including the evaluation plan, an outline of personnel and their responsibilities, a time frame, a budget, and a budget rationale, you are ready to seek funding from the financial people or, if money is in hand, to implement the work plan.

By undertaking planning steps 1–10, you prepare to carry out a program that is headed for success and to conduct an evaluation of sufficient rigor to document the extent of success.

Because of careful planning, evaluation becomes a fundamental and integral element of the program, not something tacked on at the end. If, for some reason, you find you must assess a program after it is already in operation, you will need to engage in the planning steps ex post facto by reviewing the processes that led to the program. Only then will you be able to determine how the program might be evaluated. To make that determination, you must discern the logical chain—the links from program to new behavior to related outcomes. These links must be forged and assessed if health education is to be worthy of the learners it purports to assist.

SUMMARY

In this chapter we have discussed the influence of the sponsoring organization on the health education program. We have emphasized the need to establish and use a program planning network. We have defined needs assessment and suggested some approaches to assessing needs. This chapter has also underscored the importance of using the program plan to forge a logical link from a health problem to the education to expected outcomes. Finally, we have described and discussed 11 steps that the planner must undertake to ensure that the program addresses important needs, can be evaluated, and is feasible for the sponsoring organization to undertake. A detailed discussion of cost, cost effectiveness, and cost benefit analysis is included in Appendix C for advanced discussions and courses in evaluation. The following chapter discusses qualitative evaluation methods—ways a health educator can monitor the quality of a program as it takes place.

4

Conducting Process Evaluations

"My hospital is looking for a new coordinator for our community health promotion center. What kind of skills should this person have?"

"If we use behavioral impact as the only indicator of success I think our program is in trouble. Aren't there other types of outcomes we can look at?"

"Our administrator was really pleased with our qualitative evaluation. She wants us to put more emphasis on good programs and satisfied consumers."

"I don't have the foggiest idea of how to conduct a process evaluation. How do you do it? What methods do you use?"

Professional Competencies Emphasized in This Chapter:

- definition of quality, quality control, and standards

- differentiation between efficacy and effectiveness

- specification of standards of practice

- selection and application of quality control methods

- identification and description of key program categories for program review

- identification and description of key components for conducting a process evaluation

The concept of examining program quality is not really new, in either health care or health education and promotion. Reports by Donabedian (1966) and Greene (1976) on quality of medical care, Inui (1978) on quality assurance issues in health education and medical care, and Green and Brooks-Bertram (1978) on quality assurance and health education all confirmed the need to examine the processes and skills of personnel who plan and deliver health-related programs. According to all four sources, a judgment according to an existing standard is required to evaluate the delivery process. The need to know what a program has done to and for a patient or consumer, how well it was done, and what should have been done are ongoing concerns in conducting a process evaluation. The health education promotion literature suggests a need to conduct process evaluations but provides little guidance on what elements to examine or how to proceed.

As shown in table 1.2 earlier in this text, level 1 or process evaluation usually (1) applies nonexperimental designs, (2) assesses operating procedures, (3) examines structure and process, (4) conducts observational analyses, (5) performs qualitative observations, (6) monitors program effort or activity, (7) reviews or audits data systems and records, and (8) employs formative evaluation methods. The strengths and weaknesses of a program and the processes by which participants are exposed to it or recruited are major concerns in conducting a process evaluation. Such an evaluation assesses how an outcome is produced rather than the quantitative, behavioral impact. It tries to answer questions of why the program succeeded, failed, or needs to be revised. It describes what actually happened as a program was started, implemented, and completed. A process evaluation is by definition descriptive and adaptive—a mechanism used continuously to explain the dynamics of an unfolding program. It compares what happened to what was supposed to happen, using existing standards of acceptability for comparison on each dimension. It applies standards and a level of quality defined in the literature and/or derived by professional consensus through internal or external review.

This chapter identifies normative criteria and procedures that you should strive to make integral parts of the planning and implementation of your health education/health promotion programs. At the ends of several sections, standards are suggested that you can use to assess the quality of specified program components.

QUALITY ASSURANCE

In discussing the concept of process evaluation in health education, several terms need to be defined: quality, quality assurance, quality control, and standards. By *quality* we mean the appropriateness of a set of professional activities to the objectives they are attempting to achieve. *Quality assurance* is accountability for professional activities by which consumers can know that they are appropriately performed. *Quality control* describes the methods used to produce documentation of and to ensure the quality of program procedures. A *standard* is the minimum acceptable level of performance used by experts in a specialty area to judge the quality of an individual's professional practice (Green and Brooks-Bertram, 1978).

The quality assurance review (QAR) of a health education program can be best viewed as a multidimensional process. At a minimum, it demands (1) an accurate assessment of the technical competence of the service provider, and (2) the application of policy and procedures to improve dimensions of practice that are determined to be inadequate. In discussing program quality, two concepts are frequently mentioned: efficacy and effectiveness. *Efficacy* can be defined as the power of a program, applied under *optimum* circumstances to favorably alter the history of a risk factor for individuals who comply with the intervention. Efficacy, then, is a statement about the maximum potential of a health education program to alter the health behavior of a target group. *Effectiveness* can be defined as the power of a program, applied under *practice* conditions, to favorably alter the history of a risk factor for those who comply with the intervention. It is a statement about the normal potential of a program to alter the behavior of a target group.

As an example of the contrast between efficacy and effectiveness, compare the behavioral impact of the Multiple Risk Factor Intervention Trial (MRFIT) to the behavioral impact of a typical community-based smoking-cessation program offered by a voluntary health organization at a work site or a health care institution. One purpose of the MRFIT program was to determine the efficacy of its smoking-cessation component. The intervention consisted of two parts: (1) ten sessions of 90–120 minutes with six to twelve men attending each, and (2) a continuous, individual nonsmoking maintenance program for a four-year period. A behaviorist (in most cases with a master's or doctoral degree), a nutritionist (in many cases with a master's degree), and a physician formed the intervention team. This project reported a smoking-cessation rate of 46 percent after four years among approximately 6,000 men (Hughes et al., 1981), the most successful confirmed long-term cessation results to date. MRFIT demonstrated the efficacy of a "maximum" resource intervention in altering the smoking behavior history among a sample of men aged 35 to 57. An ongoing community-based program focusing on smoking cessation over time would be expected to demonstrate an effectiveness level of approximately 25 percent cessation among men at a six-month follow-up (U.S. DHEW, 1980).

The importance of being able to distinguish between efficacy and effectiveness lies in the realization that estimates of the quality of a program reflect value judgments. Therefore, qualitative statements of expectations should be made with a degree of realism, within the context of time, resources, and empirical evidence. If one program reports a 10 percent rate of smoking cessation after six months for junior high school students, and another program for a similar population reports a 25 percent cessation, this strongly suggests a real difference in program effectiveness and the need to determine why the outcomes were different. Assuming comparable samples, data, and methodologies, the difference strongly suggests a difference in program quality, program adequacy, or provider competence. These two additional, interrelated dimensions of quality assurance—provider competence and program adequacy—need to be carefully considered when an organization is making the decision to offer such programs to consumers.

PROVIDER COMPETENCE

Provider competence can be assessed through internal or external peer review mechanisms, by examining the provider's academic and professional training, program experience, professional products, and current activities in the development, implementation, administration, and evaluation of health promotion programs. There is much concern about the need to improve the quality of professional preparation and practice in health education and health promotion. In commenting on this concern from a legal perspective, Easton et al. (1977) refer to the lack of competence as educational malpractice, and they argue that it is as serious in consequences and costs as medical malpractice.

While codification of the skills for good health education practice is still in its early stages, widely disseminated documents confirm that the profession is moving toward the identification of basic competencies (SOPHE, 1977a, 1977b; U.S. DHEW, 1978a). Using the report of the Initial Role Delineation Project (U.S. DHHS, Public Health Service, 1980a) on professional preparation in health education as a referent, two broad areas can be examined in discussing the issue of provider competence: (1) knowledge of the state of the art, and (2) technical skill.

Knowledge of the State of the Art

While the state of the art is a moving target, the literature in health education and related disciplines seems sufficiently mature to offer a body of knowledge about human behavior in sickness or health for most major diseases and risk factors. Accordingly, directors of health promotion programs need to know what has been done, what can be done, and how it should be done. While familiarity with the state of the art for a specific health problem or risk factor is necessary, it is not sufficient for health education practice. It is impossible, however, to function as "a good practitioner" without a knowledge of the most up-to-date literature germane to the program. Commonly cited reasons for program failure include lack of knowledge on the part of program staff of what is possible or probable and lack of experience in applying program skills, i.e., insufficient theoretical grounding and ignorance of previous work. These deficiencies are common, in part, because of the diverse backgrounds of individuals engaged in planning health programs, the lack of organizational clarity or direction in offering such programs, and the lack of clarity about appropriate academic and professional credentials for program personnel.

> STANDARD 1: Individuals responsible for planning and administering health promotion programs should be able to document through academic training in health education or related behavioral sciences a comprehension of and the skill to apply methods and content from the existing literature for a specific health problem, risk factor, and population.

Technical Skill

As indicated in the report of the Society for Public Health Education, "Guidelines for the Preparation and Practice of Professional Health

Educators" (1977), and the report of the Initial Role Delineation Project (U.S. DHHS, Public Health Service, 1980a), individuals involved in health education practice should be able to demonstrate competence in a number of areas (see table 1.1, earlier). More specifically, competent planners and coordinators of programs should be able to provide evidence that programs under their direction reflect high standards of practice and the state of the art, within the context of available resources.

STANDARD 2: Individuals responsible for planning and managing health promotion programs should provide documentation of training and ability to:

1. Define and interpret the extent and distribution of a selected health problem or risk factor for a selected geographical area, location, setting, and population, using available and/or derived data (assessment of need).
2. Derive and describe, from available or collected evidence and expert opinion, the behavioral and nonbehavioral risk factors associated with a specified health problem (priority setting).
3. Describe from the related literature the current state of the art of health education and promotion for the specified risk factor or health problem and the population and the degree to which it is amenable to change (definition of objectives).
4. Define and describe, from scientific evidence in the literature and from an educational-behavioral diagnosis, contributing factors found to be causally associated with the health behavior or risk factors, including:
   a. Characteristics of the target group: predisposing factors such as attitudes, beliefs, values, and channels of communication
   b. Situational characteristics of the area or setting: enabling factors such as availability and accessibility of health education services
   c. Characteristics of program or service providers: reinforcing factors such as staff attitudes, behaviors, and skill in educating consumers (specification of interventions)
5. Synthesize, interpret, and translate the information and evidence collected from steps 1 to 4 into a program plan (specification of implementation plan).
6. Design, implement, administer, and evaluate appropriate communication, community organization, and education-behavioral methods to produce change in the contributing factors and the behaviors identified in steps 3–5, in collaboration with other health professionals, organizational personnel, and consumers (specification of evaluation plan).
7. Prepare project reports of a publishable quality (preparation of program reports).
8. Conduct professional activities in an ethical manner, reflecting appreciation for human rights, quality assurance, and peer reviews established by organizations that set professional standards and guidelines.

These competencies describe the technical skills a trained person should be able to demonstrate and apply routinely in health education practice (SOPHE, 1977a; Windsor, 1980). The level of academic training that should produce a person with these competencies is the master's degree in community health education.

PROGRAM ADEQUACY

Methods for examining the adequacy of a health care program were first set forth by Donabedian (1966, 1968), modified by Starfield (1974), and described by Greene (1976) as they apply to health education and health promotion. The focus of their work was how to apply quality assessment procedures to program structure, process, and outcome. This chapter focuses on the first two aspects of a program. Chapter 5 focuses on the third.

A structural assessment of a health promotion program examines the resources, facilities, and equipment for the delivery of services, and asks: Are they adequate to deliver the service? Are those delivering the service qualified to do so? In an assessment of process, the ultimate questions are: What procedures were used to develop and implement the program? Are they consistent with normative criteria, i.e., criteria developed by a consensus of experienced peers in health education with established professional credentials? A process assessment using normative criteria is indirectly an examination of provider competence. It examines the professional activities of the provider from the perspective of peer group judgment. As in the practice of nursing and medicine, the key issue is: What constitutes good practice for a given problem and population?

In discussing the concept of normative criteria, numerous reports have confirmed that the modern practice of health education can be approached in a highly systematic and rigorous fashion. Current practice demands:

1. Exploring the causes of a health problem or risk factor presented by a group of people, i.e., conducting an educational needs and behavioral problems assessment (standard 2, steps 1–4);

2. Designing and assessing an intervention to alter the health behavior associated with a disease or undesired quality of life, i.e., planning, implementation, and evaluation of the effort and resources expended (standard 2, steps 5–6);

3. Preparing program reports that are defensible and therefore of publishable quality (standard 2, step 7); and

4. Delivering programs that reflect high ethical principles (standard 2, step 8).

Health education and health promotion practice in the 1980s will be expected to reflect these standards in special settings. For example, efforts at the work site should reflect the principles, concepts, and guidelines identified in *Managing Health Promotion in the Workplace: Guidelines for Implementation and Evaluation* (Parkinson et al., 1982). Health education and health promotion programs in health maintenance organizations (HMOs) should reflect principles, guidelines, and standards identified in "Managing Health Education in Health Maintenance Organizations," parts 1 and 2 (Deeds and Mullen, 1981, 1982) and *Guidelines for Health Promotion and Education Services in HMOs* (Mullen and Zapka, 1982b). Contemporary school health education and promotion programs should reflect discussions identified in "Promoting Health through the Schools: A Challenge for the Eighties" (Iverson, 1981). Community health education programs should apply the principles and guidelines identified in "Making Health Education Work" (Simmons, 1975). Programs interested in a generic model applicable to school, patient, community, or work site health education should reflect the approach described in *Health Education Planning: A Diagnostic Approach* (Green et al., 1980).

To achieve the principal purpose of modern health education practice—change in the health behavior of individuals—persons responsible for health education and promotion programs need to: (1) know the state of the art, and (2) be able to demonstrate the competencies described in this book.

QUALITY CONTROL METHODS

Practitioners need to conduct process evaluations of health education programs in a systematic and technically acceptable fashion. A number of techniques can be used by a project staff to gain insight into how well the program is being implemented, how it is being received by a target group, and what adjustments might be made. One quality control technique is not necessarily superior to another. Each may be useful in planning and implementing a program. Each serves a specific purpose and provides unique information about the structure and process of an ongoing program. All require allocations of resources, staff, and time. Because of this, it is important to choose the most appropriate and feasible methods for a given program. To conduct a thorough review of program quality during implementation, a combination of methods is recommended.

Six categories of approaches are discussed: (1) expert panel reviews, (2) internal audits of resource allocations, (3) program utilization and record reviews, (4) community and participant surveys, (5) observations of programs or sessions, and (6) component pretesting.

Expert Panel Reviews

The importance of specifying process evaluation procedures during the early stages of program development and introduction cannot be overstressed. A process evaluation should answer the question of who is doing how much of what to whom by when and how well. An expert panel review (EPR) is an efficient way to assess these program dimensions assuming that a written program plan exists. The plan should include the program goal and objectives, methods, activities, procedures, and tasks. It should designate the program's staff, period of time, place, and group of participants. An EPR can be conducted effectively only when the health educator has followed a systematic process to plan and implement the health promotion effort. The EPR may examine selected parts, activities, materials, and procedures of program implementation, comparing documentation of the program with a set of standards or professional ratings. The total program or specific dimensions may be reviewed, e.g., the implementation plan, evaluation design, data collection procedures, mass media components, instruments, or methods and content of the intervention. A review may be accomplished by internal and external panels.

An EPR is particularly useful during planning and early stages of implementation (Simmons, 1975; Rossi et al., 1979). A review conducted once in the first six months and again during each year of the project should provide sufficient independent insight into the program's progress. Practically speaking, it is important to have a small review panel. Two or three experts from the area or state may be asked, in many cases on a voluntary basis, to examine a program periodically, in part or in whole. While panel members must have experience with the health problem or risk factors the program is addressing, they need not be national figures. The task of the panel will depend on its purpose, but a number of generic questions should be raised by this group. Table 4.1 lists common categories used by program personnel or expert panels. The panel discusses and rates each salient program structure and procedure noted in the written implementation plan for the program. Key questions are: Were each of these activities performed? Were they performed in a timely manner? Evidence from written documents and discussions can be gathered by panel members individually and as a group from the staff. In addition to ratings, the panel provides comments on the degree of adequacy observed and suggests program revisions. This information gives the program staff an overall, qualitative judgment of the structure and process of the ongoing program. The review should be a collaborative exercise and should provide practical suggestions for immediate program improvement (Deeds et al., 1979).

Table 4.1 Key Program Categories for Program Review

Standard	Rating[a]
1. Documentation of the use of studies and reports pertinent to the problem and the population in planning the program.	1 2 3 4 5
2. Consultation with state or local officials where specific data, literature, resources, or experience is lacking.	1 2 3 4 5
3. Inclusion of representatives from the target audience and affiliated local program agencies in active program planning and implementation.	1 2 3 4 5
4. Program planning and adaptation to reflect staff input.	1 2 3 4 5
5. Program planning based on concrete needs assessment data concerning the knowledge, attitudes, practices, and social systems of target groups.	1 2 3 4 5
6. Adequate statement of objectives: (1) program, (2) behavioral, (3) educational content and activities.	1 2 3 4 5
7. Staff tasks clearly delineated and performed according to the program implementation plan.	1 2 3 4 5
8. Specification of the target group by: (1) number, (2) characteristics, and (3) proportion reached.	1 2 3 4 5
9. Well-developed outreach plans to recruit specific target groups according to priorities dictated by the objectives.	1 2 3 4 5
10. Description of the data collection plan prior to implementation.	1 2 3 4 5
11. Recordkeeping forms tested prior to the initiation of program services.	1 2 3 4 5
12. Monitoring system in place and used to monitor completeness of pre- and postprogram data.	1 2 3 4 5
13. Instruments and observation methods pretested; assessment of their validity and reliability.	1 2 3 4 5
14. Communication media and materials pretested and evaluated when implemented.	1 2 3 4 5
15. Allocation of resources according to the implementation plan; identification of costs per participant.	1 2 3 4 5
16. Description of the quality and appropriateness of formative and summative evaluation designs.	1 2 3 4 5

[a]1 = poor; 5 = excellent.

STANDARD 1: Health education and health promotion programs should document having undergone an EPR during the first six months of operation and at least once per year thereafter.

Internal Audits

All ongoing programs must audit and document allocations of staff efforts and resources. A planner, administrator, or evaluator has to

Table 4.2   Implementation Plan Worksheet

Activity: Develop a county detection and treatment center

Implementation Strategy

Who Does What	When
1. Director of ambulatory services develops proposal for detection/treatment center	1/1
2. County board of health funds proposal	3/1
3. County renovates facilities	6/1
4. Director hires staff, including administrator and medical director	6/15
5. Administrator and medical director develop protocols and procedures, including special effort to motivate residents to participate and to follow up	8/15
6. Administrator acquires equipment and supplies	8/15
7. Data specialist develops patient record forms	9/15
8. Health educator develops education materials	9/15
9. Staff and volunteers are trained by medical director, health educator, and head nurse	10/1
10. Administrator tests methods and materials with county residents	10/15
11. Staff begins detection and treatment services to county residents	11/15
12. Administrator evaluates detection and treatment services	11/15

Source: U.S. Department of Health, Education, and Welfare, National Institutes of Health, National Heart, Lung, and Blood Institute, *Handbook for Improving High Blood Pressure Control in the Community* (Washington, D.C.: Government Printing Office, 1977), p. 37.

have some idea of what proportion of time staff has been spent on implementing a program and what nonpersonnel resources are being used. The issue is accountability (Rossi et al., 1979; Squyres, 1979). While the actual time a person spends on a program may vary from month to month, most organizations require periodic assessment and documentation of the level of staff effort. Individuals in business, industry, and education routinely document monthly estimates of percentages of their time spent on categories of activities.

A program audit needs to determine the consistency between the implementation plan and reality. An example of an implementation plan for a high blood pressure program is presented in table 4.2. The number of programs developed, sessions offered, participants recruited, and participants completing the program should be routinely reported. Documentation of a staff member's performance or the program's performance might consist of data on whether the objectives of a specific instructional program were accomplished. For example, did the patients become more skilled in urine testing, or did pregnant adolescents in a school-based prenatal care program hear of or see the antismoking campaign for pregnant women? To document this, program planners must provide for assessments of immediate cognitive or performance objectives of the participants. Are there opportunities to receive feedback on participant interest and motivation and on staff performance? Since many health promotion programs are carried out in service-oriented settings, the major program objectives may be knowledge, information, or improved skill. If materials distribution is the dimension of the program that is being examined, how much of what material was distributed to whom should be documented. Procedures need to be developed to examine how well an element of a program is being applied, being accepted, and working (Simmons, 1975; Deeds et al., 1979).

> STANDARD 2: Health promotion programs should provide monthly, quarterly, and annual documentation of the type and amount of resources allocated to them, including staff time, media, and materials.

Utilization and Record Reviews

As a general rule, health education programs tend to collect too much or too little information on participants. Often the information collected is of such poor quality or so incomplete that it is not useful. Despite the difficulty, a recordkeeping system is a must for monitoring program implementation. One of the program planner's first concerns, then, is to set up a system that does not overtax the program staff, particularly if the staff is small (e.g., one person). It is essential to make all program monitoring and data collection systems compatible with ongoing data systems.

Utilization and record reviews for quality assurance encompass four topics: (1) monitoring program participation, (2) improving record completeness, (3) documenting program or session exposure, and (4) monitoring the utilization of information services.

Monitoring Program Participation. Assuming a definable target population is specified, the extent to which those people are participating in the program is of paramount concern to the program organization. Inherent, then, to setting up a monitoring system is the need to define who the program is attempting to serve and an estimated number for the target area or location. This allows a program to answer the questions: How many of those eligible were served? Were the people who participated those for whom the program was designed?

Table 4.3 Hypothetical Process Evaluation of Participation in an Employee Health Promotion Program

Compo-nent	Process	Eligible Partici-pants	Partici-pant Exposure	Percent-age Reached (A)	Program Standard (B)	Effective-ness Index (C)
1	Risk screening of employees	150	100	67	80%	.84
2	Educational diagnosis— HHA	100	88	88	90%	.98
3	Health behavior counseling	100	84	84	90%	.93
4	Group session 1	100	81	81	90%	.90
5	Behavior monitoring	100	76	76	90%	.84
6	Group session 2	100	72	72	90%	.80
7	Behavior contract	100	62	62	90%	.69
8	Group session 3	100	60	60	90%	.67
9	Follow-up 1	100	56	56	90%	.62
10	Follow-up 2	100	50	50	90%	.55

Note:

$$PEI = \frac{.84 + .98 + .93 + .90 + .84 + .80 + .69 + .67 + .62 + .55}{10} = .78.$$

Data in table 4.3 represent hypothetical results of one component of a process evaluation. Assume that this example applied to a work site with 500 employees. One of the first procedures was to conduct a brief survey screening all 500 employees, to identify the proportion with specific risk factors that made them eligible participants. Of the 500, 150 were found to be at high risk. These 150 individuals were notified by the Health Promotion Program (HPP) staff about participating in a special program to help them deal with this particular risk factor. Over a six-month period, 100 of the 150 contacted by the HPP enrolled. As noted in table 4.3, this represents 67 percent of the eligible population.

For this component and the remaining nine components, the HPP established a set of standards of acceptable utilization, i.e., performance standards. For component 1, the HPP decided that the standard would be to enroll 80 percent or 120 of the 150 employees identified as at risk in the screening survey. Only 100, or 67 percent, enrolled, however, representing an effectiveness level (EI) of .84.

Of the 100 enrollees, 88 participated in component 2, the educational diagnosis, a health risk assessment. Following the diagnosis, 84 of the individuals participated in component 3, the one-to-one health behavior counseling. An increasingly smaller proportion participated in a series of three health education and risk-reduction sessions conducted with groups of five participants each (components 4, 6, and 8). As part of the series, each participant was expected to complete two principal procedures: a self-assessment exercise between sessions 1 and 2 (component 5), consisting of recording and monitoring the frequency and sites of their smoking behavior; and discussion and signing of a behavioral contract with a significant other (component 7), between sessions 2 and 3. As noted in table 4.3, 76 percent and 62 percent of the participants participated in these two processes respectively. Two follow-up assessments and counseling sessions (components 9 and 10) were required of all participants, three and six months after the program; 56 of the participants were exposed to follow-up session 1, and 40 to session 2. This program reported a 20 percent behavior change rate—20 successes out of 100 initial enrollees for each procedure.

A program can compute its effectiveness index (EI) by dividing the proportion reached during a component by the standard the program set (using the letters of the columns in table 4.3, A/B = C). A program effectiveness index (PEI) can be computed by adding all EIs and dividing the total EI by the number of procedures:

$$\text{PEI} = \frac{.84 + .98 + .93 + .90 + .84 + .80 + .69 + .67 + .62 + .55}{10}$$

$$= .78$$

A program should specify: (1) the expected EI for individual procedures, (2) a projected total PEI, and (3) the anticipated behavioral impact.

A health promotion program of high quality should specify and confirm levels of exposure to program components. This approach enables a program to plot individual and group exposure to components. It permits a program to make clear statements about the level of implementation success. It suggests that the program is being managed well or not so well. The PEI pinpoints problem areas.

STANDARD 3: Health promotion programs should provide documentation of what proportion of eligible participants were served, the extent of participation of each individual, the program completion rate, and the effect of the program on participants' behavior.

Improving Record Completeness. For some programs standard record forms may be mandated. Programs almost always have to specify minimum demographic and psychosocial characteristics of participants. While this responsibility may seem to present insurmountable difficulties, if planners identify by consensus the types of information needed on each participant and pay particular attention to thrift in information collection, their program should be able to gather complete documentation on those served (Broskowski, 1979; Windsor, Roseman, et al., 1981).

The amount of information that can be lost by a poor instrument and recordkeeping system is illustrated in table 4.4, from a retrospective 12-month review of medical records at a 40-bed hospital to determine the quality of patient educational assessment data of admitted diabetics (Windsor, Roseman, et al., 1981). While it was hospital policy to assess each patient on admission, only 394 of 996 diabetics admitted during the review period (39 percent) had a baseline assessment on file. These 394 forms were reviewed to determine the quality of the assessments performed. From the standpoint of assessing educational needs, preparing an educational "prescription," or evaluating program effectiveness, data abstracted from the forms for this period were of no use. Serious questions about the quality, validity, and reliability of the data collected were apparent. A major problem identified, beyond nonperformance of the assessments, was the incompleteness of the data. Findings of this record review are not uncommon in health care and public health settings (Deeds et al., 1975; Baker and McPhee, 1979).

Health promotion programs can improve their recording systems by developing a monitoring mechanism that meets both staff needs and evaluation needs. It should be compatible with data processing or allow data to be aggregated by hand for quick periodic assessment, e.g., monthly or per session. A recordkeeping system is the only mechanism by which programs can confirm how many of which demographic groups of clients were served. It is an essential element to examine in a process evaluation.

Documenting Program or Session Exposure. Another dimension to consider in examining program records is participant exposure to program sessions. A baseline and follow-up assessment of all participants or a sample should be conducted. Without exception, a health promotion program must document who received how much of what and when.

The observation form in figure 4.1 was used to confirm patient exposure to a closed-circuit educational television program for diabetic patients in a 40-bed hospital. For a one-week period, patients'

Table 4.4 Completed Items in Records of Diabetic Patients,
in Rank Order

Item	Decile of Forms with Item Completed
Diabetes instructor	90–100%
Age	
Put on _____ calorie-ADA diet	80–89%
Diabetes mellitus diagnosed—year	
Demonstrated drawing up and injection of insulin	70–79%
Has been taught to use _____ urine test	
Personal hygiene and foot care items taught	
Educated in diabetic control	
After learning to use a urine test, knows how and when to test urine for sugar	60–69%
Knows how and when to test for acetone	
Knows how to use dextrostix	
Understands causes and symptoms of reactions, acidosis	
Understands need to call doctor if acidosis develops	
Attitude on admission	50–59%
Understands insulin adjustment for reactions etc.	
Attitude on discharge	40–49%
Can test urine for sugar accurately	
Knows how to use booklet to follow diet	
Patient or member of family has been taught to use glucagon	
Pretest score	30–39%
Class attendance—insulin	
Class attendance—personal hygiene and foot care	
Class attendance—reactions and acidosis	
Class attendance—diabetes	20–29%
Class attendance—urine checks	
Diet restrictions	
Knows representative foods and amount of each exchange group	
Class attendance—diet	
Patient's physical or learning handicaps	10–19%
Post-test score	0–10%
Incapable of drawing up own insulin or testing urine	

Source: R. A. Windsor, J. Roseman, G. Gartseff, and K. A. Kirk, "Qualitative Issues in Developing Educational Diagnostic Instruments and Assessment Procedures for Diabetic Patients," *Diabetes Care* 4, no. 4 (1981): 468–75.

Rm.	Patient						
	Mon.	Tues.	Wed.	Thurs.	Fri.	Sat.	Sun.
a.m.							
p.m.							

Rm.	Patient						
	Mon.	Tues.	Wed.	Thurs.	Fri.	Sat.	Sun.
a.m.							
p.m.							

Rm.	Patient						
	Mon.	Tues.	Wed.	Thurs.	Fri.	Sat.	Sun.
a.m.							
p.m.							

Rm.	Patient						
	Mon.	Tues.	Wed.	Thurs.	Fri.	Sat.	Sun.
a.m.							
p.m.							

Rm.	Patient						
	Mon.	Tues.	Wed.	Thurs.	Fri.	Sat.	Sun.
a.m.							
p.m.							

Figure 4.1 Observation Form for Closed Circuit Television Programming in the Diabetes Hospital

rooms were observed to determine whether the patients were viewing the ETV programs presented twice daily. Using this method, the staff confirmed in a very efficient manner the proportion of patients exposed to each program and the proportion of programs each patient was exposed to during the observation period. As indicated in table 4.5, on the average, only 20 percent of approximately 30 patients per day observed the closed-circuit programs, documenting a low level of patient exposure to this channel of communication. These data clearly confirmed a need to examine why so few individuals used this program medium.

Table 4.5 Patient Exposure to Closed-Circuit Television Programs

Day	Program	Patients Exposed	Potential Patients	Percentage Exposed
Monday	1	10	29	34
	2	3	31	10
Tuesday	1	5	31	16
	4	3	29	10
	5	6	27	22
Wednesday	11	6	28	21
	7	6	30	20
Thursday	8	4	30	13
	9	7	31	23
Friday	10	4	30	13
	11	10	31	32
Saturday	4	6	31	19
Sunday	13	8	31	26
	14	7	30	23
Total	14	85	419	20

STANDARD 4: Health promotion programs should document levels of participant or target audience exposure to each program component.

Monitoring the Utilization of Information Services. Some health promotion programs establish a health information or counseling service. A recordkeeping system for monitoring utilization of this component needs to be set up with concern for accuracy, quality, and consistency in completing the form. The form has to be acceptable to the program staff and participants who must fill it out or file it. A caller data form is presented in figure 4.2 as an example of a simple, two-sided instrument currently in use by the Alabama Cancer Information Service (CIS). It has proved an efficient mechanism to gather and process by computer essential and complete data on the more than 7,000 individuals who used this information service from 1980 to 1982 (Windsor, 1983).

In establishing an information service, program staff should first conduct a thorough review of existing instruments and recordkeeping systems. Staff members need to keep in mind that any form they develop may be compared to a national standard of quality for similar programs. Planners should adapt existing instruments and recordkeeping systems for their purposes. A major problem in many health education and promotion programs is the apparent neglect in setting up a system. In the development of the CIS caller data form, existing

BIRMINGHAM COMPREHENSIVE CANCER CENTER

CIS CALLER DATA FORM

CASE I.D. [ ][ ][ ][ ] 1 5   DATE [ ][ ][ ][ ][ ] 6 11

1. START (MILITARY TIME) [ ][ ][ ][ ] 12 15   2. DAY OF WEEK: [ ] 16   3. SEX (M-1, F-2) [ ] 17

4. CALLS FROM:

☐ CaPat-1   ☐ Gen Pub-4   ☐ OtherHPro-7
☐ RelCaPat-2   ☐ MD-5   ☐ StudHPro-8
☐ FrCaPat-3   ☐ RN-6   ☐ OtherStud-9
                                       ☐ Other (Specify)-10

18 19 [ ][ ]

DESCRIPTION OF CALL:
_____
_____
_____
_____
_____
_____

5. TYPE OF INQUIRY:

[ ][ ] SiteSpecInfo-01   [ ][ ] Treat-Rad-07
[ ][ ] BCCC-Info-02   [ ][ ] Referral-08
[ ][ ] CIS-Info-03   [ ][ ] Symptoms-09
[ ][ ] RiskFactor-04   [ ][ ] GenCalInfo-10
[ ][ ] Agency-Serv-05   [ ][ ] Ed-Info-Mat-11
[ ][ ] Treat-Chemo-06   [ ][ ] Other (Specify)
_____

20 21 [ ][ ]

22 23 [ ][ ]

24 25 [ ][ ]

_____
_____
_____
_____
_____
_____

6. PRIMARY SITE(S) DISCUSSED:

[ ][ ] Breast-01   [ ][ ] Skin-07   [ ][ ] Hodg-12
[ ][ ] Lung-02   [ ][ ] Melan-08   [ ][ ] Brain-13
[ ][ ] Col-Rec-03 [ ][ ] Pros-09   [ ][ ] Lym-NHodg-14
[ ][ ] Leuk-04   [ ][ ] Bone-10   [ ][ ] Pancr-15
[ ][ ] Uterus-05   [ ][ ] Kidney-11   [ ][ ] Blad-16
[ ][ ] Cervix-06   [ ][ ] Other (Specify)_____
Not applicable

26 27 [ ][ ]

28 29 [ ][ ]

_____
_____
_____
_____
_____
_____

7. PRIMARY TYPE OF SERVICE(S) PROVIDED:

☐ Info-1   ☐ Referral-3
☐ Counseling-2   ☐ MatNeeded-4
☐ Other (Specify) _____

☐ Caller emotionally upset: ☐ yes-1 ☐ no-2

30 ☐

31 ☐

32 ☐

---

8. PRIMARY (FIRST) SOURCE OF INFORMATION ABOUT CIS

[ ][ ] TV-01   [ ][ ] ACS-05   [ ][ ] RN-09   [ ][ ] HlthDept-13   [ ][ ] PrevUser-16
[ ][ ] Radio-02   [ ][ ] Rel-06   [ ][ ] ProjHELP-10 [ ][ ] LeukSoc-14   [ ][ ] BCCC-17
[ ][ ] Newsp-03   [ ][ ] Friend-07   [ ][ ] PhoneBk-11   [ ][ ] NCI-15   [ ][ ] UAB-18
[ ][ ] PrintMat-04 [ ][ ] MD-08   [ ][ ] CoopExt-12   [ ][ ] Other _____

33 34 [ ][ ]

Side 1

Figure 4.2 Birmingham Comprehensive Cancer Center CIS Caller Data Form

9. PREVIOUS USE OF SERVICE ☐ No-0   ☐ Yes-No. of times in past year

In order for us to know whether we are serving
all people in Alabama, we need to know your: Age: _____
Race: 1-B, 2-W, 3-0 _____

35 ☐
36 37 ☐☐
38 ☐

10. FOLLOW-UP SURVEY (MONTHLY)
It is very important that we evaluate our Cancer Information Service. Would you
be willing to fill out a short 1-page Questionnaire to be sent to you in the
next month to evaluate our service and the information you have just received?

39 ☐

☐ No-2   ☐ Yes-1   IF NO—TRY AGAIN

If no, why not: _____

ASK FOLLOWING INFORMATION:

Print
Name _____   Address: _____

Phone: 40 ☐☐☐ 46 ☐☐☐   County: 47 48 ☐☐   Zip: 49 ☐☐☐☐ 53

TIME ENDED CALL: _|_|_|_   TOTAL MIN. _____ _____

CLOSED OUT (X): ☐   OPERATOR NO. _____

54 55 ☐☐
56 57 ☐☐

11. FOLLOW-UP:

Mail follow-up needed?   ☐ Yes-1   ☐ No-2
Phone follow-up needed?   ☐ Yes-1   ☐ No-2

List follow-up action(s). Describe and note date completed. Include Xeroxed
materials sent.

_____
_____
_____

58 ☐
59 ☐
60 61 ☐☐

12. CLOSE OUT:

REFERRALS: _____

COMMENTS: _____
OPERATOR NO. _____

MILITARY TIME-CLOSEOUT _____

TOTAL TIME SPENT SERVICING REQUEST AFTER CALL.   MINUTES _____
73   78
DATE: ☐☐☐☐☐☐

62 63 ☐☐
64 65 ☐☐
66 ☐☐☐☐ 69
70 71 72 ☐☐☐

Side 2

CIS monitoring systems were examined, and CIS staff input was continuous and extensive during the development process. In the final record system, a quality control standard of 90 percent was set by the director of evaluation (Windsor) as the acceptable level of data completeness for each item.

Programs that are not provided the resources, that ignore the importance of the procedures described, or that plan or implement an impractical or inappropriate system either reduce or eliminate the possibility of evaluating program process and effect. From the standpoint of structure, the key question is: Does an information gathering system exist? In terms of process evaluation, the question is: How good is it? Poor recordkeeping indicates a program of poor quality. If no resources have been provided to collect the needed information, the staff should recognize that it will not be able to document who was served, how well they were served, or what changes—cognitive, belief, skill, or behavioral—occurred from exposure to the program. The documentation and evaluation expectations of staff members and program directors then must be modified accordingly. Poor data collection and recordkeeping procedures are major compromisers of program and process evaluations.

STANDARD 5: Health promotion programs should provide documentation of a 90 percent level of data completeness on all program participants and for each data record item.

Community and Participant Surveys

In addition to a participant recordkeeping system, health promotion programs may need special surveys of target audiences in a community or samples of participants. Although the purposes of a community survey vary, typically it attempts to find out whether a given program element is: (1) reaching a target audience, (2) increasing the target audience's awareness of the program, (3) increasing the level of community interest, (4) increasing the number who utilized the program or service, and (5) satisfying consumers of the educational service (Rossi et al., 1979). The representativeness and accuracy of data are crucial factors in conducting a community survey. The limitations and disadvantages of using nonrandom sampling methods need to be carefully considered by program staff; it is always preferable to select a representative sample of respondents. Nevertheless, a number of practical, less rigorous approaches can be used by a program to obtain qualitative data on audience needs and perceptions of a program prior to or during early stages of implementation.

A community assessment may use a range of methods, from a

random sample of households to a convenience sample. Of the possible techniques by which a program may systematically gather qualitative information about its progress, four are feasible as quality control methods: (1) opinion leader surveys, (2) community forum surveys, (3) network or pyramid surveys, and (4) central location surveys. Each can be conducted in a short period of time at little cost; each has advantages and disadvantages. All have a major underlying problem: They usually do not provide a representative picture of the opinions etc. of a given group. While more detailed discussions are presented in chapters 6 and 7 on sampling procedures and other technical details of data collection, in the sections that follow we describe each method, its limitations and the extent to which it gathers valid and reliable information.

Opinion Leader Surveys. Key lay or professional community informants, persons familiar with the program, are selected as participants in an opinion leader survey. This type of survey is relatively easy and inexpensive to conduct and may be particularly useful in the discussion, planning, and early implementation stages of a program when support and interest from community leaders are crucial for program success. It may also generate familiarity with awareness of, and interest in the program among these leaders. Generally data in such a survey are generated from person-to-person interviews. Using a nominal group process is also effective (Delbecq et al., 1975; Ross and Mico, 1980). Written questions are prepared to elicit key information from the leaders about their impressions of a proposed or ongoing program. An opinion leader survey usually solicits a broad range of information. Results from it reflect the degree of consensus about the program from knowledgeable community people. This method plays an important role in the politics of program introduction, and it may be invaluable to an innovative program in identifying program barriers, acceptability, and enrollee satisfaction. Using this method, program planners should be able to document community and organizational input to and support for the program.

Community Forums. In the community forum approach or conference method, several locations are selected for public meetings with a specific target audience. The meetings may be open or by invitation. They may take a few hours or a day. This method can be used to educate the participants and to gather their impressions of the diffusion of, acceptance of, and levels of participation in the program. Community forums are inexpensive and usually easy to arrange. A list of key questions is prepared as a basis for eliciting audience input (Ross and Mico, 1980, 257–72). The forum method is most efficient when the meetings are small or when the audience is divided into smaller groups with a staff member or trained layperson acting as facilitator and recorder to ensure maximum participation. A forum may encourage a wide range of community expressions about the problem. Major disadvantages are: (1) one group or individual may control the discussions or use the forum exclusively for expression of a grievance or opposition to the program, and (2) attendance may be limited or skewed.

Network Surveys. In a network survey, key individuals (e.g., those identified as "hard-to-reach"), having characteristics representative of a special target group (e.g., black, female, under 18), are selected through existing records or program contacts. A program may start off with a list of five to ten persons on file. As part of the survey, these subjects are asked to identify two personal friends with the target group characteristics who have not used the program. Each of these individuals is surveyed and in turn asked to identify one or two similar persons, until a given quota (e.g., 30 to 50) is met. This method elicits an increasingly broader selection of individuals who tend to be demographically homogeneous but not easily accessible to the program staff. The surveys can be conducted in a short period of time and provide an avenue of target audience expression about the health promotion topic, program, or community problem. This method may also provide an estimate of community awareness of the program among those with whom little contact has been made. It should help to uncover reasons why individuals with characteristics similar to program participants have not participated (Windsor, 1973; Windsor et al., 1980).

Central Location Surveys. The central location survey is another technique commonly employed to gather information quickly and efficiently from a large number of people (100 to 200) in a community. Typically, several sites are selected that are frequented by a large number of individuals who possess the characteristics of the target audience for the health promotion program. In the central location method, a shopping center, movie theater, beach, or other high movement area in a metropolitan city or rural county is selected. Interviewers then identify a specific group, e.g., females of a certain racial or age group, and conduct relatively short interviews—five minutes—of such people on the spot. Questions may concern the person's familiarity with a problem, knowledge of the availability of the program and its purpose, or interest in a special program. Views are elicited from a specific number of people, and the interviews may occur for a set number of times (U.S. DHEW, 1978b).

STANDARD 6: Health promotion programs should provide documentation of having conducted surveys of community, consumer, and participant awareness of and satisfaction with the program.

Observations of Programs or Sessions

The purpose of observational data is to describe a situation, identifying the activities that took place at a specific time and place. It describes the people who participated and examines what happened between participants and staff during a given session. A highly accurate appraisal of the interaction can be derived from observational techniques. The interpersonal skills of staff members are, in part, reflected in their interactions with an audience. The audience may be consumers of a health education program, the providers of a health care service, a group of administrators, or community leaders who play a principal role in setting organizational policy or providing community support. The quality assurance issue is the adequacy of verbal and nonverbal communication, community organization activities, and group process skills demonstrated by staff members (Axelrod, 1975).

While there are a number of ways to conduct observational assessments, almost all include some type of participant observation. These observations may be either overt or covert. The observer's activities may be totally concealed, a participant observer may be identified as an observer but not as a participant, the observer's activities may be publicly known, or the observer may act as a participant and not as an observer. Four concerns in conducting observations were noted by Lofland (1971, 136):

> First, the qualitative methodologist must get close enough to the people and situation being studied to be able to understand the depth and details of what goes on. Second, the qualitative methodologist must aim at capturing what people actually say: the perceived facts. Third, qualitative data consist of a great deal of pure description of people, activities, and interactions. Fourth, qualitative data consist of direct quotations from people, both what they speak and what they write down.

Patton (1980) has described a number of variations of participant observations that a given program may use individually or in combination. Unobtrusive measures, e.g., of discarded cigarettes at a school ground or work site, may also provide appropriate data (Webb et al., 1966). It is essential, however, to identify beforehand what is to be observed, how, and the frequency of observations. The observation process may range from a casual period of personal observation of a given session to video or audio taping of full sessions. A careful examination of the interaction between participants and staff can be performed. From this, the evaluator can assess what information was presented, how, and the quality of interactions between presenter and audience. This method is commonly referred to as *interactive analysis* (Bales, 1951; Flanders, 1960). It is often beyond the capability of the evaluator of an ongoing service project. An excellent example of an interactive analysis study of patients and physicians can be found in Roter (1977).

It is possible, however, to conduct program observations with limited resources. Observations provide an insight into what people do in a program, how they experience it, the organization of activities, and the behaviors and interactions of participants. A program may routinely apply a quality assurance system in which all instructors are evaluated by consumers. Miller and Lewis (1982) reported on a 27-item instructor assessment form that was administered to 150 program participants in the Puget Sound HMO group health cooperative. The instrument was developed by the health education department largely to offer feedback to its more than 70 facilitators per year from a sample of the 3,000 program enrollees. The form assesses technical and interpersonal competence. The items and the strength of the correlation of response to each are presented in table 4.6. An overall alpha reliability of .94 was reported, confirming an excellent level of reliability (internal consistency). A vast amount of information on observation skills and processes is available in the education, business, communications, and social/behavioral sciences literature.

STANDARD 7: Health promotion programs should document the quality of interaction between program staff and consumers.

Component Pretesting

Pretesting is one method used by health educators to assess the needs and perceptions of target audiences. It provides documentation of a quality control system. All programs should pretest selected elements prior to their application. Pretesting is a continuing problem in the field, since it requires technical skill from the staff, resources, and time that are often not available. Yet the importance and utility of pretesting cannot be overstressed. The three most common program elements that should be pretested are instruments, media, and materials, both written and visual. The following sections discuss the purposes and methods of pretesting these elements.

Table 4.6 Item-Total Correlation for Instructor Evaluation Form

Item	Item-Total Correlation
1. The instructor puts high priority on the needs of the class participants.	.51
2. The instructor makes a lot of mistakes in class.	.52
3. The instructor gives directions too quickly.	.52
4. The instructor helps me feel that I am an important contributor to the group.	.55
5. A person feels free to ask the instructor questions.	.61
6. The instructor should be more friendly than he/she is.	.58
7. I could hear what the instructor was saying.	.65
8. The instructor is a person who can understand how I feel.	.57
9. The instructor focuses on my physical condition but has no feeling for me as a person.	.65
10. Everyone who wanted to contribute had an opportunity to do so.	.57
11. There was too much information in some sessions and too little in others.	.52
12. Just talking to the instructor makes me feel better.	.60
13. The purposes for each session were made clear before, during, and after the session.	.50
14. Covering the content is more important to the instructor than the needs of the class.	.60
15. The instructor asks a lot of questions, but once he/she gets the answers she/he doesn't seem to do anything about them.	.62
16. The instructor held my interest.	.68
17. The instructor should pay more attention to the students.	.69
18. The instructor is often too disorganized.	.67
19. It is always easy to understand what the instructor is talking about.	.61
20. The instructor is able to help me work through my problems or questions.	.62
21. The instructor is not precise in doing his/her work.	.60
22. The instructor understands the content he/she presents in class.	.68
23. I'm tired of the instructor talking down to me.	.60
24. The instructor fosters a feeling of exchange and sharing between class participants.	.58
25. The instructor is understanding in listening to a person's problems.	.72
26. The instructor could speak more clearly.	.60
27. The instructor takes a real interest in me.	.62

Source: J. Miller and F. Lewis, "Closing the Gap in Quality Assurance: A Tool for Evaluating Group Leaders," *Health Education Quarterly* 9, no. 1 (1982): 55–66.

Instruments. In conducting a process evaluation, the quality of the evaluation instrument (questionnaire) should be determined. A deficiency well documented in the literature is the failure of many health education programs to establish the reliability and validity of their instruments and data. All instruments should be examined to determine their relevance to the specified objectives of the program. In the development and pretesting of an instrument, program planners must demonstrate concern for the consumer. The instrument should be kept to a manageable length; the shorter the better. Only essential information should be collected from participants.

Instruments should be pretested for characteristics such as: time of administration, ease of comprehension, readability, sensitivity, reactivity of questions, organization of questions, and standardization of administration and scoring. The first step is to select a sample of individuals who are representative of the population for whom the instrument is prepared. Then the instrument is tested under conditions comparable to those in which it will be applied in the program setting. Procedures for developing instruments (Windsor, Roseman, et al., 1981) are:

1. Formulation of program objectives; review of the literature

2. Definition of objectives in behavioral or performance terms

3. Review of existing and available instruments and recordkeeping systems

4. Identification of essential cognitive, affective, and psychomotor skills, and descriptive information needs by internal review

5. Preliminary construction of the instrument and agreement on procedures

6. Identification of measurement methods and coding; interviewer training

7. Pilot testing with 30–50 individuals from the target group to determine essential characteristics of the instrument:

   a. Validity

   b. Reliability

   c. Adequacy of questions

   d. Ease of administration

   e. Degree of standardization

   f. Efficiency; time required

8. Repetition of the internal review and modification; external review

9. Formal clinical testing of the instrument with 100 target group members to reexamine the characteristics in 7a–f.

10. Repetition of the internal review; revision of the measurement process and the instrument for clinical or field application

As a preliminary refinement step, to eliminate glaring problems of omission or commission, four or five individuals from the target group can be asked to review and complete the instrument before a formal pilot test. Dimensions such as ambiguity of questions, lack of clarity, or insensitivity in word choice should be identified by the target group. To assure distribution of responses across characteristics, 30 to 50 people are frequently used in a pilot test. If the pilot test is self-administered, a set of written instructions on how to complete the form needs to be provided. Respondents should be able to provide reactions and suggestions for changes.

Pretesting is an important first step to ensure data quality. One of the most useful suggestions is to rely heavily on instruments that have been used by comparable programs; no program should develop a new instrument unless absolutely necessary. Seven evaluation handbooks, products of a recent project funded by the Center for Health Promotion and Education of the Center for Disease Control, should be examined for their applicability to the program. These handbooks include instruments to measure common outcomes of health education and health promotion programs (Walter Gunn, personal communication, 1982). If, for example, the program is attempting to change the participants' personal health practices or beliefs, the staff should adapt forms identified in the handbook or available from national agencies for surveying health risk factors, practices, knowledge, and beliefs. The procedures listed above should be used to modify an existing instrument to fit the objectives of the program. After applying these procedures, program planners are in a better position to make appropriate modifications of the instrument. In its final form, the instrument should facilitate the aggregation of data for hand tabulation or keypunching and data processing.

STANDARD 8: Health promotion programs should document pretesting of their instruments, providing information on data accuracy (validity) and reproducibility (reliability).

Media and Messages. Pretesting can systematically gather target audience reactions to written, visual, or audio messages and media. In assessing the quality of media, program staff should be able to document having followed procedures that meet professional standards (Squyres, 1979). Program planners who do not pretest media lose the opportunity to gain valuable insights into the quality of those methods of communication (Bertrand, 1978; U.S. DHEW, 1978b; U.S. DHHS, National Cancer Institute, 1980). A very thorough review of formative evaluation of instructional media is provided by Cambre (1978, 1981), who emphasizes ascertaining the effectiveness of a product during its development.

The ultimate purposes of pretesting media (formative evaluation) are to improve means of communication before their diffusion and to predict which alternatives will be most efficient and effective in the field. The concept of pretesting is relatively simple; it involves measuring the reactions of a group of people to the object of interest (e.g., a film, a radio spot, or a poster). Pretesting should be done not only with members of the target audience but also with in-house staff. Obviously, the sophistication and funding that can be applied to conducting a pretest are almost unlimited. The resources expended by the advertising industry each year confirm this fact.

In developing health information programs and revising existing messages and media, pretesting is an essential tool to assess ease of comprehension, personal relevance, audience acceptance, ease of recall, and other strengths and weaknesses of draft messages before they are produced in final form. A pretest can establish a target audience baseline and help to determine if there are large cognitive, affective, perception, or behavioral differences within the target audience (Knutson, 1952; U.S. DHHS, National Cancer Institute, 1980).

Programs should design pretests of media to provide information on the following components of effectiveness (Windsor, 1977; Bertrand, 1978; U.S. DHHS, National Cancer Institute, 1980):

1. *Attraction*: Is the presentation interesting enough to attract and hold the attention of the target group? Do consumers like it? Which aspects of the presentation do people like most? What gained the greatest share of their attention?

2. *Comprehension*: How clear is the message? How well is it understood?

3. *Acceptability*: Does the message contain anything that is offensive or distasteful by local standards? Does it reflect community norms and beliefs? Does it contain irritating or abusive language?

4. *Personal Involvement*: Is the program perceived to be directed to persons in the target audience? In other words, do the consumers feel that the program is for them personally or do they perceive it as being for someone else?

5. *Persuasion*: Does the message convince the target audience to undertake and try the desired behavior? How favorably predisposed are individuals to try a certain product, use a specific service, or initiate a new personal health behavior?

The following general suggestions were made by Hecht (1978, 4) to planners of instructional media:

1. State briefly what the program is to be about

2. List the primary and secondary program audiences

3. State why a program is important

4. Specify what the program is expected to accomplish for consumer and provider

5. Specify what the viewer should know and be able to do as a result of exposure to the media   ·

6. State the attitudinal or belief changes the media are attempting to influence

7. Prepare a 10- to 30-minute instructional program

8. Choose the medium, providing information on why this is an important health information source

9. Prepare a script with content based on relevant characteristics of the audience

10. Plan visual materials

11. Develop a story board

12. Describe the evaluation procedures that will assess cognitive, belief, skill, and behavioral impacts

13. Conduct the program

14. Evaluate the program

15. Revise the product

In designing a pretest or field trial, no absolute formula can be used. A pretest should be tailored to the object of interest in terms of time, cost, resources, and availability of the target audience. Planners may have to decide which media will be formally pretested and which may undergo only internal staff review. The decision must be tempered by the risk of creating active opposition to a program by not assessing audience or organizational responses beforehand.

All ongoing programs need to examine their media carefully before applying them to a given program audience. A wide range of highly technical and costly procedures are available. The acceptability and memorability of selected media may often be improved without a major allocation of time or resources, however (Windsor, 1978).

Written Materials. Written materials are commonly employed in educational programs. The major concern is: Can people read and under-

stand the material? While written materials are almost always evident
in health promotion programs, using them as principal elements of
the program is archaic. They should serve as information transfer ad-
juncts. Written materials should clarify and reinforce the principal
messages specified in the program objectives. A vast number of pro-
fessionally developed and field tested written materials are available
for most health problems and risk factors. Program materials should
be assessed by a three-step process: (1) analysis of content, (2) assessment of reading level, and (3) review by health education specialists
(U.S. DHEW, National Institutes of Health, National Heart, Lung, and
Blood Institute, 1981).

First and foremost, the program staff must be involved in gathering materials and reviewing them thoroughly to determine which
ones might serve the program objectives. Some can be modified for
the specific target audience. Written materials should be designed for
efficient distribution at a low cost. They must be capable of capturing
the interest of the audience and be presented in an imaginative yet
simple fashion. It is important that the terms, word choice, and other
characteristics be chosen to promote reading. Pretesting can be used
to gather words, phrases, and vernacular from target audiences,
so that appropriate language can be used in materials, and to determine the most effective method for communicating information. For
preparing written materials, Manning (1981) offers the following
suggestions:

1. Use one- and two-syllable words if appropriate

2. Write short, simple sentences with only one idea in a sentence

3. State the main idea at the beginning of each paragraph

4. Break up stretches of narrative with subheadings and captions

5. Use the active voice

6. Highlight important ideas and terms with boldface or italic type

7. Leave plenty of white space on the printed page

8. Add the phonetic pronunciation of key technical terms

9. Define difficult words

10. Summarize important points in short paragraphs

In assessing the quality of materials, program evaluators should
ask a number of major questions: What are we trying to accomplish?
Why are we using this particular medium to communicate this information? For whom is the written material intended? Under what
circumstances will people read it? What languages do we need to

consider in preparing our materials? These issues must be resolved during the development of written material, before significant resources are spent. In constructing materials the writer needs to select a succinct title, prepare a written text in some format, and consider the number and type of illustrations to be used. The staff also needs to reach agreement on when, how, and how often the written materials will be introduced to participants in the health promotion program. Programs should have a mechanism to document the distribution of written materials, e.g., monthly or quarterly by type. *Printed Aids for High Blood Pressure Education: A Guide to Evaluated Publications* and *Pretesting in Health Communications* are excellent resource documents produced by the National Heart, Lung, and Blood Institute, and the National Cancer Institute, respectively, both of the National Institutes of Health (U.S. DHEW, NIH, NHLBI, 1981; U.S. DHHS, NIH, NCI, 1977). They provide current information on the content, methods, and instruments for assessing printed materials.

If a program uses written materials extensively as aids or reinforcement to its educational efforts, planners may want to assess whether participants are using the information. In a study by the Rand Corporation for the Food and Drug Administration on informing patients about drugs, study participants were asked seven questions to determine their behavioral responses to a written insert in a medication package (Winkler et al., 1981, 32):

1. Do you remember a leaflet that came with your prescription?
2. Did you read it before you started taking erythromycin?
3. (If no): Did you get a chance to read it later?
4. After you read it, did you ever go back and read it again?
5. (If yes): Why did you read it again?
6. Did you keep the leaflet, did you throw it away, or what?
7. Did anyone else read the leaflet from your prescription?

The results from 879 men and women using 69 pharmacies in Los Angeles County in 1979 and 1980 provided evidence refuting the myth that "no one reads those things." As indicated in table 4.7, across experimental conditions a very large proportion of subjects read the leaflet before starting to take their prescription, a significant proportion read it more than once, a majority kept the leaflet, and approximately one in four showed it to someone else. The questions, documentation, and formative evaluation design applied in this study could be used by many ongoing programs that use written information. They determine in a formative fashion how effective written components of a program are in communicating information to program participants.

Table 4.7   Behavioral Responses to Leaflets, Study 1

Response	Experimental Condition			
	Low Expla-nation, No Instructions	Expla-nation	Instruc-tions	Explanation and Instructions
Read leaflet	77.6%	84.6%	70.3%	80.6%
Read before starting medication	67.2%	65.3%	64.1%	59.7%
Read more than once	36.2%	32.7%	31.3%	33.9%
Kept leaflet	53.4%	63.5%	51.6%	61.3%
Showed leaflet to someone else	22.8%	25.0%	29.7%	27.4%

Source: J. Winkler, D. Kanouse, S. Berry, B. Hayes-Roth, W. Rogers, and J. Garfinkle, *Informing Patients about Drugs* (Santa Monica, Calif.: Rand Corporation, 1981).

Note: Based on the responses of 236 men and women who received leaflets in study 1. Cell sample sizes ranged from 44 to 64. Effective sample sizes were slightly lower, because of missing data.

While a large number of other questions were examined in this study (e.g., variations in format, length, content, and style), the basic process was to determine what type of document worked best. The study used methods that have broad applicability to health programs. It conducted a qualitative effectiveness assessment of participants' reactions to the package insert using a semantic differential scale. Individuals were asked to rate different pamphlets on the basis of their thoroughness and clarity of explanation, degree of stimulation, quality of stimulation, simplicity or complexity, level of reassurance, and factuality. Such studies have also been performed by other investigators, such as Ligouri (1978), Dwyer and Hammel (1978), Hladik and White (1976), and Wilkie (1974).

Readability is another important aspect of pretesting written materials. Interpreted pretests for readability are available and easy to apply. Readability tests essentially determine the reading grade level required of the average person to understand the written materials. Readability estimates provide evidence of only the structural difficulties of a written document, that is, vocabulary and sentence structure. They indicate how well the information will be understood but do not guarantee the effectiveness of the piece. While a large number of readability formulas exist (Dale and Chall, 1948; Flesch, 1948; Fry, 1968; Klare, 1974–75), one of the most commonly applied is the

SMOG grading formula for testing the readability of educational material (McLaughlin, 1969). It is generally considered the best method of assessing the grade level that a person must have reached to understand the text, since it requires 100 percent comprehension of the material read. To calculate the SMOG reading grade level, McLaughlin advises program personnel to use the entire written work that is being evaluated and follow these four steps (1969, 639):

1. Count off 10 consecutive sentences near the beginning, in the middle, and near the end of the text.
2. From this sample of 30 sentences, circle all of the words containing three or more syllables (polysyllabic), including repetitions of the same word, and total the number of words circled.
3. Estimate the square root of the total number of polysyllabic words counted. This is done by finding the nearest perfect square, and calculating square root.
4. Add a constant of three to the square root. This number gives the SMOG grade (reading grade level) that a person must have completed if he or she is to fully understand the text being evaluated.

Sentence and word length and difficulty affect the readability score. The SMOG formula ensures 90 percent comprehension, i.e., a person with a tenth grade reading level will comprehend 90 percent of the material rated at that level. This procedure can be applied to all texts prepared by a program for public consumption. Klare (1974–75) and the National Cancer Institute (U.S. DHHS, NCI, Office of Cancer Communications, 1979) present useful extensive discussions of readability in general and in health-related literature.

Visual Materials, Radio, and Television. In pretesting visual aids, e.g., posters, a principal focus is their ability to attract. In general, they are designed to be attention getters, conveying one single idea. The extent to which they are comprehensible, acceptable, and promote audience involvement should also be assessed. If a major fiscal expenditure is being made, a sample from the target audience may be needed. To pretest a poster, however, a small number of people may be sufficient—five to ten, for example. While many questions can be asked, ten are presented here that can be used by an interviewer or in a self-administered questionnaire to determine an individual's response to a visual aid:

1. What is the most important message presented?
2. Is this visual aid asking you to do anything in particular?
3. Is there anything that is offensive to you or other people who live in your community?
4. What do you like about it?
5. What do you dislike about it?
6. In comparison to others that you have seen before, how would you rate it?
7. Is the information new to you?
8. How likely are you to do what the visual aid recommends?
9. Do you think the average person would understand it?
10. How would you improve it?

These questions and others that a program staff may consider appropriate should be asked as the visual is shown to the individual. The responses will provide insight into the attractiveness, comprehensibility, and acceptability of the visual portrayal (U.S. DHHS, National Cancer Institute, 1980; U.S. DHEW, National Institutes of Health, 1980).

The pretesting of radio and television spots follows the general principles outlined for other categories of media. One difference, however, is the limited opportunity to test a produced spot. Cost is a major factor to be considered. While a radio spot can be easily taped on a recorder and a poster designed in rough form, the expense of producing a TV spot or program, even in preliminary form, can be high. Figure 4.3 is an instrument used to pretest a radio spot and illustrates the questions that might be asked.

Health Message Testing Service. For programs on a number of specific health problems (e.g., smoking cessation, breast self-examination, physical fitness), the staff may choose to use the Health Message Testing Service of the National Cancer Institute and the National Heart, Lung, and Blood Institute. This service provides a standardized system of assessing audience response to radio and television messages about health to gauge the communication effectiveness of these messages (U.S. DHEW, National Institutes of Health, 1980). The system informs program planners of the audience's message recall, comprehension, and sense of the personal relevance and believability of the message, as well as identifying strong and weak communication

Case number: _____

Radio spot (identification): _____

Code

1. In your own words, tell me what the spot said.

   _____

2. Was the spot asking you to do something in particular?

   1. ____ Yes   2. ____ No   9. ____ Don't know

   2a. If yes: What? _____

3. Did the spot say anything that you don't think is true?

   1. ____ Yes   2. ____ No   9. ____ Don't know

   3a. If yes: What? _____

4. Did the spot say anything that might bother/offend people who live here in _____ (name of community)?

   1. ____ Yes   2. ____ No   9. ____ Don't know

   4a. If yes: What? _____

5. Do you think this spot is intended for someone like yourself, or is it for other people?

   1. ____ Self   2. ____ Others   9. ____ Don't know

   5a. If "others": Why? _____

6. Was there anything about the spot that you really liked?

   1. ____ Yes   2. ____ No   9. ____ Don't know

   6a. If yes: What? _____

7. Was there anything about the spot that you didn't like?

   1. ____ Yes   2. ____ No   9. ____ Don't know

   7a. If yes: What? _____

8. In comparison to the other spots on the radio these days, how would you rate this spot on _____ (topic)?

   1. ____ Excellent   2. ____ Good   3. ____ Fair

   4. ____ Poor   9. ____ Don't know

9. What do you feel could be done to make it a better spot?

   _____

   _____

Figure 4.3 Questions for Pretesting Radio Spots

points. In testing a message, the major concern is its appropriateness for its intended subgroup. To measure communication, a testing service examines the attention-getting ability of the message and audience recall of the main idea. Overall, the Health Message Testing Service can provide invaluable insights for refinement of rough or draft message announcements, choosing between alternative messages, and planning future health promotion campaigns.

Television Program Evaluation and Analysis by Computer. One of the most recent powerful advances in the evaluation and research of television productions has been the application of microcomputer technology. Electronic analyses can be made of the effects of a TV presentation, documenting an audience's reaction second by second. With this technology, it is possible to observe the effects of minute changes in the presentation on the audience's attitudes, knowledge, and skill. This information gives program personnel the opportunity to manipulate covertly what audience members see and to analyze their responses instantaneously. The technology, referred to as the Program Evaluation Analysis Computer (PEAC), is a product of PEAC Developments, Toronto. It allows program personnel to collect instant feedback data on an infinite number of visual, graphic, verbal, and other configurations. Time series analyses are often used.

While most service programs are not capable of applying this highly sophisticated method of assessing audience response, it is a new useful and powerful technique for conducting formative evaluations of media during the production stages. Discussions by Nickerson (1979a, 1979b), Sullivan (1977), and Baggaley (1982a, 1982b), and Baggaley and Smith (1982), the latter three works a collection of papers from four International Conferences on Experimental Research in Television Instruction (1979–82) from the Memorial University of Newfoundland, provide a thorough insight into this computer technology. Given the increased impetus to use television as a major medium in health promotion and education via the Public Broadcasting System and Cablevision, the PEAC technology may be of particular relevance to national or multisite efforts where considerable formative evaluation of products is essential. Before investing in production costs that easily could run into six or seven figures, agencies will need to perform careful preliminary assessments.

STANDARD 9: Health promotion programs should document pretests of their media and materials for the following effectiveness components: (1) attraction, (2) comprehension and readability, (3) acceptability, (4) audience involvement, and (5) persuasion.

SUMMARY

Numerous quality control methods, standards, and guidelines are available to use in conducting a process evaluation of an ongoing health education program. Standards exist in the fields of education and communications that apply to all of the elements discussed in this chapter. Program planners, evaluators, and administrators must seek out, comprehend, and be able to apply these established techniques.

5

Evaluating Program Effectiveness

"We have to figure out what's the best design to evaluate our program."

"My health officer said he wants us to evaluate our smoking-cessation program. I don't know how many people we will need to do a good job."

"When I read other evaluation reports I'm not sure what to look for or what questions to ask."

"Our consultant really helped us. She made sense and she managed to explain the important problems with internal validity."

Professional Competencies Emphasized in This Chapter:

• selection of an evaluation design

• identification of factors affecting internal and external validity

• application of a standard notation system

• determination of sample size

• description of strengths and weaknesses of common designs

• establishment of a control or comparison group

• critiquing of the methods and results of published reports

Although systematic evaluations of health promotion and education programs are essential, they are often neglected because of lack of time, resources, and staff. Even when resources are available for an evaluation of program effectiveness, program staff may lack the technical expertise or experience to plan and evaluate the success of the program. Despite these problems, federal, state, and other agencies that support health promotion programs are increasingly demanding that evaluation be an integral component of the planning and delivery of services. Before expending significant resources, all program organizations need to establish systems to examine the extent to which their programs have produced desirable changes in participants.

The setting and type of a health program may work against conducting an evaluation of high quality. A common constraint is the difficulty of employing the classical experimental model, i.e., a randomized trial with treatment and control groups. Realistically, every intervention program and component cannot and should not be evaluated as if it were a trial. While the value of the experimental model should continue to be stressed in planning health program evaluations, this design may not be feasible for some programs and settings. Often, adjustments to the constraints of a given situation can be made. Evidence from the literature confirms that several good designs can be adapted to special circumstances. The adaptation of these designs and methods to your setting is one of the most creative exercises for a health education specialist (Weiss, 1972; Green and Figa-Talamanca, 1974; Rubin, 1974; Kenny, 1975; Shortell and Richardson, 1978; Windsor et al., 1980).

You will need to gain competence in selecting, applying, and adapting program evaluation designs and methods. You should be able to choose from among alternatives, basing your decisions on factors such as (1) the objectives of your program, (2) the purposes of the evaluation, (3) the availability of evaluation resources, and (4) the characteristics of your setting and population. Before preparing an evaluation plan you need to be aware of and attempt to control for the numerous possible sources of bias that affect the interpretation of impact data. You need to be able to determine what is and is not possible in your particular setting, time period, and resource constraints.

The purpose of this chapter is to translate evaluation theory into practice by: (1) increasing your awareness of the problems and methodological issues common to health program evaluation, (2) stressing the need for more careful and rigorous assessments and documentation of health promotion and education programs, (3) demonstrating the importance and utility of evaluations early in program development and throughout implementation, and (4) confirming that frequently more rigorous and analytical methods can be used than the uneducated or inexperienced eye can see (Cook and Campbell, 1983; Rossi et al., 1979; Windsor et al., 1980; Windsor and Cutter, 1981).

In order to begin an evaluation of a program's effectiveness, you need a number of components, including a written plan for the program, objectives, specification of the intervention, program methods, procedures, and activities to document program implementation. Experience and the literature suggest that these components cannot be assumed; evaluation consultants are often asked to help evaluate programs in which several of the components are lacking or not well defined. So, before you can design an evaluation of program effectiveness and address related methodological issues, you may have to go back to step one to specify program elements and methods (see chapter 3).

To conclude that a program has been effective, you must deal with a number of methodological issues. You will need an appreciation of evaluation principles, procedures, and methods described in the literature to answer two questions commonly asked about a program: Did it work? Can the observed impact (if any) be attributed to the program intervention(s)? Two broad issues that need to be considered to answer these questions are: What design will be used? What is its purpose?

SELECTING A DESIGN FOR EVALUATION

A design is a guide that specifies when, from whom, how, and by whom program components will be applied and measurements will be gathered during the course of program implementation and evaluation. A design creates the infrastructure for a well-organized evaluation. A design delineates the rationale for and methods of gathering comparative information, so that program results can be judged within an appropriate context for magnitude and programmatic importance. A design allows the evaluator to draw conclusions with varying degrees of certainty about the effect of a program. It helps the evaluator to hypothesize with varying degrees of confidence how things would have been if the program participants had not been exposed. A good design accomplishes this by specifying that the measurement instruments, test questionnaires, or observations will be administered to comparison groups not receiving the program. This description of the utility and meaning of a design needs to receive much broader dissemination (Fitz-Gibbon and Morris, 1978; Spector, 1981).

Three levels of design are important for this discussion: (1) experimental, (2) quasi-experimental, and (3) nonexperimental. An *experimental design* includes random assignment, a control and a treatment group, and observations of both groups, usually prior to and always after application of the intervention. Results derived from an experimental design usually yield the most interpretable, definitive, and defensible evidence of effectiveness. Designs of this type assert the greatest degree of control over the major factors that influence the validity of results. *Quasi-experimental* designs usually include the establishment of a treatment and a comparison group by methods other than random assignment. Such designs include observations of both groups both prior to and after application of the intervention. Results from this design may yield interpretable and supportive evidence of program effects. Quasi-experimental designs exercise varying degrees of control over several but usually not all factors that affect the internal validity of results. A *nonexperimental design* does not include random assignment or a control group and asserts little control over the major factors that confound interpretation of an observed effect.

FACTORS AFFECTING VALIDITY OF RESULTS

Several common factors influence the internal and external validity of an observed program outcome. *Internal validity* can be described as the extent to which an observed effect (e.g., improved cognitive, skill, behavioral, economic, or health status indicators) can be attributed to a planned intervention. In selecting a design to evaluate a program, a major question is: Did the planned intervention produce the observed effect or was the change produced by other factors?

External validity can be defined as the extent to which an observed impact can be generalized to other settings and populations with similar characteristics, e.g., workers in a similar business, patients using a comparable clinic, or high school students in an adjacent county school system. External validity, as noted in chapter 1, tends to be an issue addressed by evaluation research. Although program personnel should be concerned with both internal and external validity, generally speaking, ongoing health education services tend to be more concerned about internal validity. External validity is frequently beyond their scope. Their attempts to create a program that has broader applicability may dissipate the unique characteristics and synergy of program personnel and participants at a given site, so that no or little effect is produced. Moreover, improving the internal validity of results should be the major focus of an ongoing program because it enables the program staff to make optimal use of resources, time, facilities, and personnel to produce a desired change among program participants.

In selecting an evaluation design, you need to consider eight common factors that influence the internal validity of an observed behavioral impact. Each factor may confound an interpretation of program effectiveness by independently producing all or part of an observed outcome. The factors are:

1. *History*: significant, unplanned national, state, local, or internal organizational events or exposure occurring at the program site during the evaluation study period that result in change by participants.
   Example—a principal and school board impose a schoolwide ban on smoking on school grounds.

2. *Program or participant maturation*: natural, biological, social, behavioral, or administrative changes occurring among the participants or staff members during the study period, such as growing older, becoming more skilled, or staff becoming more effective and efficient in program delivery.
   Example—a child of 10 matures socially and psychologically to an adolescent of 13 in an urban setting where peers encourage drug use.

3. *Testing or observation*: the effect of taking a test, being interviewed, or being observed on outcomes.
   Example—an adult in a screening is interviewed by a nutritionist about her amount of fiber intake; she may be prompted to give socially and programmatically desirable responses and might change her fiber intake behavior over a short period of time.

4. *Instrumentation*: bias produced by changes in the characteristics of measuring instruments, observation methods, or data collection processes, i.e., factors affecting the reliability and validity of instruments.
   Example—evaluators use a carbon monoxide method of ascertaining smoking levels at baseline and a behavioral report at follow-up.

5. *Statistical regression and artifacts*: selection of a treatment or comparison group on the basis of an unusually high or low level of a characteristic that may yield changes in subsequent measurements.
   Example—a program selects and studies a group of employees at least 30 percent overweight at the beginning of a weight-reduction program.

6. *Selection*: identification of a comparison group not equivalent to the treatment group because of demographic, psychosocial, or behavioral characteristics.
   Example—a group of 100 smoking community residents is chosen as a comparison group to 100 smoking university employees.

7. *Participant attrition*: nonrandom or excessive attrition (10 percent or more) of the treatment or control group participants, which introduces a bias in the outcome data.
   Example—in a stress management course, 20 of 100 participants from the control group and 6 of 100 from the intervention group drop out of the program; those experiencing high stress levels drop out in greater numbers because they feel unable to devote time to the program, due to other commitments.

8. *Interactive effects*: any combination of the previous seven factors (Campbell and Stanley, 1966; Kerlinger, 1973; Cook and Campbell, 1983; Windsor et al., 1980; Windsor and Cutter, 1981).

You need to become familiar with factors that confound results and learn how best to control for their effects. With increased competence and confidence, you can select an appropriate design, one that allows you to rule out plausible alternative explanations for an impact. Problems with any of the confounding factors will limit your ability to observe an impact or attribute it to the program interventions. The literature and our experience confirm that factors 4, 6, and 7 (instrumentation, selection, and attrition factors) are the most frequent major compromisers of evaluation results (Porter and Chibocos, 1975; Bernstein, 1976; Windsor and Cutter, 1981).

EVALUATION DESIGN NOTATION

It is important that you learn the hieroglyphics of evaluation. A specialized set of notations is used to portray different elements of a design. Although no full consensus exists on the notations to be used to diagram a design, the following are reasonable and common choices:

R = random assignment of an individual to a group.

E = an experimental, treatment, or intervention group; may be expressed as E_1, E_2, E_3, to portray exposure of a group to different elements or types of treatment.

C = a control or equivalent group established by random assignment; the group not exposed to an intervention or exposed to only a minimum or standard intervention.

$\underline{C}$ = a comparison group established through any means other than randomization.

N = the number of subjects or participants in an E, C, or $\underline{C}$ study group.

O = an observation to collect data; may employ methods such as a test, interview, visual or audio rating, or record review; O_1, O_2, O_3, . . . , O_n signifies multiple observations at different times.

T = time; specifies when an observation, assignment to a group, or application of a treatment or program element has taken place; T_1, T_2, T_3, . . . , T_n describes the period of time between observations.

X = the treatment or intervention applied to a study group; X_1, X_2, X_3, . . . , X_n, signifies that the treatment consisted of different elements or types of interventions.

These notations will be used in discussions in the following sections of the book.

DESIGNS FOR PROGRAM EVALUATION

There are numerous designs that you might select to evaluate your program. The number of designs that are administratively feasible and produce interpretable results are few, however. Five designs are frequently used to evaluate program effectiveness. Each will allow you to attribute observed outcomes to the application of your program to some degree. The methodological and analytical issues in selecting these designs and their strengths and weaknesses in interpretability and internal validity are specified in the sections that follow. These five designs have the widest applicability to planning evaluations of health promotion and education efforts. While more sophisticated designs, e.g., multifactorial designs, are possible, they are usually beyond the resources of an ongoing program. More complex designs are likely to fall within the domain of evaluation researchers, who can meet their demands for expertise, resources, and time.

Table 5.1 presents information on the internal validity of these five common evaluation designs. The eight factors that threaten internal validity represent potential independent sources of effects. Each factor may be a plausible explanation for an observed impact. To control for them, you should select a design appropriate for the purposes of your evaluation and adapt the design to what is possible. Program staff members often do not fully recognize what is possible, and, as a result, do not perform more rigorous, more powerful, and methodologically stronger evaluations. You should start with the most rigorous design that might be possible and then adapt it to your situation. The assumption is that, if you start off in a compromising mode, you lose opportunities to examine the total program or program elements before you have thoroughly explored all possibilities. The best plan is one that is tempered with a good sense of reality, derived from a careful individual and internal peer review process.

Design 1: One Group Pretest and Post-Test

Design 1 in table 5.1 is the simplest design (nonexperimental) for program evaluation. It should not be your choice to assess program *effectiveness*. The information in table 5.1 confirms that a number of factors will prevent you from attributing an observed change among program participants to the intervention using this design. It raises many problems of inference and may control for only one or two of the eight factors that threaten interpretation of observed changes. Interpretation is largely a factor of what pattern emerges between the two observation periods. While you might be tempted to attribute an observed change that occurred between 0_1 and 0_2 to the intervention (X), a number of alternative explanations might be equally plausible. For example, other events, unplanned exposures, or unexpected activities involving program participants between 0_1 and 0_2 may have played a role in producing the observed change. The longer the time between 0_1 and 0_2, the more probable it is that historical events or other such factors will influence program results. This design, then,

Table 5.1 Internal Validity Strengths and Weaknesses for Five Evaluation Designs

Design	Threats to Internal Validity							
	History	Maturation	Testing	Instru- mentation	Regres- sion	Selection	Attrition	Interactive Effects
1. One group pretest and post-test E O X O	–	–	–	–	?	+	+	–
2. Nonequivalent control group E O X O C O O	+	+	+	+	?	+	+	–
3. Time series E OOO X OOO	–	+	+	?	+	+	+	+
4. Multiple time series E OOO X OOO C OOO OOO	+	+	+	+	+	+	+	+
5. Pretest and post-test with control group R E O X O R C O O	+	+	+	+	+	–	?	?

Source: T. D. Cook and D. T. Campbell, "The Design and Conduct of Quasi-Experiments and True Experiments in Field Settings," in *Handbook of Industrial and Organizational Psychology*, ed. M. D. Dunnette (New York: John Wiley & Sons, Inc., 1983). Reprinted by permission of the publisher.

Note: E = experimental group; C = control group; C̲ = comparison group; O = observations; X = intervention; – = weakness; + = strength.

has serious weaknesses (Campbell and Stanley, 1966; Windsor and Cutter, 1982).

Design 1 may be useful in the formative stages of a program, however, if the interval between observations is short and you can reasonably rule out other significant historical or maturation effects. It may be useful to assess the immediate educational impact of an information or in-service training program. It is important to control for the fact that an observation or pretest may have an impact on participants; a reasonable expectation is that data collection procedures may independently produce a behavioral impact. If the baseline observation is minimal and occurs prior to the intervention, e.g., one week earlier, it may not pose a plausible threat to the interpretation of short-term program impact. To control this threat, regardless of the size or purpose of your evaluation, you should routinely assert maximum control over the quality of the instruments and the data collection processes. You should conduct reliability and validity checks.

The weakness in design 1 in terms of regression is the extent to which individuals selected for the program are uncharacteristic of those in an organization, community, or clinic. The extent to which regression compromises results can be examined by determining the comparability of those who participate and those who do not. How individuals are selected for a program and variations in characteristics between those who do and do not participate are the central issues.

In the aggregate, then, design 1 has a number of major weaknesses. With careful attention, however, a program might assert some control over several of the threats to internal validity. This design might be used to conduct a *formative assessment* of immediate program effects, particularly knowledge and skills.

Example of Design 1—A maternal–child health (MCH) program is conducting a smoking behavioral assessment. The staff observes that there is a 15 percent quit rate between the onset of pregnancy and childbirth for women under 30. On their entry into an MCH clinic for pregnant women, 50 smokers are comprehensively interviewed (0_1) on their level of smoking knowledge, health beliefs, and practices. One week later they begin an education program in groups of five. The program consists of four one-hour, peer-led, peer-developed discussions on smoking cessation for pregnant women (X_1), conducted over two weeks. One week after program completion, a follow-up interview (0_2) is performed at the participants' monthly visit, using the same instrument on the 50 patients. The health educator reports the following effects: (1) an increased health belief score—from 60 percent to 95 percent; and (2) a decrease in smoking practices—from 50 smokers to 35 smokers. This level of immediate effect (a 30 percent quit rate versus the normal 15 percent quit rate without the program), with the threats to validity acknowledged, provides the program with some encouraging feedback on program impact.

Design 2: Nonequivalent Control Group

Design 2 builds on design 1 by adding a comparison group ($\underline{C}$). This usually improves the chances of being able to attribute observed effects to the program. The dotted line in table 5.1 between the intervention group (E) and the comparison group ($\underline{C}$) signifies that the groups were established by a method other than randomization. A comparison of the strengths and weaknesses of designs 1 and 2 suggests that the comparison group improves the evaluator's ability to rule out some alternative explanations of impact, such as the effects of history, maturation, testing, and instrumentation.

The extent to which this design controls for regression is questionable. This can be dealt with by ensuring that neither the comparison nor the treatment group is selected because of an extreme trait. Careful matching of individuals in the two groups may increase the precision of the design. As noted, baseline (0_1) and follow-up observations (0_2) are necessary for both groups.

A continuing problem with design 2 is the difficulty of selecting the most appropriate method for statistical analysis of results. There is still much discussion about what analytical technique is the most appropriate for results produced by nonequivalent control group designs (Rubin, 1974; Kenny, 1975; Windsor et al., 1980). An example of the application of this design is presented in case study format later in this chapter (Perry et al., 1980).

Design 3: Time Series

You might select design 3 if your program is able to: (1) establish the periodicity and pattern of the outcome variable being examined; (2) establish the degree of stability of the outcome measurement; (3) collect outcome data unobtrusively; (4) observe at multiple data points, in many cases six months to one year before and after the intervention; and (5) introduce an intervention that can be applied in a specific time period and withdrawn abruptly. In using a time series design (TSD), many data points are required for the most sensitive statistical tests. Multiple data points increase the power of the design to make causal inferences, so a principal need for application of a TSD is that there be an adequate number of observations. Some recommend a minimum of 50 data points for assessing an effect (Glass et al., 1975; Ostrom, 1978). The observation points must occur at equal intervals and must cover a sufficient period of time to confirm preintervention and postintervention variations for the outcome variables.

While you should be sensitive to the statistical issues in choosing a TSD, you may use one with fewer data points. Observation and analysis of a behavior change trend over time, even with fewer than 50 data points, usually represents a significant gain over design 1. Because the principal issue in applying a TSD is to determine the significance of a trend, the treatment must be powerful enough to produce shifts in the dependent variable considerably beyond what you would normally expect in your setting (Campbell, 1969; Cook and Campbell, 1983; Windsor and Cutter, 1981, 1982).

If you apply a time series evaluation, you must examine the extent to which you can control for the principal threat to internal validity—history. Did historical, nonprogram events or activities confound the observed results? You need to establish the pattern of the program impact variables being used. The plausibility of effects from factors such as weather, seasonality, shifts in personnel, and changes in resources must be examined. The threat of extraneous historical effects increases with the duration of the evaluation. Design 3 may provide a range of evidence of effects from suggestive to very good. It does not usually produce definitive evidence about intervention effects. Only through replication of an evaluation using a TSD and reports of consistently significant and programmatically important evidence of impact over time can you make conclusive statements about effectiveness (Windsor and Cutter, 1981, 1982). An example of the application of this design is included in the case studies section later in this chapter (Windsor, Cutter, et al., 1981).

Design 4: Multiple Time Series

The quasi-experimental design 4 can be more powerful than the non-experimental design 1 and the quasi-experimental designs 2 and 3. Multiple time series (MTS) describes a design in which outcomes are studied at differing points in time for a treatment (E) and a comparison group (C). The addition of the comparison group strengthens the program's control over possible historical effects. The MTS design is particularly appropriate in situations where retrospective and prospective data bases are easily accessible or where an organization can observe program participants periodically, for example, each month.

As noted in table 5.1, the MTS design improves your control over the major factors that confound or compromise your interpretation of observed program results. A major inhibitor to use of this design is the need for multiple observations of the comparison group before and after the program. These observations are time- and resource-intensive. Like the simple time series design, the MTS design demands a number of baseline and follow-up observations, depending on what factors affect these observations. Your main concern is to be able to say with reasonable assurance that, before the program, a stable pattern of outcome measurements was confirmed for both the comparison and the treatment group. Time series analytical techniques, as noted for design 3, require a large number of data points to produce sensitive statistical analyses. You need to be concerned about this trade-off, and choose the number of observations to optimize your ability to rule out extraneous factors that may bias your results (Cook and Campbell, 1983; Spector, 1981; Windsor and Cutter, 1982).

Design 5: Randomized Pretest and Post-Test with Control Group

There are several methods to conduct an experimental study of program effectiveness. If you have a large number of participants strongly interested in participating in your program, you usually can assign them by random selection to different intervention groups. Assignment may be done all at once if participants enter the program together, or you may assign persons randomly as they enter the program over time. Assuming no major implementation problems, this design usually produces strong control over the major factors that confound interpretation of program impact. The principal concept behind this experimental design is that the evaluator establishes two groups that are not significantly different for any salient outcome characteristic at baseline, e.g., E_1 has 33 percent smokers, C_1 has 31 percent smokers. Programs that use random assignment assert optimum control over the threats to internal and external validity. Confirmation that the randomization process has in fact established equivalent groups is essential, however (Cook and Campbell, 1983). Case study 3 presented later in this chapter discusses the application of this design (Hughes et al., 1981).

The literature and training programs need to give much more attention to methodological, analytical, and design issues related to evaluation of program effectiveness. In selecting a design, it is crucial for you to consider what is possible within the constraints of time, resources, and characteristics of the situation. The designs we have discussed form a hierarchy, in ascending order from design 1 to design 5, representing increasing ability to provide defensible evidence of program effect. Even when a randomized design such as design 5 is used, however, the evidence may not be conclusive.

DETERMINING SAMPLE SIZE

Two questions frequently asked in planning an evaluation are: How large should the control (comparison) and treatment groups be? How should we select each group? Knowledge of what the sample size should be for each study group is of paramount importance. To ensure sufficient statistical power in data analysis and interpretation you should, prior to implementation, estimate the minimum number to be recruited in each group. *Statistical power* is defined as the probability of being able to reject a null hypothesis (H_0) if it is false (committing a Type I error). (The null hypothesis is the hypothesis of no significant differences between the E and C groups.) Since the objective of a program is to have an impact, i.e., to reject H_0, you must establish large enough E and C groups to have the opportunity to do this. Regardless of the total number in a group, the groups should be approximately the same size, e.g., E = 77 and C = 80.

To determine the most efficient sample size for each study group, you must define certain parameters. One of the first concerns is to select a level of statistical significance. An accepted convention for this parameter is: alpha = 0.05. *In a formative evaluation of effects, you might decide that 0.10 is an adequate level.* In other words, if alpha = 0.05, you are willing to accept a null hypothesis when the probability of being wrong is less than 5 percent. Having specified the alpha level, you must also consider the beta level, the probability of accepting a null hypothesis when it is false (committing a Type II error)—in other words, concluding that a program could not produce a significant effect when it can in some cases. The literature specifies that beta should be equal to 1 minus approximately four times alpha; or 1 − beta = 4 times alpha. Thus, where alpha = 0.05, beta = 1 − 4(0.05) = 0.80 (Cohen and Cohen, 1975). Given these two conventions, you have to estimate either from the literature or from ongoing program data, the current median level of expected effectiveness, i.e., the *effect size*, for your program.

The process of estimating effect size can be described by using a smoking-cessation example. The literature indicates that the self-initiated cessation rate (P_1) among smokers is approximately 10 percent (or P_1 = 0.10). Available evidence also confirms that a reasonable expectation of impact for a smoking-cessation program (P_2) at a six- to twelve-month follow-up is approximately a 30 percent cessation (or P_2 = 0.30). With these four parameters, alpha = 0.05, beta = 0.80, P_1 = 0.10, and P_2 = 0.30, you can use standard sample size tables to find out how many participants you need in both E and C groups to test the significance of a difference (Fleiss, 1981).

Data presented in table 5.2 for a two-tailed test on proportion specify the sample sizes needed for a treatment and control group for various alpha, beta, P_1 and P_2 parameters. Using the parameters of our smoking-cessation example, the data in table 5.2 indicate that the program would need 71 participants per group to confirm the hypothesized difference between P_1 and P_2 as statistically different. Data

Table 5.2 Sample Sizes per Group for Two-Tailed Test on
Proportions Where $P_1 = 0.10$

P_2	Alpha	Beta (Power) 0.95	0.90	0.80	0.50
0.20	0.01	471	397	316	189
	0.05	348	286	219	117
0.25	0.01	238	202	162	98
	0.05	177	146	113	62
0.30	0.01	149	126	102	63
	0.05	111	92	71	40
0.35	0.01	104	88	72	45
	0.05	77	64	50	29
0.40	0.01	77	66	54	34
	0.05	58	48	38	22

Source: J. Fleiss, *Statistical Methods for Rates and Proportions* (New York:
Wiley, 1981), p. 262.

in table 5.2 also belie the common statement that 30 or 50 individuals
are needed per group. In the smoking example, the literature suggested that 10 percent of smokers stop on their own, and the median
level of effectiveness for smoking-cessation programs at six- and
twelve-month follow-ups is approximately 30 percent. The use of 50
subjects per group would require a program to produce an impact of
at least 35 percent cessation, a greater magnitude than that hypothesized, to confirm the effect statistically. The likelihood, then, of finding a statistically significant difference between the E and C groups
with samples sizes of N = 50 each where $P_1 = 0.10$ and $P_2 = 0.30$, is a
little higher than chance—not very good odds.

The underlying step, then, in deciding on sample sizes is to determine what level of impact you expect. If the literature and empirical evidence suggests that your program will have a small effect, e.g.,
$P_1 = 0.10$ and $P_2 = 0.20$, and if a small impact is programmatically or
organizationally important, then, using the data in table 5.2 and the
same alpha, beta, and P_1 values, each of your sample groups will need
approximately 219 persons. If you anticipate a moderate level of impact, e.g., $P_1 = 0.10$ and $P_2 = 0.30$, then approximately 71 subjects per
group will be needed to satisfy statistical power demands. If the evidence suggests that the impact of your program will be large, e.g., P_1
= 0.10 and $P_2 = 0.40$, then a sample size of 38 per group may be
sufficient.

There is almost no discussion in the health promotion and education literature on the logic and methods used to determine treatment and control group size. Much more consideration needs to be given to this issue to improve the quality of future evaluations. Because of the complexity of determining sample size and selecting appropriate analytical techniques, health educators should seek biostatistical consultation (Cohen and Cohen, 1975; Anderson, 1976; Windsor et al., 1980; Fleiss, 1981).

ESTABLISHING A CONTROL OR COMPARISON GROUP

The key issue in establishing a control group is: Does it adequately control for the effects of other factors (e.g., age, education) that might produce or explain part of an observed impact? An equivalent control group is used to assert control over the independent variables so that extraneous sources of error are minimized. It does this by distributing individuals with particular characteristics equally between E and C groups. A control group is used to determine whether program participants have improved as a result of exposure to the treatment, by comparing them to those not exposed or to those exposed to something else. An assumption in making a comparison between E and C groups is that the groups were equivalent before introduction of the treatment. This assumption must be tested; random assignment does not always produce equivalent groups at baseline.

In selecting a design, you face the immediate problem of identifying and selecting a control group. While there is no magic formula for establishing a control group there are a number of common methods. In this discussion, *control group* means a group established by random assignment (C), while *comparison group* means a group established by nonrandom assignment (C̲). A major constraint in designing an evaluation may be the availability of individuals who can be used as control or comparison subjects; this is always dependent on the characteristics of the situation. Ideally C and E are identical for all of the dependent (outcome) variables and independent variables associated with the dependent variables.

A crucial issue limiting control groups in the practice of health education (particularly in patient education settings) is that the staff cannot withhold the health education program from participants. While this may seem an insurmountable problem at first glance, in practice it need not be. Since human nature and all programs are fallible, program improvements are usually needed. Although you cannot withhold the basic or standard program, you can vary the intensity, duration, methods, materials, or frequency of program elements to see which are most effective. Or you can compare the standard program (X_1) to $X_1 + X_2$ (where X_2 is systematic reinforcement). Or you can devise other alternatives. The central issues are how effective the existing program is and what practical methods could be applied that might raise that level of effectiveness.

Random Assignment

Randomization of participants into E and C groups is the most desirable method for establishing groups for evaluation purposes. It is the best method to control for the major threats to internal validity. If a program has the opportunity to assign participants randomly as they are recruited, assignment may take a number of forms. If the numbers of confirmed participants are large, e.g., 100 to 200, then simple random assignment may be adequate to establish equivalent groups. To achieve greater precision, however, a program may choose a stratified system of randomization. In such a system individuals with selected demographic characteristics are grouped by a given characteristic, e.g., age or sex, paired with another individual of similar characteristics, and then randomly assigned to a treatment group or a control group.

Delayed Treatment

A common misinterpretation of classical experimental design is that the administration of a treatment is an all or nothing affair. In the simplest of delayed approaches, about half the individuals from an applicant pool are randomly selected to serve as a control group. The rest of the applicants are exposed to the program initially, while the control group is delayed in its participation. In this way eligible candidates are randomly assigned to immediate or delayed treatment, with each having an equal opportunity to participate. Randomization may be the fairest and most equitable method of selecting initial program participants in a case where all who are interested in participating cannot be served at the same time.

Table 5.3 shows how a delayed treatment method would look on paper. At T_1, a group of individuals agree to participate in a program. Using the parameters alpha = 0.05, beta = 0.80, $P_1 = 0.10$, $P_2 = 0.35$, a sample size of 50 per group is chosen (see table 5.2 earlier). Of 100 individuals who agreed to participate, 50 are randomly assigned to group E and 50 to group C. A baseline observation (O_1) is performed during the recruitment period prior to the start of the program. At T_2 those assigned to group E are exposed to the program (X_1); those assigned to group C are not exposed. Observations (O_2) are made of

Table 5.3 Establishing a Control Group via Delayed Treatment

Time 1 (T_1) Recruitment-Baseline	Time 2 (T_2) Program 1 Starts	Time 3 (T_3) Program 2 Starts	Time 4 (T_4) Follow-up
O_1 R E (N = 50)	X_1 O_2	$-O_3$	O_4
O_1 R C (N = 50)	$-O_2$	X_1 O_3	O_4

both groups. At a predetermined time in the future, T_3, those in group C are exposed to the program.

This approach is particularly useful in confirming immediate and short-term estimates of program effectiveness, because of randomization and replication. It cannot be used for assessing intermediate or long-term impacts, however (impacts after six months or one year or more), because people who expect to receive the program will probably be unwilling to wait much longer than three months. This design and method would be very useful in conducting formative evaluations of different program elements in the early stages of a program (Campbell, 1969; Boruch, 1976).

A Multiple-Component Program

In some situations, you may choose to apply combinations of different interventions to some individuals and withhold them from others. In other words, if you have a captive audience of individuals who want to participate in a health promotion program, you may elect to conduct a randomized microevaluation study in which selected program elements are applied or withheld. You might examine such factors as program duration, program reinforcement, and intensity, to determine which individual or combined elements are the most efficient in producing a level of effect.

You may be interested in determining the differential effects of elements of the program. To do so, you can establish an applicant pool and design the program with multiple components. You then expose subsamples to different components. As indicated in table 5.4, the initial pool of 210 recruited applicants may be randomly assigned to three "equivalent" groups (N = 70) (the equivalence should be tested, not assumed). Participants in each of these groups may be exposed to single or combinations of parts of a program. The control group might receive either nothing or, more likely, a minimum standard intervention.

Table 5.4 Establishing a Control Group in a Multiple-Component Program

Time 1 (T_1) Recruitment-Baseline	Time 2 (T_2) Program 2 Starts	Time 3 (T_3) Program Ends	Time 4 (T_4) Follow-up
O, R E, (N = 70)	X, X_2 O_2	O_3	O_4
O, R E_2 (N = 70)	X, X_3 O_2	O_3	O_4
O, R C, (N = 70)	X_1—O_2	O_3	O_4

Table 5.5 Establishing a Control Group for a New Program

Time 1 (T_1) Recruitment-Baseline	Time 2 (T_2) Programs Start	Time 3 (T_3) Programs End	Time 4 (T_4) Follow-up
O, R E, (N = 70)	X, O_2	O_3	O_4
O, R E_2 (N = 70)	X_2 O_2	O_3	O_4

A New Program

If your organization has an opportunity to develop or present a totally new program or a new version of an ongoing program, assuming your resources are sufficient to offer both programs simultaneously, you could randomly assign participants to be exposed to either the standard program (X_1) or the new, enriched program (X_2) for purposes of comparison. An evaluation of which program was the most effective may then be made. As indicated in table 5.5, having recruited and established baselines for a pool of participants, you randomly assign individuals to participate in program X or program Y. Follow-up observations are conducted as in other group designs. A medium effect size ($P_2 = 0.30$) is posited for this example.

To the extent that the randomized experimental design is compromised, the study's results and conclusions are weakened. Perhaps the most important point to be made about establishing a control group is that you must grasp the rationale, purposes, strengths, and weaknesses of each method and design.

COMPARABILITY OF STUDY GROUPS

Establishing the comparability of the treatment and nontreatment groups in a quasi-experimental or experimental evaluation cannot be

Table 5.6 Baseline Data for Treatment and Comparison Groups

Variable	Experiment (E) (N = 280)	Comparison (C) (N = 170)	Significance Level (P)
		Group	
Age (years)	45.7	44.1	NS
Annual income	$9,077	$8,776	NS
Years in school	11.3	11.5	NS
Black female	25%	28%	NS
White female	75%	72%	NS
Has a family doctor	79%	84%	NS
Has had uterus removed	24%	23%	NS
Has had a physician's visit in the last six months	74%	77%	NS
Mean cognitive score	71.8	70.9	NS
Mean belief score	1.45	1.47	NS
Breast self-examination practices in the last three months			
None	33%	23%	< 0.01
One	20%	23%	
Two	19%	14%	
Three or more	27%	40%	
Pap smear practices			
None	22%	14%	NS
Fewer than 12	55%	56%	
More than 12	23%	30%	

Source: R. A. Windsor, J. Kronenfeld, M. Ory, and J. Kilgo, "Method and Design Issues in Evaluation of Community Health Education Programs: A Case Study in Breast and Cervical Cancer," *Health Education Quarterly* 7, no. 3 (1980): 203–18.
Note: NS = not significant.

overstressed. In identifying a comparison group, you must give considerable attention to selecting individuals or groups who are as similar to the treatment group as possible. The rationale for identifying individuals or groups to serve as a comparison group must be well examined and described in detail. While randomization is the best choice, a nonequivalent comparison group may represent the only reasonable alternative in the circumstances. The objective of comparing baseline data on the treatment and control or comparison groups is to confirm that no major differences existed between these groups prior to the program. Data in tables 5.6 and 5.7 portray the com-

Table 5.7   Mean Values of Selected Variables among MRFIT
Participants Assigned to Special Intervention (SI) and
Usual Care (UC)

	Units	SI (N = 6,428)	UC (N = 6,438)
Values at first screen			
Serum cholesterol	mg/dl	253.8	253.5
Diastolic blood pressure	mm Hg	99.2	99.2
Cigarette smokers	%	63.8	63.5
Cigarettes smoked per day	No.	33.7	34.2
Framingham 6-year risk of CHD death	%	3.12	3.15
Values at second screen			
Age	years	46.3	46.3
Diastolic blood pressure	mm Hg	91.2	91.2
Systolic blood pressure	mm Hg	136.0	135.8
Percentage on blood pressure medication	%	19.6	19.1
Weight	lb	189.3	189.1
Height	in.	69.2	69.3
Drinks/week	No.	12.5	12.7
Serum			
Fasting glucose	mg/dl	99.5	99.3
Thiocyanate	μmole/liter	131.0	131.1
Plasma			
Total cholesterol	mg/dl	240.3	240.6
HDL cholesterol	mg/dl	42.0	42.1
LDL cholesterol	mg/dl	159.8	160.3
Triglycerides	mg/dl	194.7	193.9
Values at third screen			
Diastolic blood pressure	mm Hg	90.7	90.7
Cigarette smokers	%	59.3	59.0
Cigarettes/day smoked	No.	32.4	32.8
Flat or downsloping ST depression ≥0.5 mm post exercise	%	2.48	2.35

Source: R. Sherwin, K. Kaelber, R. Kezdi, M. Kjelsberg, and H. Thomas,
Jr., "The Multiple Risk Factor Intervention Trial (MRFIT), II: The Development of the Protocol," *Preventive Medicine* 10, no. 4 (1981): 402–25.

parability of treatment and nontreatment groups participating in two
published studies.

In table 5.6 baseline statistics for 450 female participants in a rural
cancer control program are presented (Windsor et al., 1980). Randomization was not possible in this program. The comparison group was
identified using a peer-generation method—participants were asked
to identify a nonparticipant friend of the same age and sex. The data
indicated that the two groups were relatively comparable at baseline
in terms of sociodemographic factors, physician utilization, cognitive

and health belief scores, and behavioral reports. The noted exception was the higher level of breast self-examination reported by the comparison group at baseline. Another problem was the difference in sample size between the E and $\underline{C}$ groups.

Data are presented in table 5.7 on the Multiple Risk Factor Intervention Trial (MRFIT) (Sherwin et al., 1981). This national effort established two groups, one to receive a special intervention (SI) or (E) and one to receive usual care (UC) or (C). Three screening procedures took place before the program intervention began. The data confirm that the mean values of the quantitative measures performed for the SI and UC groups were highly comparable. No significant differences were noted for the screening variables.

These two studies—the first a small demonstration project in a rural community with limited resources, and the second a randomized clinical trial of national significance with resources over $125 million—confirm that program resources, scope, and duration play a significant role in the ability of investigators to establish comparability of study groups. While the amount and type of data collected will vary dramatically according to a program's purpose and resources, all programs must establish the baseline characteristics of treatment and comparison group participants and their comparability.

ESTABLISHING A COMPARISON GROUP

The opportunity to perform randomized experimental studies occurs far more often than is suggested in the literature. In a number of program evaluation situations, however, a classical, experimental model may not be feasible. This is particularly true in a field setting where a program does not have easy access to a "captive" audience. It may then be necessary for an evaluator to select a comparison group. Where a comparison group ($\underline{C}$) and not a control group (C) is established, the potential level of effect (P_2) of a program is likely to be reduced (Boruch, 1976).

The definition of a comparison group, as noted, is any group not formed by random assignment. The goal, then, is to identify comparison groups that are highly comparable to the group exposed to the program. In essence, in using a nonequivalent comparison group, you are attempting to replicate an experimental study in every way with the exception of randomization. In setting up a $\underline{C}$ group, you must document the similarities and differences between the comparison and the experimental groups prior to exposure to the program. The following methods are suggested for selection of the comparison group to improve your chances of identifying your program's effectiveness.

Participant- or Peer-generated Groups

One method found to be useful is to have individuals match themselves with a friend. In the participant-generated method, a participant identifies one or two friends or neighbors very much like himself or herself in age, sex, race, socioeconomic status (SES), etc. You request participants to provide the names and phone numbers of these people to be contacted by the program staff. This method may establish a nonrandomized comparison group at little cost (Windsor, 1973; Wang et al., 1975; Windsor et al., 1980). It was used to establish the $\underline{C}$ group reported in table 5.6. One problem with participant generation, as observed in table 5.6., may be the failure of a significant proportion of treatment group participants to identify a comparison friend. Using this method may also result in interaction between E and $\underline{C}$ subjects, increasing the potential for contamination of $\underline{C}$ subjects.

Matching by Unit

You may have the opportunity to match program data in your area to program data in a comparable area where the intervention you are applying was not introduced. This design is most feasible in a situation where a uniform data base exists or can be introduced at alternative locations. Examples include clinics, hospitals, schools, or work sites. In identifying subjects to serve in a comparison group, you should seek approximately the same number of individuals as you have in the treatment group. If the comparison site already has a monitoring system, you may be able to identify a number of units whose participants are highly comparable to your treatment group in demographic traits. The greatest difficulty in using this method is gaining the cooperation of intact groups in other settings. Some type of longitudinal design, often a time series, is the most appropriate evaluation method to use with this type of $\underline{C}$ group (Windsor and Cutter, 1982).

CASE STUDIES: THEORY AND APPLICATION

Three case studies are presented to illustrate the strengths and weaknesses of the quasi-experimental and experimental designs discussed in this chapter. They have been selected because they are part of the current literature and represent programs with different purposes, settings, and populations. The discussion in the case studies focuses on five main components of concern to planners and evaluators of health promotion and education programs: (1) background and objectives, (2) intervention, (3) evaluation design, (4) program impact, and (5) internal validity of results.

Case Study 1: Rural Cancer Screening Program

Source: R. Windsor, G. Cutter, and J. Kronenfeld, "Communication Methods and Evaluation Designs for a Rural Cancer Screening Program," *American Journal of Rural Health* 7, no. 3 (1981): 37–45.

Background and Objectives

In 1974 the Alabama Department of Public Health established a Cancer Screening Program (CSP), initially with National Cancer Institute support, to remove barriers to service use in local rural communities: availability, accessibility, acceptability, and cost. At the end of 1981 this project had 50 clinics in operation and had screened approximately 110,000 women, 90 percent of whom were members of families below the poverty level. Of those newly screened, 57 percent reported that they either never had had a Pap smear, had not had one within the last two years, or did not remember ever having one. The CSP has a continuing interest in determining methods to increase service utilization, particularly by women who have never used the program.

In 1978, a collaborative effort with representatives from the University of Alabama-Birmingham faculty, the Alabama State Health Department, and the Cooperative Extension Service was initiated to develop, implement, and evaluate a community-based Cancer Communications Program. The objective of the program was to increase during the second quarter of 1979 and 1980 the number of women using the CSP who were over 35 years of age and had never before used the CSP in Alabama. The Hale County screening program was selected as a demonstration site because it had a large pool of high-risk females over 35 years of age (approximately 3,500), it was similar to a number of counties in south central Alabama, and it had been operational since 1977. As indicated in table 5.8, residents in this county were predominantly black, poor, and rural, with limited access to primary health care services and personnel.

Intervention

As shown in table 5.9, five elements were identified as the principal components of the community intervention. A multiple-component intervention was used because the literature and the experience of the investigators strongly confirmed that no single source of exposure could be expected to have an appreciable behavioral impact on the target group. Combinations of messages from multiple salient channels, particularly interpersonal sources at repeated intervals, were applied.

Two community health education programs were implemented in Hale County during the second quarter, April–June 1979 and 1980. The principal messages communicated by the programs during the three-month interventions were: (1) women over 35 who had never had a Pap smear were at higher risk for cervical cancer and therefore should contact the CSP, and (2) cervical cancer was highly curable if detected in its

Table 5.8 Selected Demographic Characteristics of Hale County and Alabama

Location	Estimated Population (1977)	Percentage Black	Percentage Rural	Population per Physician	Percentage Below Poverty Line	Percentage Without Adequate Plumbing	Socioeconomic Status Index
Hale County	15,500	63	79	3,972	55	51	50
Alabama	3,600,000	26	42	1,860	25	16	100

Sources: Southern Regional Council, *Health Care in the South: A Statistical Profile* (1974); U.S. Department of Agriculture, *Indicators of Social Well-Being for U.S. Counties*, Rural Development Research Report no. 10 (Washington, D.C.. Government Printing Office, 1979). U.S. mean = 100: standard deviation (SD) = 20.

Table 5.9 Elements, Channels, and Purposes of the
Hale County Intervention

Element	Channel of Communication	Purpose
1. Community organization	Local lay and professional leaders	Increase acceptance and support Demonstrate and increase program credibility
2. Mass media	Electronic and print media: radio, local newspaper, church and club newsletters, posters, and bulletin boards	Increase awareness of and interest in program message Reinforce program message
3. Lay leadership	Leadership training—standardized package	Increase assumption of responsibility by locals in community or group Decrease misinformation Increase program acceptance by groups through peer participation and pressure Increase standardization of messages
4. Interpersonal group sessions	Group process: 1- to 2-hour standardized cancer education program session	Increase efficiency of networking Increase adaptability to personal evaluation and responsibility Increase motivation and social support Increase personalization of messages Increase legitimacy of at-risk role
5. Interpersonal individual sessions	Individual word-of-mouth diffusion	Increase persuasion Increase efficiency of diffusion Increase salience of messages Increase trial and adoption

early stages. The first intervention, element 1 in table 5.9, was applied in 1979. This community organization effort recruited and trained 39 female lay leaders, 21 white and 18 black, from existing community groups. The leaders were trained to conduct programs for women's groups throughout the county. They held 45 cancer communications meetings with about 15 to 20 participants each. Approximately 750 women were documented as having been directly exposed to the Cancer Communications Program. Considerable emphasis was placed on word-of-mouth diffusion by participants to friends. The second intervention, in 1980, utilized elements 2 and 5.

Evaluation Design

A time series design with a repeated treatment was chosen to evaluate the behavioral impact of the Cancer Communications Program. The computerized data system of the CSP of the Alabama Department of Health was used to confirm unobtrusively the pattern of new users by quarterly report. These data were examined to determine the extent to which the two interventions increased CSP use by new users beyond what one would normally expect. In applying a time series design, this project: (1) established the periodicity of the pattern of behavior being examined, (2) collected outcome data unobtrusively, (3) confirmed multiple data points one year prior to and one year following the intervention, and (4) applied and abruptly withdrew the intervention during a specific time period. This design was selected because it was the highest quality quasi-experimental design that was feasible to evaluate a program of this type in a field setting.

Program Impact

The frequency (number) of new users by quarter and by year for Hale County is illustrated in figure 5.1. A new user was defined as an individual who had not previously used the Alabama CSP. A look at the pattern of figure 5.1 for the three-year period suggests a significant difference in CSP use during the two intervention periods. The frequency of CSP new users for the five baseline quarters prior to intervention 1 was relatively stable although the increase in the frequency of new users in the second quarter of 1978 suggested a seasonal variation. An increase of 345 percent in new users, from 20 to 89, was observed for the second quarter of 1979, the intervention quarter. In other words, 89 new clients used the service during this period, compared to an average of 15 in 1978 and a maximum of 20 for the second quarter baseline in 1978.

As noted in figure 5.1, another increase in client use, from 20 to 50 (approximately 150 percent), was observed during the second intervention period. In the aggregate, an estimated 100 more new users were motivated to use the CSP than would be expected from the pattern observed during the nonintervention periods in 1978 and 1979. Throughout the three-year period, the demographic characteristics of the new users remained relatively stable, suggesting that the two interventions had an effect on similar women. An analysis of the new user increase using a linear regression model found that the observed frequencies for the intervention quarters were significantly higher ($P > 0.01$) than the observed frequencies for the nonintervention quarters. An examination of utilization data from a contiguous, matched county revealed no

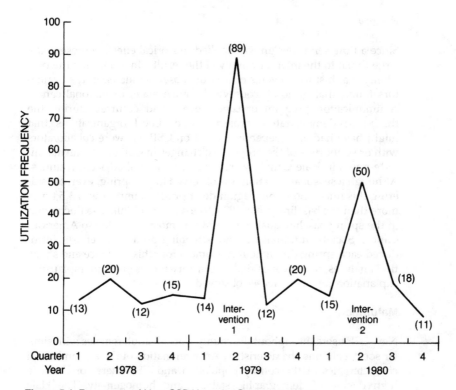

Figure 5.1 Frequency of New CSP Users by Quarter and Year

Source: R. A. Windsor and G. Cutter, "Methodological Issues in Using Time Series Designs and Analysis: Evaluating the Behavioral Impact of Health Communication Programs," in *Progress in Clinical and Biological Research*, vol. 83: *Issues in Screening and Communications*, ed. C. Mettlin and G. Murphy, 517–535 (New York: Alan R. Liss, 1981).

changes in CSP use by new users of the magnitude noted in Hale County. From the available evidence, it was concluded that the increases in new CSP users in Hale County were *primarily* due to the two interventions.

Internal Validity of Results

As noted in previous discussions in this chapter, program evaluators should consider the plausibility that a number of factors other than the intervention produced an observed impact. Using the Hale County project data, each of the major factors noted in table 5.1 is examined with regard to the plausibility that it produced the increases observed. The main question to ask for each factor is: Could this factor have produced the observed change?

History

Since a time series design was applied, historical effects represented a large threat to the internal validity of the results. In examining the possibility that historical events caused the observed increase, the evaluators found that no local, countywide, area, state, or national cancer communication program or cancer event had occurred during the three-year demonstration project period. Local organizations that might have had an independent effect on CSP use were collaborators with or supporters of the project. No changes in CSP use of the magnitude noted in Hale County were evident in several adjacent counties. Although a seasonal variation was observed in the spring, even considering this fluctuation, the magnitude of program impact was 3.5 times more than the baseline use in 1978 (89 users versus 20). The fluctuation in the spring baseline quarter of 1978 was most likely due to American Cancer Society fund-raising and screening-promotion efforts introduced each spring throughout Alabama. From this evidence and statistical analyses, it was concluded that history represented an implausible explanation for the increases observed.

Maturation

New CSP users throughout the county were all adult females with similar socioeconomic characteristics. An examination of the age and racial characteristics of the county population and CSP users confirmed a high degree of demographic stability and homogeneity. The Hale County CSP was selected because it had been operating for two years and was considered a stable and mature program. No significant social, biological, or psychological changes among female residents of this county were apparent. A maturation effect, therefore, was felt to be an implausible explanation for the noted impact.

Baseline Observations and Testing

Because the data observed were unobtrusive measures of behavioral impact (CSP use), this factor could not be a plausible explanation for the observed change during the intervention periods. No direct contact occurred between study personnel and clinic users. The time series design controlled for the effects of multiple observations by using unobtrusive measurement.

Instrumentation

An examination of the instruments and data collection procedures used by the CSP confirmed a high degree of standardization. No documentation errors were apparent to the investigators during the three-year observation period. CSP instruments and personnel remained constant, and the endpoint, i.e., increased service utilization by new users, was easy to confirm. All CSP users were confirmed as Hale County residents. No significant administrative or staffing changes occurred during the study period. It was concluded that instrument and measurement errors did not represent a plausible explanation for the observed behavior changes.

Statistical Regression

The evaluators assessed the extent to which the observed change was a statistical artifact. The demographic characteristics of the users for the three-year period were very stable. While it was confirmed that more women used the service, those new users were not significantly different from previous new users. The level and type of new CSP users were relatively stable during the nonintervention period. Hale County was selected because it is generally comparable to a number of counties in south central Alabama and not because of any extreme characteristic or screening problem. The evidence suggested that the observed impact was not due to a regression effect.

Selection

No comparison group was used in this study. In addition, the demographic characteristics of those motivated to use this service were comparable to new and previous users. The age distribution and racial makeup of the new users was also very stable. The information available suggested that selection did not play a significant role in producing the observed change.

Participant Attrition

Since the impact variable of this study was CSP use by new users, attrition by study participants was not an issue. While this factor frequently represents a problem in studies and might have represented a problem in this study if a concern had been repeat user attrition (missed appointments), it could not have compromised the internal validity of the observed results in the present study.

Summary

Considering the discussion of the case material relating to the principal threats to internal validity, it was felt that the observed behavior changes in CSP use were produced by the Cancer Communication Program applied in the spring of 1979 and 1980. This conclusion was strengthened by the replication included in this field experiment. The observed increases were statistically and programmatically important in that the methods and issues examined were useful to ongoing community health education efforts (Windsor and Cutter, 1982; Windsor, 1983).

Case Study 2: High School Smoking-Cessation Program

Source: C. Perry, J. Killen, M. Telch, L. A. Slinkard, and B. G. Danaher, "Modifying Smoking Behavior of Teenagers: A School-based Intervention," *American Journal of Public Health* 70, no. 7 (1980): 722–25.

Background and Objectives

In 1978, a special program was implemented to reduce the smoking behavior of tenth grade students from five high schools near Palo Alto, California. As part of their regular tenth grade health education classes, 498 teenagers in three schools (E) received a special smoking prevention/cessation program (X_1). In two other high schools, 399 teenagers (C) received traditional tenth grade health class materials emphasizing the long-term harmful effects of smoking (X_2). These five schools represented all of the high schools in two local school districts. The schools were matched according to socioeconomic status and then randomly assigned to the X or Y group. The purpose of the study was to compare the effectiveness of a multi-component smoking-cessation program to the traditional antismoking sources. The new course emphasized the immediate physiological effects of smoking and the social cues that influence adoption of the smoking habit. It was hypothesized that the multi-component smoking program would be more effective than the traditional antismoking curriculum in reducing the incidence of smoking among high school students.

Intervention

Adolescents in the three treatment schools received a special smoking prevention/cessation program consisting of 45-minute sessions on four consecutive days in their regular health education classes during the fall of 1978. Regular teachers trained by project staff implemented the program. The experimental classes focused on identification of the social pressures to adopt the smoking habit and skills to deal with them. Another focus of the experimental program was on the immediate physiological effects of smoking. Slide shows, films, and other media presenting promotional techniques and other marketing strategies to encourage smoking were discussed in the sessions. The teachers emphasized the development of verbalization skills that the students could use to counter the effects of cigarette advertising, and students led discussions on peer group influences on individual behavior. Methods of resisting these pressures, including modeling, were applied. In addition, students in the special program were exposed to simple behavioral techniques, such as recording and monitoring the frequency of their own smoking behavior and relaxation methods to help deal with urges to smoke [see table 5.10].

To demonstrate the physiological effects of smoking, students from Stanford University performed physiological measures and performance tests (carbon monoxide [CO], skin temperature, blood pressure,

Table 5.10   Experimental Program in Smoking Prevention/Cessation

Session	Intervention
1	The teacher-facilitator introduces the topic of smoking prevention: the pressures for young people to smoke tobacco, the immediate negative effects of smoking, and how to help others quit. Student small groups discuss social pressures to smoke and methods to handle social pressures. Student groups present their ideas to the class on ways to handle social pressures. Students see a brief slide show on the pressures to smoke tobacco.
2	The teacher-facilitator presents the topic: How advertising affects adoption of smoking by adolescents. The students see the movie: *Too Tough to Care.* The students see a slide show on cigarette ads; the students identify to whom the ad is addressed, what it is really selling, and how to counteract advertising. The class discusses each slide.
3	Topic: The immediate effects of smoking. Students form three teams and measure their own levels of carbon monoxide in the breath, blood pressure, pulse rate, lung capacity, and skin temperature. The teacher-facilitator shows the results of the self-measures by comparing smokers to nonsmokers in the class. The teacher-facilitator leads a discussion on the effects of smoking, emphasizing the implications of the physiological measures. The teacher-facilitator completes the discussion on the immediate effects of smoking and distributes articles from *Licit and Illicit Drugs* and *Reader's Digest.*
4	The teacher-facilitator leads a discussion on how to help other people quit smoking. Students conduct brainstorming sessions in small groups on how to help others remain nonsmokers, quit smoking, or build a non-smoking community. Student groups present their ideas to the class.

Source: Adapted from C. Perry, J. Killen, M. Telch, L. A. Slinkard, and B. G. Danaher, "Modifying Smoking Behavior of Teenagers: A School-based Intervention," *American Journal of Public Health* 70, no. 7 (1980): 722–25.

pulse rate, and lung capacity assessments) on the high school students. Feedback was provided to smokers and nonsmokers in the course of program discussions.

Students in the comparison schools received the standard lecture material on the harmful effects of smoking with no instruction on social skills to deal with peer pressures to smoke.

Evaluation Design

A nonequivalent comparison group design was used to evaluate the behavioral impact of the two interventions. Data collected on all subjects for both programs included knowledge and attitude questionnaires,

Table 5.11   Percentage of Subjects Reporting Smoking Cigarettes

	Experimental Program (N = 477)		Control (N = 394)	
	Pre	Post	Pre	Post
Smoked in past day	13.9	9.7[a]	14.5	13.1
Smoked in past week	19.5	16.3	21.6	21.9[b]
Smoked in past month	29.2	23.6[a]	26.3	30.4[b]

Source: C. Perry, J. Killen, M. Telch, L. A. Slinkard, and B. G. Danaher, "Modifying Smoking Behavior of Teenagers: A School-based Intervention," *American Journal of Public Health* 70, no. 7 (1980): 722–25.
[a] Within-treatment differences, P < 0.05.
[b] Between-treatment differences, post-test only, P < 0.05.

self-reported incidence of smoking, and CO samples at baseline and follow-up. Individual subjects were not identified in the data collection process. Baseline assessments were conducted in September 1978 and follow-up assessments approximately six months later in February 1979.

Program Impact

Self-reported smoking behavior by the experimental and comparison groups is reported in table 5.11. As noted, individuals in the experimental program were comparable to the controls at baseline for assessments of having smoked in the past day, week, or month. No significant improvements were noted between baseline and follow-up for the comparison group. Between-group differences in subjects reporting smoking were not significant at baseline. Differences between the experimental and the comparison group at follow-up indicated, however, that a significantly greater proportion of the treatment subjects reported abstaining from smoking.

Differences between the groups at follow-up for several knowledge questions are noted in table 5.12. Participants in the experimental program scored significantly higher than those in the standard program on five items relating to immediate physiological effect, one item relating to the best way to quit, and one item relating to the best way to prevent others from smoking. The two groups did not differ in general attitudes toward smoking. The published report noted that the data strongly suggested the superiority of the experimental program in positively affecting subjects' knowledge and attitudes, reported smoking behavior, and CO levels.

Table 5.12   Percentage of Subjects Responding Correctly on Smoking Knowledge and Attitude Survey

Survey Item	Treatment (N = 524)	Control (N = 399)	χ^2
1. What happens to your blood pressure if you smoke?	89	62	91 1[a]
2. What happens to the carbon monoxide in your blood?	87	60	91 0[a]
3. What happens to your pulse rate?	81	52	88.3[a]
4. What happens to your skin temperature?	65	12	268.0[a]
5. What happens to your lung capacity?	88	69	49.8[a]
6. What are the reasons people your age smoke?	80	65	NS
7. Is it difficult for people your age to quit?	50	52	NS
8. What is the best way to quit?	41	26	26.6[a]
9. What can a high school student do to prevent others from becoming hooked on cigarettes?	88	52	66[a]
10. What is your general opinion about smoking?	68	65	NS

Source: C. Perry, J. Killen, M. Telch, L. A. Slinkard, and B. G. Danaher, "Modifying Smoking Behavior of Teenagers: A School-based Intervention," *American Journal of Public Health* 70, no. 7 (1980): 722–25.

Note: The discrepancy in the number of treatment subjects reported in the text and in the table in this study is discussed under Participant Attrition in the section on internal validity of results.

[a]$P < 0.001$

Internal Validity of Results

In assessing the quality of this investigation and its reported results, it is important to examine the plausibility of alternative explanations for the results reported by the authors. Each factor that might compromise the validity of the results is examined next.

History

When a nonequivalent control group design is applied, particularly when the subjects reside in the same locale, as they did in this study, exposure to events or activities external to the program is most likely to occur among both experimental and control subjects. In addition, since this was an exploratory study conducted over a short period—six months—it seems unlikely that historical events were a plausible explanation for the reported results. Logic, grounded in the literature, also suggests that smoking behavior is not easily changed and would not likely be influenced by episodic or single exposures to media or admonitions by adults to stop smoking. From the available evidence, it seems reasonable to conclude that history did not play a significant role in producing the observed results.

Maturation

Given the short duration of the program, it is unlikely that maturation among the subjects played a significant role in producing the observed change. No significant social, biological, or psychological changes could be expected to have occurred in this period. Maturation is an implausible explanation for the noted impact.

Baseline Observations and Testing

The design and methods discussed in this report prevent clear assessment of the extent to which the baseline observations affected the follow-up assessments. In general pretest or baseline observations tend to have a slight effect on subsequent observations. While anonymity was guaranteed in this study, the subjects were aware that they would be reassessed and aware of what answers were more socially desirable. These factors play a role in the direction of the observed results. This factor is controlled to some extent by the fact that the influence the pretest had would reasonably be similar on both groups. Since individuals were not randomly assigned to groups, however, this is not fully controlled. The design does not establish the effects of baseline assessment on study participants. Evidence in table 5.11 that smokers in the control group decreased from 14.5 percent to 13.1 percent might be interpreted as a behavior change due to effects of the baseline observation or a reflection of the tendency to give a more socially desirable response. The differences observed between baseline and follow-up in the comparison group may be due to measurement error, pretesting effect, response bias, or chance variation.

Instrumentation

This study used both self-reports and CO levels to confirm smoking behavior. The accuracy of these data were examined by computing a correlation between CO levels and reported smoking from the preceding day. A correlation coefficient between these two variables of $r = 0.53$ was reported. No evidence on the reliability or validity of the knowledge and attitudes questions was provided. The report confirmed a high degree of standardization in the data collection process.

With regard to the accuracy of the data derived from the subjects, several small concerns are apparent. While a correlation of 0.53 is statistically significant, it indicates some measurement error and some lack of congruence between the CO levels and self-reports. CO levels are increased by a number of other factors, including air pollution and marijuana smoking; on the other hand, CO has a short half-life, thus preventing detection of some smokers in this and other studies. While the addition of the CO post-test measure added considerably to the quality of the data derived in this study, some students in the experimental group may have provided responses that were more socally desirable than accurate. Not being able to link baseline and follow-up observation data to individual students represents another possible source of error. It is plausible that instrument measurement error played a small role in explaining the observed change. The evidence suggests that some error was apparent in the collection of the outcome data. Errors or measurement variations of the magnitude of the effect reported in this study (5 percent) would not be uncommon in adolescent smoking studies.

Statistical Regression
The data suggest that regression is not a likely explanation for the observed changes. All study participants were from the same local geographical area and the same grade level. However, no background demographic data are presented to provide unequivocal evidence of comparability. The baseline observations and discussion in the report provide evidence that the groups were relatively comparable. The evidence suggests that neither group was selected because of any extreme characteristics or inherent quality that would make its members predictably more receptive to a smoking-cessation. The relative stability of the dependent measures among control group members suggests that statistical regression was probably not a good explanation for the observed results.

Selection
The selection of the schools to receive the experimental control conditions was performed by random assignment. Individual subjects, however, were not randomly assigned to an intervention. The report indicated that the schools were matched by socioeconomic status, all individuals were students in the tenth grade, and an equal proportion of males and females participated in both groups. The information provided suggests that selection did not play a significant role in producing the results. In the absence of random assignment of subjects to treatment, however, it is possible that preexisting characteristics of subjects in the schools assigned to each group may have produced part of the observed changes. Selection represents a notable threat to internal validity in this study.

Participant Attrition
Available information indicates that baseline and follow-up data were collected on all subjects. This suggests no participant attrition. However, the data in table 5.11 confirm a loss of 21 subjects in the experimental group, from 498 to 477, and a loss of 5 subjects in the comparison group, from 399 to 394. This suggests either participant attrition or an error in reporting. There may have been a loss in both behavioral

reports and CO measurements for some subjects, particularly in the treatment group. If this interpretation is accurate, it suggests a small possible bias. Since most literature indicates that individuals lost to follow-up in smoking studies are more likely to be smokers than non-smokers 5 percent or less of the observed reduction in smoking levels at follow-up for the experimental group may be due to the loss of subjects and not to program effectiveness.

A confusing aspect of this report is the discrepancy in the number of experimental group subjects reported in table 5.11 (477), in table 5.12 (524), and in the text (499). The rates of attrition and turnover within groups (students leaving and coming into the schools) are small for a study of this type, but these changes may account for some of the reported behavioral impact.

Summary

The study report indicated that conclusions about the long-term effectiveness of the experimental program would be premature, although the overall post-test results were somewhat encouraging. An alternative conclusion for the observed results might be that measurement error, selection, and participant attrition produced all or most of the observed effect. A more rigorous assessment of the data suggests that less enthusiasm about the superiority is warranted. The study was a well-designed investigation and produced some useful data, but it is not conclusive because of design and methodological problems and because the observed differences between and within the groups were only approximately 5 percent. A larger impact and less equivocal evidence are needed to show that the multi-component smoking program was more effective than the traditional anti-smoking curriculum in reducing the prevalence of smoking among tenth grade students.

Case Study 3: National Smoking-Cessation Program (MRFIT)

Source: G. Hughes, N. Hymowitz, J. Ockene, N. Simon, and T. Vogt, "The Multiple Risk Factor Intervention Trial (MRFIT), V: Intervention on Smoking," *Preventive Medicine* 10, no. 4 (1981): 476–500.

Background and Objectives

The Multiple Risk Factor Intervention Trial (MRFIT) was a six-year evaluation research study designed to investigate the effects of reducing cardiovascular risk in a group of 12,866 asymptomatic men between 35 and 57 years of age who were at high risk of cardiovascular disease. A three-part screening process was used to recruit participants. The first screening visit (S_1) was used to determine interest in and eligibility for the trial on the basis of three risk factors and to check for major exclusionary criteria such as the existence of other medically diagnosed problems. A second screening visit (S_2) was used to apply exclusionary criteria not addressed in the first screening, to explain in greater detail the purposes and requirements of the trial, and to develop an impression of the subject's intent to participate. A third screening visit (S_3) was used to confirm final eligibility, collect additional baseline information, assign participants randomly to either the special intervention (SI) or the usual care (UC) group, and initiate the intervention with those assigned to SI. Twenty-two clinical centers were used to screen over 361,662 possible participants at S_1. Of those, 12,866 were randomly assigned to the SI and UC groups. Data presented in table 5.7 earlier confirm the comparability of the treatment and control groups at baseline.

In this case study, only the smoking-cessation component of the MRFIT will be examined. The major purpose of the smoking intervention was to motivate those assigned to the SI group to stop smoking for the duration of the trial, a four-year period. As noted in table 5.7, 59 percent of the SI and UC groups were smokers at the onset of the intervention (S_3).

Intervention

The smoking-cessation program for MRFIT used a variety of behavioral techniques. The initial cessation program, immediately following assignment to the SI group, consisted of (1) a strong antismoking message from a physician, who discussed the effects of smoking on the cardiac and respiratory systems, and (2) an interview with the smoking specialist. Intensive intervention groups were formed, consisting of 6–12 SI participants, approximately two-thirds smokers and one-third nonsmokers. These groups met with an intervention team usually consisting of a behaviorist, a nutritionist, and a physician for ten sessions of 90 minutes each. The group sessions included presentations about smoking, nutrition, the relationship of blood pressure to cardiovascular disease, and techniques for changing patterns of behavior. Participants in the treatment groups were given pertinent information about cigarettes and smoking and their harmful effects. Smoking-cessation films and written materials were also developed and applied. The long-term benefits of not smoking were emphasized. Control of the behavior modification process by the participants and individual responsibility were emphasized during the special intervention.

In addition to the special intervention, a maintenance program was applied by staff to selected participants. The frequency of contact depended on the individual's success in remaining a nonsmoker. While there was variation among participants, after the first intervention year those who maintained nonsmoking status were generally seen at annual follow-up visits. A newsletter was another constant feature of the maintenance program. Occasional group meetings were also part of the maintenance effort. For those who were unsuccessful in stopping smoking after the special intervention, an extended intervention program was available. The methods used in the extended intervention effort varied across intervention sites. In the aggregate, the special intervention program, the maintenance program, and the extended intervention program represent probably the most powerful interventions yet applied to a smoking population. The program was designed to provide evidence of the efficacy of smoking-cessation efforts. This study offers the best evidence to date on long-term effects of a multi-component smoking-cessation program for adult males using maximum resources. It should be noted that the interventions and personnel used in this study were highly resource-intensive and, therefore, beyond the capability of all but a select few (wealthy) health promotion and education programs.

Evaluation Design

Following an intensive screening of over 360,000 individuals, a total of 12,866 men were randomly assigned to the special intervention (SI) or usual care (UC) group. Extensive baseline data were established for treatment and control group participants (presented earlier in table 5.7). Randomization and establishment of comparability of the two groups produced a rigorous model for evaluating effects. While it is obvious that many of the parameters assessed in this trial are beyond the means of an ongoing program, the procedures used and the theory underlying the protocol have broad application in the practice of health promotion and education. The study represents one of the best for large-scale smoking-cessation trials.

A randomized pretest and post-test with control group design (identified in table 5.1 earlier as design 5) was used. As noted, this is the most powerful method for determining the effectiveness of an intervention. The design used in the MRFIT controlled for many of the major problems noted in the smoking-cessation literature by using randomized experimental and control groups, long-term follow-up, structured group follow-up, and both self-reported and objective measures of smoking status (saliva thiocyanate, or SCN). The methods and design dramatically increased the power and utility of the reported results. As the researchers noted, "The design of the cigarette smoking control portion of MRFIT is itself a notable and outstanding accomplishment that will be a standard against which smoking studies of the present and future will have to be measured" (Hughes et al., 1981, 500).

Program Impact

Table 5.13 presents an abbreviated summary of the reported smoking data during screening and follow-up for the SI and UC groups for this randomized trial (Sherwin et al., 1981). As indicated in the table, the percentage of smokers in the treatment and control groups was the same at the S_3 baseline (59 percent). The SI group dropped to ap-

Table 5.13 Reported Cigarette-Smoking History for SI and UC Participants at Each Screening Visit and Month of Follow-up

	Special Intervention				Usual Care			
		Cigarettes/Day					Cigarettes/Day	
Visit	N[a]	Mean	SD	Percentage Smokers	N[a]	Mean	SD	Percentage Smokers
S_1	6,428	21.5	20.3	63.8	6,438	21.7	20.5	63.5
S_2[b]	6,428	NA	NA	62.0	6,438	NA	NA	61.3
S_3	6,428	19.2	19.9	59.3	6,438	19.3	20.3	59.0
12 months	6,114	8.3	14.2	35.9	6,080	16.8	18.8	55.5
24 months	6,000	8.6	14.6	35.2	5,922	16.2	18.9	52.2
36 months	5,896	8.7	14.6	35.1	5,794	15.8	18.8	50.5
48 months	5,804	8.5	14.6	33.9	5,721	15.0	18.6	48.2

Source: J. Neaton, S. Broste, L. Cohen, E. Fishman, M. Kjelsberg, and M. Schoenberger, "The Multiple Risk Factor Intervention Trial (MRFIT), VII: A Comparison of Risk Factor Changes between the Two Study Groups," Preventive Medicine 10, no. 4 (1981): 519–43.

[a]Each entry includes all participants for whom a cigarette-smoking history was obtained.
[b]The number of cigarettes smoked was not obtained at screen 2 (NA, not available).

Table 5.14 Percentage of Unadjusted and Adjusted Quit Rates for MRFIT SI Participants

Follow-up Visit (Months)	Unadjusted Quit Rate (Percentage)	Adjusted Quit Rate (Percentage)
4	47.3	43.9
12	43.1	40.2
24	44.1	40.2
36	44.4	39.7
48	45.9	40.3

Source: G. Hughes, N. Hymowitz, J. Ockene, N. Simon, and T. Vogt, "The Multiple Risk Factor Intervention Trial (MRFIT), V: Intervention on Smoking," *Preventive Medicine* 10, no. 4 (1981): 476–500.

proximately 36 percent at 12 months as confirmed by behavioral report. The group maintained this level throughout the 48 months, dropping slightly to 33.9 percent smokers at four years. In the control group a small reduction in smoking was observed during the first year of the trial and a reduction of equal magnitude occurred each successive year of the four-year period. The percentage of smokers in the control group at the 48-month follow-up was 48.2 percent, a significant improvement over the four years.

Two measures were made of the percentages of SI participants reporting that they had quit smoking cigarettes. Data in table 5.14 show the reported quit rate at the first follow-up visit (at four months) and at each annual visit for the four years. Data at the four-month visit represent the impact of the intensive smoking intervention, a 47.3 percent decrease. The overall quit rate at 48 months was 45.9 percent. The adjusted quit rate data reflect estimates of participants for whom there were missing data; an assumption was made that the missing data indicated that the person was a continuing smoker. Assuming the men who missed visits were smoking at the same level as at the previous visit, these adjusted quit rates were calculated. They reflect a conservative estimate of overall cessation at 40.3 percent.

Internal Validity of Results

Because this study used a randomized pretest and post-test with control group design and established comparability using multiple objective and subjective measures at baseline, considerable control over the threats to internal validity was asserted. It is necessary, however, to examine the major threats in light of actual application of the design to confirm the plausibility that each affected the observed quit rates.

History

The design controlled for historical effects that might occur during its course by the initial comparability of the groups, since whatever effect history might have would be of equal magnitude on both groups. The progressive societal shift toward interest in health and the incremental reduction in the production of adult males who smoke played a significant role in the overall decrease in both the SI and the UC groups. As noted, the quit rates of the UC group each year confirm an incremental trend toward abstinence. Part of the observed quit rate in both groups can be accounted for by the national trend, the participants' intensive contact with MRFIT staff, and self-initiated programs.

Maturation

The experimental design of this study controlled for maturation effects. If biological, sociological, or psychological shifts occurred over time, they would have influenced the behavior of both groups. Published reports present some evidence that quit rates in the male population have increased in recent years. Male smokers, as they mature, tend to be more receptive to internal and external cues to action and, therefore, more likely to quit on their own. This increased tendency to initiate or maintain cessation, however, seems to be of a considerably less magnitude than that observed among the SI group. Because the equivalence of the SI and UC groups was established by screening and randomization, maturation over the six to seven study years produced a comparable effect on both groups. Maturation probably played some role in producing the quit rates for both groups.

Baseline Observations and Testing

The multiple observations of SI and UC groups may have had a significant impact on quit rates throughout the study. Individuals in both groups were sensitized to the objectives of the study and influenced by the program observations and contacts over four-year period. Their continuing relationship with the study may have affected their behavior. Testing and observation probably had a significant effect on the quit rates of both groups.

Instrumentation

The instrumentation, measurements, and data collected by MRFIT on smoking cessation reflected a high standard of quality. The combination of behavioral reports and serum thiocyanate tests improved the investigators' ability to confirm quit rates. The validity and reliability of the instruments and the quality of the data collection process provided strong evidence of implausibility that instrumentation effects had produced the observed quit rates. The errors noted with the SCN values were relatively small and because of randomization could be expected to have a roughly equivalent and probably nonsignificant effect on the observed smoking behavior changes over time.

Statistical Regression

As discussed in the Background and Objectives section of this study, males between the ages of 35 and 57 who were at high risk for coronary heart disease from a combination of risk factors represented the target population for this clinical trial. Participants were selected on the basis of their high-risk characteristics. Regression did not seem to represent a problem, however, because of the extensive screening process, randomization, and the confirmation of group equivalence. Whatever pattern is expected for either cardiovascular risk or changes in smoking behavior would occur at approximately equal levels in the treatment and control groups. While this design asserted strong control for regression effects, it should be noted that both groups of smokers (SI and UC) regressed 5 percent between S_1 and S_3.

Selection

Selection may represent a plausible explanation for a significant part of the quit rates observed in the SI and UC groups. The MRFIT group was made up of health-conscious men. It is reasonable to assume that those who participated in the four-year trial were not characteristic of adult male smokers who participate in formal smoking-cessation programs. While all smoking-cessation programs reported in the literature use volunteers, it is likely that MRFIT participants were different from other volunteers because it clearly took highly motivated persons to go through the screening process and continue throughout the study.

While the experimental design asserted excellent control for the main effect of selection relating to group assignment, it, like all studies, was unable to assert control over those who chose to participate. Selection may have played a role in producing part of the observed quit rates.

Participant Attrition

An examination of the data on attrition indicated that 90.3 percent of the participants in the SI group and 88.9 percent of the UC group had a complete history for the duration of the project. Approximately 10 percent of the participants in the SI and UC groups were lost during the course of this study. A comparison of the characteristics of lost and remaining members between and within the groups suggested random or equivalent attrition in both groups. The randomized design markedly improved the investigators' ability to control for participant attrition effects. In this case attrition was not dramatic, and it occurred in approximately equal numbers of individuals with similar characteristics in both treatment and control groups.

Of the individuals who appeared for the third screen, 1,245 or 8.8 percent, were not randomized because of refusal to participate. A comparison of the characteristics of those 1,245 with the 12,886 who were randomized confirmed almost identical levels for age, serum cholesterol, diastolic blood pressure, number of cigarettes smoked per day, and percentage of smokers. This information suggested that those who were eligible to be randomized but who did not participate were very similar to those who did participate in the study.

The design and reported results confirmed that the observed attrition at the third screen and in the two study groups had little effect on the internal validity of the observed quit rates.

Summary

The randomized pretest and post-test with control group design, the quality of instrumentation and data collection, the comparability of groups at baseline, and the objective measures applied consistently at baseline and follow-up produced a very high degree of internal validity for the effect on the SI group. The observed increase exceeded previous reports in the literature for smoking cessation over an extended period of time. The design, methods, and interventions used for this study have broad application to programs attempting to motivate individuals to stop smoking. Many aspects of this study can serve as excellent guides for future smoking-cessation efforts by health promotion and education specialists.

SUMMARY

In evaluating the effectiveness of health promotion and education programs, there are a number of critical issues to be dealt with. The time frame, resources, and capabilities of your program must be considered prior to making a final decision about the specific design or methods you will propose and implement. In making a decision about a design, you must consider the potential factors that affect internal validity—factors that will compromise or bias estimates of program impact. A number of designs exist, but only a few are really useful for program evaluators. The five designs identified in this chapter—(1) a one group pretest and post-test, (2) nonequivalent control group, (3) time series, (4) multiple time series, and (5) randomized pretest and post-test with control group—are the most likely choices for 95 percent of ongoing health promotion and education programs. In deciding what design to implement for your program, you need to fully appreciate the strengths and weaknesses of each.

Considering the prominent role designs play in increasing the probability of your demonstrating an effect and determining whether what you observe is significant, you must estimate an effect size and decide on the needed sample size during the planning of an evaluation. There are a few good ways to establish a control or comparison group. You must consider what problems will arise in implementing an evaluation that includes two or three study groups. Although at first glance it may seem impossible to use a randomized design, more careful thought about the key questions to be answered, combined with a consultation and literature review, may provide the inexperienced evaluator with an insight into the use of a control group instead of a comparison group in evaluating a program. Regardless of the type of design or group that is used, you must establish the baseline comparability of study groups. In summary, the theory and applications discussed in this chapter represent an essential body of information that you need to know and be able to apply to plan, manage, and evaluate a health promotion and education program.

6

Issues in Data Collection

"Of course this measures what I want—just read the sentences and you can tell."

"I don't have the time or space to assess reliability. Let's assume it's reliable."

"I don't care how the program works, just if it produced changes in outcomes."

"We'll collect all the measures we can and figure out what to do with them later."

Professional Competencies Emphasized in This Chapter:

• ability to identify and provide mechanisms to assess selected educational methods

• ability to establish the scope of a program evaluation

Selecting the right approach to measurement for a particular study can be a confusing task. A person looking at the smoking-cessation literature will find self-reports of the number of cigarettes smoked per day, measures of attitudes toward smoking, measures of serum thiocyanate (a by-product in the blood that varies with the number of cigarettes smoked), possibly even tests of knowledge about smoking. A person looking at the weight-loss literature will find measures of weight, calories consumed, and energy expended. A person looking at the sex education literature will find measures of knowledge, self-reports of frequency of copulation with and without contraception, and measures of attitudes toward certain erotic topics. In evaluating practically every aspect of a health promotion program, you will have to select what to measure from a variety of alternatives.

Along these lines, the initial Role Delineation Project (U.S. DHHS, Public Health Service, 1980a) identified two skills:

III. C. 4. The health educator must be able to provide mechanisms to assess selected educational methods.

V. A. 2. The health educator must be able to establish the scope for program evaluation.

A broad variety of issues must be considered in establishing the scope of, and developing mechanisms for, evaluating health promotion programs. In most cases, the selection of dependent variables should be based on the objectives of the program. If a program has been designed to promote weight loss, weight measured by a standard calibrated scale is appropriate. If a program has been designed to promote positive attitudes toward heavy people among spouses of the obese, an attitudinal measure is appropriate. If a program attempts to influence what a person is *able* to do (as opposed to what a person actually does), a measure of capability to perform the behavior, i.e., a skills test, is appropriate.

Most health education programs attempt to influence the frequency of a particular behavior. Methods for measuring the targeted behaviors are often not readily available, however. For example, an explicit goal of your sex education program might be to reduce the number of teenage pregnancies in your community by promoting either sexual abstinence or effective contraceptive behavior. The primary indicator of the effectiveness of such a program is the number of teenage pregnancies in a particular community. A lack of reduction in pregnancies, however, does not necessarily mean that your sex education program was ineffective. The incidence of teenage pregnancies may have been rising over the last five years, and your program may have slowed the level of increase; or the program may be reaching only a segment of the population of sexually active teenagers who are abstaining or using contraception while the rest are not; or the program may have unintentionally misinformed the teenagers. In either of the latter two cases, you may want more behavioral data from the teenagers. Since it is not feasible for you to follow all the teenagers 24 hours a day to observe their sexual habits and contraceptive practices, you might ask for self-reports of these practices. Alternatively, the teenagers might be asked to demonstrate effective contraceptive techniques on a plastic model. While these latter two methods are reasonable approaches to collecting data, who can say that the self-reports are accurate, or that the teenagers practice what they can demonstrate in the classroom?

As this example shows, the area of measurement is fraught with complexities and pitfalls. This chapter generally discusses the possible measures and issues in selecting variables, including development of a model, assessing the validity and reliability of the instruments, secondary selection criteria, and threats to validity.

CONCEPTS AND VARIABLES, INSTRUMENTS AND MEASURES

Evaluation is most useful when it is built on a conceptual foundation. You cannot understand a program, or evaluate its effectiveness, unless you have some conceptual basis for understanding how it is supposed to work. The term *conceptual basis* means that a theory or, at a less formal level, a model hypothetically explains how the program is supposed to work. Any theory or model has variables. Variables define specific concepts. The model proposes that the variables are related in specific ways. Each variable in a model should be measured.

Take, for example, a model that identifies how people learn to lower the amount of salt in their diet. At a simple level, a model based on social learning theory (Bandura, 1977; Parcel and Baranowski, 1981) proposes that the likelihood that an individual will reduce salt in his or her diet is directly related to that person's behavioral capability (knowledge and skills) to do so and self-efficacy (or perceived self-confidence) at being able to do so. Figure 6.1 shows three vari-

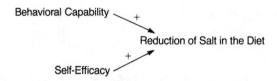

Figure 6.1 A Simple Social Learning Theory Model for Reducing Salt in the Diet

ables: behavioral capability to reduce salt, self-efficacy at reducing salt, and reduction of salt in the diet. The model specifies two relationships among these variables, both with a positive sign. The positive sign indicates that the greater the behavioral capability the more likely it is that the person will reduce salt. Similarly, the more self-confidence the person feels the more likely it is that the person will reduce salt. According to this model, a program interested in reducing salt in some target group's diet would attempt to increase the behavioral capability and self-efficacy of salt reduction in members of the target group.

The direct approach to evaluating the effectiveness of a program based on this approach would be to measure the dietary salt consumption of people in the target group. If you wanted to know whether the program was working according to the hypothesized model, you would also need to measure the group's behavioral capability and self-efficacy for dietary salt restriction. Measuring these variables requires instruments and measurements.

The word *instrument* has been used to identify something that produces a measure of an object. In the physical sciences, instrument usually refers to a machine (simple or complex) designed to produce meaningful numbers about particular objects. For example, a thermometer produces numbers in the form of degrees Fahrenheit or Celsius pertaining to the heat in some object. A flame spectrophotometer produces numbers in the form of percentages of the volume of one type of chemical contained in a solution.

Behavioral and social scientists do not usually use physical machines as instruments to obtain measures. Instead, they usually have some sequence of questions (usually with precoded response alternatives) to measure a concept. These sets of questions are their instruments. The numbers that come from applying the instrument to a particular person are called *measures*. Two or more instruments may produce or attempt to produce the same measure. To produce the measure, the instrument includes not only the specific questions but also instructions to an interviewer in applying (asking) the questions or in probing initial responses and procedures for taking the responses and producing the numbers. The terms *instrument* and *measure* are often used interchangeably in discussions of various categories of mea-

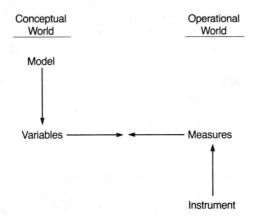

Figure 6.2 Relationships among a Model, Variables, Measures, and an Instrument

surements. In this chapter *instrument* will be used primarily to refer to the questions and procedures for obtaining *measures* on individuals.

Figure 6.2 shows the stated relationships among models, variables, measures, and instruments. A model and variables exist in the conceptual world. That is, variables are ideas that exist in the mind. They are abstractions about human experience. Referring back to figure 6.1, no one has ever seen behavioral capability or self-efficacy to reduce salt in the diet. They are useful ideas, however, to organize our understanding of what may account for the fact that some people are able to reduce salt in their diet and others are not. A model is based on theory and specifies expected relationships between two or more variables.

An instrument and measures exist in the operational world, that is, they embody the operations and methods people employ. An instrument is the set of questions (or observational categories, or other operations and methods) and all the procedures to maximize the accuracy of those questions. Applying an instrument to a particular person (or other object, as appropriate) will produce measures. Under the best of circumstances, there will be a close correspondence between the variables in the model and the measures resulting from the instrument. How to achieve the highest degree of this correspondence is the subject of validity, discussed later in this chapter.

TYPES OF VARIABLES

Many types of variables exist. In the "human factors" area, Alluisi (1975) has described psychobiological, psychophysiological, sensorimotor, and performance variables. In the personnel counseling area, there are ability, performance, and social-psychological adjustment variables. Obviously, in each area of inquiry certain kinds of variables are more appropriate than others. In health education and promotion, the following variables seem to be most frequently used: demographic, informational, cognitive, value or motivational, attitudinal (belief), personality, capability (skill), performance (behavioral), service utilization, and physiological.

Demographic

Demographic variables concern general social characteristics of people, such as age, sex, race/ethnicity, occupation, and education. These data are useful for characterizing the people in a program and comparing them to groups in other programs or to the population at large (through census data). Demographic variables separate people into common groups that are useful in testing for differences in the effectiveness of a program or in defining the population to which a study's findings can be generalized. For example, the percentage of mothers breastfeeding their infants upon departure from the hospital varies by ethnic group, income level, and family structure (Baranowski et al., 1982).

Informational

Informational variables have usually been labeled *knowledge* variables. Measures of information usually assume that some answers are right and others are wrong. The greater the percentage of right answers, the more knowledgeable the person is considered. Informational data are often used to confirm levels of community awareness about a problem, program, or activity. Whether people know that a service exists is an essential piece of data in designing a public information campaign.

Cognitive

Cognitive instruments measure the results of mental processes by which a person arrives at a conclusion. Cognitive processes of concern to a health promotion program may include attributional processes about illness, judgmental processes about achieving health, and problem-solving processes. *Attributional processes* deal with how people infer certain characteristics about themselves or about other people or events. Attributions are involved when a person uses symptoms to infer that he or she is sick. *Judgmental processes* refer to how people use various sources of information to arrive at a quantitative estimate of some characteristic of others or events. Judgments are often made about "how sick" a person is. *Problem-solving processes* refer to how a person defines a particular problem, identifies alternative solutions to the problem, and selects the most appropriate solution. The goal of a health education program may be improvement of any of these processes in regard to health phenomena. For example, knowing which symptoms people use, and how they are used, to decide to seek medical care can be useful in educating patients about the appropriate use of medical services.

Value or Motivational

Value or motivational variables concern the factors that attract or repel a person and thereby influence the person to act. There are different levels of value and motivational data. At the most abstract level are enduring values, e.g., beauty, truth, health, and religious faith, which can be major influences in a person's life decisions. At another level are more immediate motivations or incentives or expectations, e.g., wanting a reward for having lost ten pounds, or wanting to avoid a penalty imposed by a program for not having lost ten pounds. Value data can be a primary dependent variable (e.g., increasing the concern for health in a person's life) or a mediating variable (e.g., a program may have the greatest impact on those who value health the most).

Attitudes

Attitudinal or belief instruments measure the opinions of people. Attitudes are typically considered to have three components: a belief about a particular content area; a value about that belief (good or bad); and a predisposition to behavior. Knowing whether clients like or dislike group meetings can assist in the design of an approach to smoking cessation. Whether attitudes toward fat people change may be an important outcome for a training program for spouses of fat people.

Personality

Personality instruments measure characteristics that differentiate individuals from one another. There are a broad range of personality measures. Two commonly used within health education are internal-external locus of control (Lau and Ware, 1981), and Type A behavior (Jenkins et al., 1974). Personality variables have been used as dependent measures (e.g., in attempts to promote internal control), as mediating measures (e.g., where a program is expected to be effective with the internally controlled, but not others), and as screening variables (e.g., in identifying Type A's to participate in a stress-reduction program).

Capability

Capability or skill variables concern a person's ability to perform a task. In the sex education example, a teenager may or may not be capable of effectively performing a contraceptive task, such as putting on a condom. A person who is not able to put on a condom in a measurement session is very unlikely to do so at the height of passion. Persons with diabetes need to know how to monitor sugar in their urine and how to inject their insulin. Capability measures are useful because people cannot effectively perform the behavior or task routinely in other settings unless they can demonstrate the skill in an assessment setting. Just because they know how, however, does not necessarily mean they usually do the task in the desired circumstances.

Performance

Performance or behavioral variables concern whether, or how frequently, people perform one or more behaviors or tasks in their daily life. Most health promotion programs are concerned with specific health-related behaviors. Is the hypertensive patient consuming fewer high-salt foods? Is this family doing more exercise? Although these data are crucial for measurement in evaluating health education programs, they present many problems. Of greatest concern is the fact that not all of a person's behaviors are readily available to outside observation.

Utilization

Service utilization variables are used to describe patterns among clients in the use of a service. This is a subcategory of behavioral measures, i.e., whether and what kinds of people use a particular service.

Physiological

Physiological variables may be used for three purposes: as an outcome measure; to check whether a person is performing a desired behavior; or to assess a change in an important aspect of health or health risk. For example, blood pressure is often used as the primary outcome measure of hypertension patient education programs. Urine sodium tests measure the amount of salt consumed by an individual and thus can be used as a check on a person's self-report of that. Serum thiocyanate measures the by-products in the blood from cigarette smoking and therefore tests a person's self-report of smoking. High levels of high-density lipoprotein (HDL) cholesterol in a person's blood protect against heart attacks and reflect the amount of exercise the person habitually gets. An evaluator may want to assess the impact of an intervention on the person's risk for heart attacks by assessing serum HDL cholesterol.

SELECTING VARIABLES: A MODEL

Given this vast panoply of variables, how do you know which are most appropriate to your project's concerns? The primary step in selecting measures is to have a conceptual model. Three kinds of models may be useful: a model explaining how the behavior occurs; a model explaining how the health education service is produced; and a model explaining how the service affects or interacts with the ongoing behavior to promote change.

Model of Behavior

The model of behavior should identify the important variables related to a behavior and how they relate among themselves and to the behavior. The variables and relationships in a model should reflect the latest understanding of the phenomenon available in the literature. For example, in a weight-loss program, a model is needed of the variables affecting the weight of obese people. Figure 6.3 shows a simple weight-loss model. Weight is affected by the amount of food consumed (calories ingested) and the activity level (calories burned). How much a person eats is in turn affected by several factors. There is reason to believe that people have a mechanism, perhaps like a ther-

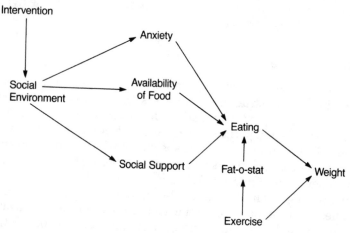

Figure 6.3 A Simple Model of a Weight-Loss Program

mostat, that is sensitive to the amount of fat in the fat cells. This mechanism can be called a *fat-o-stat*. It either decreases appetite to maintain a certain level of fat in those cells (Morley and Levine, 1982) or varies the rate at which energy is extracted from the food consumed (Sukhatme and Margen, 1982). Exercise may be one of the few things that can reset the regulator on the fat-o-stat. Eating patterns may also be affected by social support. Important people in the obese person's environment may encourage that person to overeat or to undereat. In some cases, obese people overeat when they are anxious or when food is too readily available. The availability of food and a person's anxiety level are both, in turn, reflections of the obese person's social environment (family, friends, coworkers, etc.). How much exercise a person gets probably reflects the amount of social support the person receives for exercise.

Such a model of behavior is valuable for three reasons. First, the model identifies the ideas underlying a program. It enables the program staff and evaluators to arrive at a common understanding of the behavior of concern, or at least enables the evaluator to understand explicitly the concepts of the program staff. Second, a model poses a clear direction for action. The model in figure 6.3 points up the importance of the social environment in weight gain or loss and the need to design a program that at least takes the social environment into account if it does not actively involve members of the social environment, e.g., the family. Third, such a model identifies variables for which measures need to be found. To evaluate the outcome of the intervention, measures of eating, exercise, and weight are necessary. Depending on the approach to intervention, the evaluator might also want to assess anxiety, food availability, and social support, to see if the intervention is having a desired impact on each of these hypothesized intervening variables.

Model of Service

A model of how a service is produced identifies other kinds of variables: the inputs, structures, processes, and service outputs. Figure 6.4 presents a simple conceptual model of a service system. In the inner box are the unspecified structures and processes for producing output. All programs have inputs, some of which come from the immediate environment and some from elsewhere. The output must return to some environment. The most common inputs to a program are participants, staff time, and other resources, e.g., training materials. The structure for a program usually consists of the organizational structure (i.e., the positions and qualifications for positions in the or-

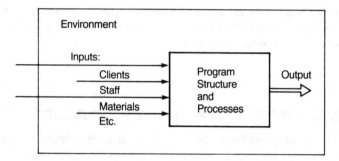

Figure 6.4 A Model of a Program as a Production System

ganizational hierarchy) and the activity structure (i.e., the sequence of service activities provided to a participant). The processes of a program refer to what is actually done to or for a participant. The desired output of such a program may be changes in knowledge, behaviors, skills, attitudes, values, or health status. The environment refers to the physical and social aspects of the surroundings within which the program operates and the participants live and work. Two questions in regard to the environment are of particular importance: Are the necessary resources available for the program from the immediate surroundings? Is the output of the program in turn accepted by the surroundings? For example, it would not make sense to develop a smoking-cessation program in an area where few people smoke. Alternatively, it makes little sense to produce nonsmokers who must return to groups of smokers, because they are likely to be seriously tempted and thus return to smoking in a short period of time.

A health promotion service model is valuable for several reasons. It explicates the necessary resources, the program structures, the processes for service delivery, the desired outputs, whether the inputs are available in the environment, and whether the environment will accept the outputs. Each of these concerns could be the focus of a program evaluation. A study of the inputs to such a system is often called a needs assessment (see chapter 3 and Baranowski, 1978a, 1978b). A study of the availability of service structures has been called a resource inventory (Bosanac et al., 1982).

Model of Change

The model of how a service interacts with behavior to promote change simply shows at what points in the ongoing behavior the program would intervene and what changes would be expected as a result of such intervention. Such a model identifies points in the ongoing behavior process at which it is useful to measure or document the expected effects of program efforts.

SELECTING THE MOST APPROPRIATE INSTRUMENTS

Once the model has been developed, instruments must be selected to measure the specified variables. The twin issues of reliability and validity are extremely important in selecting and developing instruments. You should locate existing instruments to use as models.

Reliability

Reliability is the extent to which an instrument will produce the same score if applied to an object two or more times. Imagine using an oral thermometer three times on the same person. On the first administration, a temperature of 105° F is obtained. This is clearly a sign of serious fever. Worried, you apply the thermometer again, one minute later, and obtain a temperature of 93° F. This temperature defines hypothermia, an equally serious problem. Still worried that something is wrong, you immediately reapply the thermometer and obtain a temperature of 98.6° F, normal body temperature. If a thermometer produced measures with that much variability it would be considered "unreliable." That is, the instrument produced different results on each administration. These differences were so large that you could not distinguish normal from pathological states without being concerned that the results were due to chance or to a defect in the instrument rather than to a serious illness in the person.

The reason that the medicine cabinet thermometer is such a useful instrument is that it is highly reliable at what it measures. Using this instrument allows a person to decide with reasonable confidence whether the body is diseased or not. This does not mean that the medicine cabinet thermometer has no unreliability; that is *not* the case. If you use such a thermometer three times, you may get readings something like this: 98.6°, 98.4°, and 98.7°. The results are clearly different, but the differences are insignificant for the purpose for which you are using the thermometer. If, however, you need to make distinctions of one-tenth of a degree, say between 98.4° and 98.5°, or you need to measure temperature beyond one decimal place, the medicine cabinet thermometer is unreliable. Thus, one instrument can often be quite reliable for one use yet highly unreliable for another.

Methods of Assessing Reliability. Before using an instrument to collect program data you should be concerned about its reliability. Does the instrument enable you to make distinctions between two or more behaviors with a reasonable level of confidence? For a few instruments, the reliability has already been calculated with many different groups. For most, it has not. There are several approaches to assessing the reliability of an instrument. Those used in the behavioral and social sciences can be classified using two factors: the type of instrument (observer versus self-report), and the times at which the instrument is applied (same time versus different times). The four possibilities are shown in figure 6.5.

Interobserver Reliability. If several observers are used to collect data at the same time, you can estimate reliability by having two observers rate the same performance. This is called interobserver or interrater reliability. This tells you whether two people are seeing and interpreting the same thing in the same way at the same time. Windsor (1981) used this technique in evaluating a diabetes patient education program.

Intraobserver Reliability. If an observer is used to assess the same person at two points in time, comparison of the consistency of the results is called intraobserver reliability. This kind of reliability test is not frequently performed because it assumes no difference in the phenomenon being assessed (performance or whatever) between the two points in time. Such a technique might be used if little change is expected, e.g., on mass assembly lines in factories or about perceptions of physical environments. Since an amount of change is usually the phenomenon of concern, observer reliability is usually assessed at one time using two observers (interobserver reliability).

Time Instrument Applied

Type of Instrument		Same Time	Different Times
	Observer	Interobserver Reliability	Intraobserver Reliability
	Self-Report	Split-Half Reliability Multiple-Form Reliability Internal Consistency	Test–Retest Reliability

Figure 6.5 Types of Reliability

Split-Half Reliability. Several techniques are available to assess the reliability of self-report instruments applied at the same time. If a large number of items measure the same concept or construct, you may conduct a split-half reliability assessment. You randomly assign items in the instrument to two groups, sum the scores of the two groups, and correlate the two sets of scores. This correlation should be reasonably high, 0.80 or higher, because both halves are supposed to be measuring the same construct.

If a multi-item scale is used to test split-half reliability, a statistical technique called *Cronbach's alpha* can also be applied to establish the internal consistency of the instrument (Nunnally, 1978). In theory, Cronbach's alpha produces the average of all the split-half reliabilities possible on a group of items. (The KR–20 is a form of Cronbach's alpha for discontinuous measures.)

Multiple-Form Reliability. Another approach to assessing the reliability of self-report instruments administered at the same time is to create two instruments (or two forms of the same instrument) that theoretically measure the same thing, and have the respondents answer both sets at the same measurement session. A correlation of 0.80 or higher should be obtained between the two sets of measures, because they are supposed to be measuring the same thing.

As a continuing monitor on the reliability of an instrument, you can simply repeat the same items at two points in a questionnaire. If these items assess important concepts, asking the same question twice will provide a continuing monitor on how reliably a selected number of items are measured over the course of the evaluation.

Test–Retest Reliability. Measuring reliability by using the same test at two points in time is called test-retest reliability. Reliability scores from this method are expected to be lower than from the split-half or multiple-form methods, because time has elapsed between the first and the second assessment. The longer this interval is, the more likely it is that something will happen to some of the people that induces a real change in the measures the test is providing.

There are many related issues in reliability assessment, and you should consult appropriate texts (Nunnally, 1978) before using one of these methods.

Managing Reliability. We have reviewed several concepts of or approaches to measuring reliability; we also need to review the sources of random errors that produce unreliability. Six general sources of unreliability have been identified: instructions, the instrument, the person making the measurement, the environment, the respondents, and data management problems. Unreliability can enter from any and all these sources, and often does. For example, the instructions may be confusing to the respondents. The instrument items may not be clearly understood by the target group. The person making the measurement may be slovenly in his or her use of the instrument. The environment in which the instrument is applied may be too noisy or otherwise distracting to the respondents. The respondents may be suffering from hangovers, headaches, or other factors that divert their attention. Errors can be made in coding, keypunching, or editing the data. Each of these sources of error adds to unreliability. The kinds of things that go wrong in data collection fully support Murphy's law. Careful attention must be paid to anticipating possible sources of error and developing contingency plans to avoid or deal with them as they occur. Concern for and assessment of reliability should occur each time an instrument is used.

Validity

Validity is the degree to which an instrument measures what the evaluator wants it to measure, that is, the underlying variable. It is possible to have an instrument that measures something you do not think it is measuring. This might happen because not enough thought went into creation of the instrument, because recent research has changed the complexity of the variable being measured, or because the instrument was not used with care and attention to detail. In many ways study of the validity of an instrument is more difficult than study of its reliability. Using the same instrument at two points in time or with two observers at the same time is relatively easy. Studying validity requires you to obtain or develop some more accurate measure of the variable of concern. Four general approaches to studying validity have been proposed. These are listed in table 6.1.

Face Validity. Face validity describes the extent to which an instrument *appears* to measure what it is supposed to measure. Thus, the question, "How many minutes of running/jogging did you do today?" appears to measure one important component of a person's aerobic activity for a particular day. For most adults, this question should work fairly well. For children, however, it probably will not. Children do not usually wear watches; they have their time organized for them (e.g., by bells or buzzers at school); and they do not have a well-developed concept of time. Thus, there is little reason to believe that accurate durations of running/jogging would be assessed by asking this question of children.

The question may lack validity even for adults. If you are inter-

Table 6.1   Definitions of Alternative Types of Validity

Type	Definition
Face	The extent to which the instrument appears to be measuring what it is supposed to measure
Content	The extent to which an instrument samples items from the full breadth of content desired
Criterion	The extent to which an instrument correlates with another more accurate (and usually more expensive) instrument (the criterion)
Concurrent	The criterion is an instrument administered at the same point in time as the instrument being tested for validity
Predictive	The criterion is an instrument administered at some time after administration of the instrument being tested for validity
Construct	The extent to which the measure of concern correlates with other measures in predicted ways, but for which no true criterion exists
Convergent	The measure correlates with the items with which it is predicted to correlate
Discriminant	The measure does not correlate with the items with which it is expected not to correlate.

ested in *aerobic* activity, which has cardiovascular benefit, there are other criteria to apply. Typically, to obtain cardiovascular benefit, a person must engage in aerobic activity for a minimum of 15 minutes at a time (without stopping), for a minimum of three times every week (American College of Sports Medicine, 1980). Furthermore, the activity must reach a certain intensity to promote cardiovascular fitness. Sufficient intensity would produce a heartbeat that is 60 percent or more of the person's maximum heart rate (calculated from commonly available tables for age and sex groups). You may, therefore, have a difficult time interpreting a response to the above question. Suppose the answer given is: "20 minutes." Was the activity sufficiently intense to merit the label "aerobic"? Did the person cover 4 miles (tremendous cardiovascular benefit) or 1½ miles (less cardiovascular benefit) in those 20 minutes? Were the 20 minutes in one continuous block of time or broken into two 10-minute segments, or four 5-minute segments, or some other division without cardiovascular benefit? Each of these qualifications raises issues about whether the question really gets at the construct of concern. A measure, therefore, must be carefully specified to assess the desired variable. You could create a self-report measure for adults that assesses distance traveled, intensity (e.g., heart rate), and continuous duration of activity (segments in minutes). On the other hand, people may not be able or motivated to keep track of or remember all this information. In such a case, the validity of the instrument is again in question. The more complex questionnaire may work with marathon runners in training (who are highly motivated to keep such records to assess their progress) but may not work for the casual early morning jogger. The validity of the instrument thus may be high with one group (the marathon runners) but not another group (the casual joggers).

This discussion should serve notice that a concern for validity requires more than attention to the face validity of the instrument. A valid measure should have other characteristics as well.

Content Validity. Another desirable characteristic is content validity. Some instruments are expected to cover several domains of content. To have content validity, an instrument must sample items from each of these content areas. For example, Windsor, Roseman, et al. (1981) developed an instrument to measure the ability of diabetic patients to care for themselves. Diabetic self-care is a complex activity requiring knowledge and skills in many areas. The Windsor team used a consulting body of experts and identified a broad variety of content areas for diabetes self-care, including foot/skin care, urine testing, diet, self-administration of insulin, safety measures, complications, and general information. Within each area, multiple knowledge and performance items were developed. Because of its comprehensiveness, this instrument currently has high content validity. It has sampled items within each major area of concern in diabetes self-care. As the years pass, however, and more is learned about diabetes, diabetics will be expected to do more or different things for themselves. The content validity of this instrument will then decrease, and the instrument will need further development and refinement. Thus, the content validity of an instrument may be time-limited.

Criterion Validity. On occasion, there are instruments that produce highly accurate measures of a characteristic but are very costly or difficult to apply. The objective of the evaluator faced with this situation may be to develop a less costly measure. The costly instrument is considered the criterion against which a less costly instrument can be assessed. If the correlation between the two instruments is high, the criterion validity of the second instrument is considered high. Criterion validity may be assessed by using the two instruments at the same time (concurrent criterion validity), or by using the less costly measure at one time to predict the measures of the more costly instrument at the second time (predictive criterion validity).

The assessment of sodium in the diet provides an interesting example. With mounting evidence that sodium intake is related to high blood pressure, many health education programs are interested in instruments to measure habitual sodium intake. A relatively accurate measure is an assessment of the sodium excreted in the urine. Given the high day-to-day variability in an individual's consumption of sodium and the lag time between episodes of unusually high sodium ingestion and the body's achievement of sodium balance, Liu et al. (1979) have estimated that an evaluator needs seven consecutive days of 24-hour urine samples to estimate a person's habitual sodium consumption. Many difficulties arise in obtaining such samples. People do not want to carry urine sample bottles to work, play, or other activities, because it is embarrassing. People forget to provide every sample, for a variety of reasons. It is costly to furnish the many containers necessary to collect so much urine, not allow it to become contaminated, and pick it up at intervals. Studies are now being conducted to assess whether an overnight urine sample, testing for both sodium and creatinine, can obtain similar information and replace the tedious and expensive 24-hour samples. Other investigators are using self-report measures of dietary consumption. In both cases, however, the seven consecutive days of 24-hour urine samples provide the criterion against which the other measures are assessed.

Construct Validity. One final type of validity needs to be mentioned: construct validity. As knowledge of a variety of phenomena increases, investigators learn more about how particular measures should relate to other measures. In part these relationships come to define the underlying construct. For example, people who are experiencing a high degree of anxiety are expected to experience a wide variety of physiological responses (e.g., more rapid heartbeat and breathing, higher blood pressure, changed galvanic skin response) and are expected to be less efficient at certain cognitive tasks (e.g., memory, judgment). If an investigator believes that the existing measures of anxiety are inadequate because they are highly related to some other variable that is not related to anxiety, she or he might decide to develop and test the construct validity of a new instrument. The investigator would expect two things. First, the new measure should correlate more highly with the physiological and cognitive performance changes (convergent validity) than the old measure. Second, it should correlate less well with the variable that is not related to anxiety (discriminant validity) than the old measure. If the new instrument demonstrates such convergent and discriminant validity, it is considered to have higher construct validity than the old measure. Such a demonstration indicates a greatly increased capacity to define and measure an important construct. If the new instrument, however, costs considerably more to use than the original measure, it may not be used frequently unless an evaluator needs to avoid the newly identified sources of error.

Relationships between Validity and Reliability

Validity is a more important issue than reliability. If an instrument does not measure what the investigators think it is measuring, it hardly matters that the measurement is reliable. Reliability, on the other hand, is much easier to assess. Formulas exist for measuring various aspects of reliability. The procedures for using an instrument at two times are relatively straightforward. Furthermore, reliability sets an upper bound to validity; that is, assuming that an instrument really is measuring what it is supposed to be measuring, the instrument can be no more valid than it is reliable. Thus, if a squared reliability coefficient is 0.5, the validity coefficient can never be higher than 0.5. This makes sense. If a measure cannot be consistently reproduced from one occasion to the next, there is no way it can accurately measure some underlying construct. Developers and users of instruments must be concerned about both validity and reliability. A means for estimating reliability should be employed every time an instrument is used. Tests of validity should be used prior to an investigation, to confirm that the instrument is measuring the desired variable in the selected sample of participants.

Threats to Validity: Bias

Measurement errors reduce the reliability and validity of instruments. For example, if a person did not carefully read the numbers on a thermometer, he or she could not get the same reading at two times, even if the temperature did not change. Error thus decreases reliability and, by implication, decreases validity. Health program evaluators are concerned with two types of error: random error and systematic error (also called *bias*).

Random Error. Random error is like "noise" on the radio. It gets in the way of clearly receiving a message that was sent. Random errors include any effects that give something other than a true response *and* produce responses that are distributed around the true response. For example, suppose a person takes the same test on ten different days and the ten scores are distributed as shown in figure 6.6. Assume that the true response is depicted in the figure by the vertical line. The ten measures vary around the true response for many reasons, e.g., the person got up late one day and was rushed, was too tired another day, and was anxious about an incident at home another day. The important characteristic is that, in random error, the obtained scores vary around the true response; if an infinitely large number of measures were taken, the mean of the obtained measures would equal the true response.

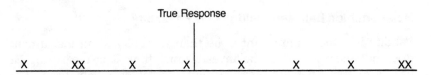

Figure 6.6 Distribution of Scores of Multiple Applications of a Test with Random Error

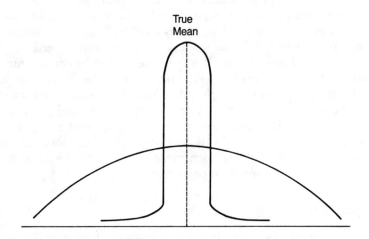

Figure 6.7 Two Distributions of Scores around the True Mean

Figure 6.7 shows the curves from two distributions of scores. If these curves were obtained from applying an instrument many times in two different ways, we would say that the taller curve has less random error, because more of the scores on that curve are closer to the true mean than those on the flatter curve. The way in which the test was administered to give the taller curve is more desirable because it produces less error.

Random errors decrease reliability. We may not reach different conclusions using a measure with high versus low random error, but it would be more difficult to obtain relationships between the high random error measure and other measures, or it would take a greater number of subjects to detect differences between groups using this measure.

Systematic Error (Bias). Systematic errors produce a systematic difference between the obtained scores and the true scores. For example, assume that a person took the same test on ten occasions and the scores are distributed as shown in figure 6.8. If the true response is

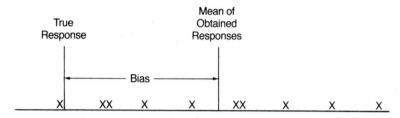

Figure 6.8 Distribution of Scores of Multiple Applications of a Test with Systematic Error

the vertical line at the left, figure 6.8 indicates that there was a bias in the test. The bias is the distance between the true response and the mean of the obtained responses. Of course, evaluators do not usually know what the true response is, although they may sometimes learn it from other information. With systematic errors, the mean of the obtained scores is always systematically different from the true score by one or more units: a systematic bias.

Bias threatens validity. A biased measure may induce you to conclude something completely different from a set of data than you would if you had the true measure. For example, if you were interested in attitudes toward smoking and you used a five-point scale, you might find the mean values shown in figure 6.9. The difference between the true score and the mean of the obtained scores is only a point and a half. The mean of the data obtained may lead you to believe that these subjects are unsure about, or even slightly dislike, smoking. If the true score were known, however, you would conclude that they have positive feelings about smoking. Somehow a bias crept into the data and led you to an erroneous conclusion about the attitudes of this group.

What factors might introduce bias into data collection procedures? There are many potential sources of bias. Some authors have tried to catalogue these to help develop ways of avoiding them. Webb et al. (1966) have identified 12 common biases in human measurements:

1. *The guinea pig effect—awareness of being tested*: People aware that they are being measured may respond in uncharacteristic ways. Some experience heightened anxiety and perform a variety of otherwise irrational acts. Others become defensive and distort their behavior or reports of behavior in other ways. In some cases, the awareness of being measured is hard to detect, because the effects are so subtle. A bias will occur if awareness of being measured induces a large number of people to report answers that deviate systematically in one way or another from the responses they would have given if they were not aware they

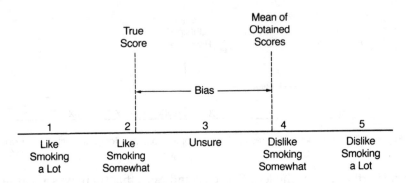

Figure 6.9 Effect of Bias on Conclusions

were being studied. The guinea pig effect is the basis on which instruments are divided into *obtrusive* and *unobtrusive* categories. These categories are discussed in chapter 7. The guinea pig effect also leads to many of the following biases.

2. *Role selection*: The awareness of being measured may influence people to feel that they have to play a special role. They ask, "What is expected of me in this situation?" and act accordingly. Others, angry at being measured, react by not conforming to what is expected of them and even displaying the opposite behavior.

3. *Measurement as a change agent*: The act of taking a measurement may affect the subsequent behavior of those being measured. For example, merely keeping track of what a person eats on a daily basis will affect what she or he eats during the recordkeeping period. People who are keeping track of their intake of high salt foods and who know that salt may have deleterious effects on their health will begin to lower their consumption of these foods for at least a short period. This may happen because the measurement instrument informs them of the many sources of salt in their diet, focuses their attention more clearly on their eating behaviors, or makes it obvious that they consume vast quantities of these foods, which they now believe they should not. The reduction in consumption is an obvious bias from the subjects' normal, premeasurement eating.

4. *Response sets*: Several investigators have shown that people respond to questionnaires, and even interviews, in predictable ways that have little or nothing to do with the questions posed. One such response set is *yea-saying*, which means that people are much more likely to say "yes" than say "no" to any particular

question in an instrument. Another response set is *social desirability*, the fact that people tend to answer a question the way they think the interviewer or tester wants the question answered, rather than according to their true feelings or thoughts about the issue. These response sets are not conscious strategies to distort responses; they work at a subtler level.

5. *Interviewer effects*: Characteristics of the interviewer may affect the receptivity and answers of the respondent. For example, a male interviewer may have difficulty obtaining accurate sexual information from female subjects. Interviewers of a lower socioeconomic status may elicit snide or uncharitable reactions from higher status respondents and vice versa. You can imagine many characteristics of an interviewer that might bias responses.

6. *Changes in the research instrument*: Any time an instrument is used more than once, there is the possibility of a learning effect. Interviewers may become more proficient in implementing an interview schedule the longer they use it; they may ask more probing and sensitive questions in later interviews than in earlier ones. Or at some point they may get bored and ask less probing and sensitive questions. Similarly, if a respondent answers the same set of questions at different points in time, the later answers may be deeper and richer because the questions have greater depth of meaning from repetition, or the later answers may become more shallow and mundane because of respondent boredom.

7. *Population restrictions*: The method of data collection may impose restrictions on the populations to which the results can be generalized. For example, telephone interviewing requires the respondent to have a telephone. Although most people have telephones, those who do not, those with new unrecorded telephone numbers, and those with unlisted numbers may be different in some characteristic from people with current telephone numbers in the public directory. Thus, estimates of this characteristic of the total population is biased in a telephone survey, because the method does not get at the total population. Other ways of collecting data may impose similar kinds of restrictions.

8. *Population stability over time*: An instrument administered at different points in time may be collecting the same data on differing populations. In a hypertension control project in one rural community, three random sample surveys were conducted at yearly intervals to document the impact of the program on the community. Between the second and third interviews, however, three of the five coal mining companies in the area closed, due to difficult economic circumstances. The younger miners who lost their

jobs were geographically displaced. Fewer younger miners were, therefore, included in the third random sample survey. These were exactly the people least likely to comply with their hypertension medication regimens and on whom the greatest amount of information was desired. In addition to this sampling bias, the loss of health insurance coverage by unemployed miners may have sensitized those remaining in the area to health care issues, probably making them value the hypertension control program more and thereby biasing their responses.

9. *Population stability over areas*: The same way of collecting data in two different geographic areas may tap different kinds of people. For example, users of small clinics in rural Appalachia are different in many ways from users of small clinics in inner cities. Users of one rural clinic may be very different from users of another rural clinic in demographic, ethnic, social class, and other characteristics. Comparisons of data on clinic users in differing areas are very difficult to interpret, because of these many possible biases.

10. *Restrictions on content*: There is a limited range of data that can be reported by each method. Self-report questionnaires, for example, cannot be used to study the cognitive mechanisms of moving information from short-term to long-term memory. Observational data cannot be used to study relationships among a person's values. Each method of data collection has a restricted range of data to which it can be applied. Using observational data to infer values will probably introduce several biases because of the assumptions observers make about the meaning of the observed behaviors.

11. *Stability of content over time*: If a program restricts a study to naturally occurring behavior, the content of the studied phenomenon may differ over time. For example, a study looking at the impact of health related messages on television may find that the sophistication of these messages changes significantly over time, or that certain events with higher priority (e.g., a governmental scandal, or an assassination) force health programs off the airwaves. The content, thus, is not stable over time. If investigators do not take these differences in both frequency and content into account in their analyses, their estimates of the effects of exposure to health messages will probably be biased.

12. *Stability of content over an area*: A program may not be uniform in content throughout the area in which it is applied. The study of the effects of televised health messages on children's behaviors is a good example. The content and sophistication of a television

message will vary in differing areas of the country, depending on what the producers perceive to be the most effective appeals to regional audiences. Comparisons across areas, therefore, have to take content differences into account in making inferences, or the inferences will be biased.

Any evaluation in which data are collected is subject to some forms of bias. While it is impossible to control all sources of bias, it is important to minimize each major source in a particular evaluation. From experience, you must take steps to select an instrument and method of data collection that minimize the likely biases. Other issues in selecting methods and instruments are discussed next.

CRITERIA FOR SELECTING A DATA COLLECTION METHOD

Each instrument is based on a particular method for collecting data, e.g., interviewing, self-recording, observing, or taking data from medical records. How do you select an instrument and, by inference, a method for data collection? Your primary concern is to select an instrument and method that have high reliability and validity for the groups, situations, and purposes of your study. Instruments without validity and reliability can produce nonfindings or even negative findings that are not warranted. There are, however, other issues in selecting a method.

Cox and Snell (1979) have identified four criteria or issues in the selection of variables and measures for a particular study: the nature and purpose of the study, sequential modifiability of the design, economy, and comparisons with other studies. Feinstein (1977) has noted a further consideration in the selection of measures: hardness of data. Webb et al. (1966) have identified three other considerations: dross rate, access to descriptive cues, and ability to replicate. These issues are relevant to the selection of variables and measures in evaluative studies.

Nature and Purpose of the Study

A method for data collection must be selected that most clearly meets the nature and purposes of a study, within resource constraints. An evaluative study can be conducted for a variety of purposes. For a smoking-cessation program (a service production system like that depicted earlier in figure 6.4), you might conduct an evaluation to assess the output (stopped smoking or not), the acceptance of the output by the environment (social support for continued nonsmoking), the availability of resources in the environment (number of smokers willing to pay for a smoking-cessation program), the quality of the resources, the appropriateness of the structure (is the program well designed), whether the processes are occurring as planned (is the program being conducted according to the design), or whether the processes are related to outputs (are people who attend more sessions more likely to quit). Each of these topics can be the focus for an evaluation in a particular program. The type of question posed by the evaluation should determine the method of data collection. This criterion for method selection is similar to our strong emphasis on the role of a model in conducting an evaluation, but here we focus on one specific aspect of the evaluation.

Sequential Modifiability of the Design

An important aspect of instrument and method selection is whether a preliminary study can be performed to select and develop measures. As noted earlier, a variety of instruments might be used for any particular variable. If you have the time and resources to conduct a preliminary study, you can make multiple measures of the same variable in your study. Some thought must go into developing criteria for the selection of the appropriate measures, e.g., greater reliability, or higher correlations with other variables of interest. If you cannot make a preliminary study, you must pay greater attention to selecting the instrument and method without the benefit of pretesting. The two primary issues are validity and reliability of the instrument and method for the population you are studying.

Economy

Economy of measurement has several characteristics:

Dollar cost

Time spent by the evaluation staff

Time spent by respondents

Ease of setting up instruments

Difficulty of getting individuals to participate

Loss of accuracy due to increased workload

Availability and quality of official statistics

You can imagine an instrument that measures exactly what you want. All instruments cost money, however, and some may be too costly. (Think of sending observers to record clients' behaviors all day, every day.) Some approaches may not be feasible. (Think of supplying a personal computer to everyone in a health education program.) Some approaches may produce other problems. (Think of how hostile clients can get if they have to complete an hour of paperwork every day for a month.) The key to selecting good measures is to choose a set that is sufficiently valid and reliable for your study's purposes yet is developed at minimal cost to the project and the respondents.

An important aspect of economy is collecting no more data than are necessary to achieve the purposes of the particular study. Many investigators collect data on every conceivable variable. For example, one investigator developed a 124-page questionnaire requiring three hours to complete. This strategy creates many problems. The program must bear tremendous costs in time, printing, collating, key-punching, and data processing. Respondents must bear considerable costs in completing the questionnaire. They may become hostile to such a questionnaire and refuse to participate at all, select only questions of personal interest to answer, or actively subvert the data collected. It is a common finding that investigators collect more data than they can reasonably analyze; that is, the parties incur the costs of collection, but nothing is ever done with the data. All these reasons argue for the greatest economy in selecting measures.

Comparisons with Other Studies

In some cases, program personnel may want to compare the results they obtain with evaluations done elsewhere or at another time. If so, they must assess the same variables with the same instruments; otherwise comparisons cannot be made. If a particular measure has a major flaw, the evaluator should include both the original measure (so comparisons can be made), and an alternative measure, to see if a different pattern is obtained with the new measure.

Hardness of Data

Another criterion in selecting measures is often discussed: the hardness of data. There is a feeling among investigators that certain kinds of data are "harder" than others (which are called "soft"), and therefore more important to collect. According to Feinstein (1977), the following characteristics are typically associated with data hardness: (1) the data are obtained objectively (e.g., physiological measures) rather than subjectively (e.g., self-reports); (2) the primary data can be preserved for repeated analyses (e.g., a videotape of an encounter, which can be reobserved and checked); and (3) the measurement is on a dimensional scale (i.e., a ratio or interval scale).

Feinstein has debunked many of these ideas, however. For example, physiological measures often considered hard data can be highly unreliable. There may be rapid changes in the values of the physiological measure; the variable may not be clearly and precisely related to the phenomenon of concern; or there may be problems of mechanical determination of the physiological values by the laboratory. Certain variables, e.g., eye contacts, may be very difficult to quantify from a videotape because they are not precisely specified or because they require too much judgment and interpretation on the part of the observer. Having a ratio or an interval scale does not ensure reliability. Feinstein has argued that the criterion of primary concern in hardness is reliability; he has also shown how a wide variety of ostensibly soft measures can provide useful and reliable data in clinical trials. His admonition is to collect all variables that are directly relevant to the concerns of a project, regardless of hardness, while paying particular attention to the reliability of data collection.

Dross Rate

The dross rate is the ratio of useless to useful information obtained by a particular method for a unit of time. Methods with a high dross rate are obviously inefficient approaches to collecting data. If a program is interested in behavior that does not occur frequently or with some regularity, the amount of useful data obtained per unit of data collection time can vary widely. For example, an observational study of total eating behavior is inefficient to perform, because subjects may snack at many times during the day. Some may have small meals and eat candy bars or potato chips at work or at school. Thus, observers would have to follow subjects for a whole day to be there when eating occurred, but only a small percentage of the full day would be spent in observing eating behavior. A questionnaire is a more efficient approach. In 15 to 20 minutes of directed questioning, an entire day's eating behavior can be assessed. But can subjects accurately remember everything they ate that day or the previous day? The observational approach obtains more dross per unit of data collection time than does the questionnaire or interview, but it may be a more valid instrument, depending on the issue of concern.

Access to Descriptive Cues

The extent to which a method is used to check on which population has been included in a study is considered access to descriptive cues. Questionnaires and interviews can ask specific questions to achieve this access; observational methods are limited to characteristics easily observed, which may be misleading.

Ability to Replicate

An investigator is able to replicate a study more easily using certain methods than others. For example, a questionnaire can be used and reused at multiple points in time with differing groups. A review of medical records before and after a particular event (e.g., a continuing education course) may not be replicable at a later time period, because the medical records will differ due to historical factors.

SUMMARY

Health program evaluators should have a conceptual model underlying the evaluative study they are planning. Instruments should be selected to measure the variables in the model. The instruments selected need to be valid and reliable measures of the variables of concern; be as inexpensive as possible; permit comparisons with important related evaluations; have as small a dross rate as possible; permit the collection of descriptive data; and be replicable. The various threats to the validity of a particular instrument should be anticipated and steps taken to counter the threats that are preventable. This is a tall order and requires much effort, but it is not an insurmountable job.

The instruments for measuring the desired variables use many kinds of methods. A broad spectrum of the more commonly used methods are discussed in the next chapter, in light of the considerations presented here for instrument selection.

7

Methods of Data Collection

"Physiological measures are always more accurate than that social and behavioral stuff."

"If I could only get access to that doctor's records, think of all the evaluation I could do!"

"Let's just jot down some questions, and send them around for people to answer."

"It won't take much time!"

Professional Competencies Emphasized in This Chapter:

• ability to provide mechanisms to assess selected educational methods

• ability to assist in specifying indicators of program success

• ability to help develop methods for evaluating programs

• ability to participate in the specification of instruments for data collection

• ability to train personnel for evaluation as needed

• ability to collect data through appropriate techniques

• ability to use survey techniques to acquire data

• ability to evaluate results of the skill development process

Should the health education program evaluator use self-reported statements of numbers of cigarettes smoked, observations of actual smoking behavior in certain settings, or physiological indicators of recent smoking behavior, to assess whether a smoking-cessation program worked? Which would be best for a smoking-prevention program in a junior high school? Should an evaluator use self-reported frequencies of high-salt food consumption, a 24-hour dietary history obtained by interview, observations of consumption of all foods, or overnight urine sodium tests, to determine dietary sodium restriction among hypertensives?

These are the kinds of decisions with which evaluators of health education programs constantly struggle. Since rights and wrongs are rarely clear-cut, evaluators must become familiar with a broad variety of methods and select the best of good methods or the least bad of unpalatable approaches. In becoming familiar with the strengths and weaknesses of many methods, the evaluator should develop skills identified by the Initial Role Delineation Project (U.S. DHHS, Public Health Service, 1980a) in four areas: (1) assessment and selection of methods:

> *III. C. 4.* *The health educator must be able to provide mechanisms to assess selected educational methods.*
> *V. A. 1.* *The health educator must be able to assist in specifying indicators of program success.*

(2) development of methods for a specific evaluation:

> *V. A. 3. The health educator must be able to help develop methods for evaluating programs.*
>
> *V. A. 4. The health educator must be able to participate in the specification of instruments for data collection.*

(3) training of those employing the instruments:

> *V. B. 2. The health educator must be able to train personnel for evaluation as needed.*

and (4) use of a variety of methods:

> *V. C. 1. The entry-level health educator must be able to collect data through appropriate techniques.*
>
> *VII. A. 3. The health educator must be able to use survey techniques to acquire data.*
>
> *VII. F. 5. The health educator must be able to evaluate results of the skill development process.*

This chapter promotes the above skills by taking each method of data collection, identifying its strengths and weaknesses (biases), considering the other issues in method selection, and outlining straightforward steps for developing an instrument and implementing the method. The various methods are considered within two categories: obtrusive and unobtrusive methods.

OBTRUSIVE MEASURES

The term *obtrusive* implies that the person being studied is aware of being measured, assessed, or tested. The term *unobtrusive* implies that an individual is not aware of being studied. Methods usually included in the obtrusive category are self-report questionnaires, interviews, and direct observations of behavior. The methods usually included in the unobtrusive category are record abstractions, physiological measures, and behavior trace methods. Behavior trace methods include such things as measuring the thickness of a shoe sole to assess how much walking a person has done. Since many of the behavior trace methods require much greater development and validation, they are not further considered in this chapter.

Obtrusive measures raise validity and reliability questions, because becoming aware of being studied affects a person's behavior and thought processes. Unobtrusive measures are valued because they are supposed to produce less random error and bias, since subjects are not aware of being measured. The differences between obtrusive and unobtrusive methods, however, are not always so clear-cut. For example, a skillfully designed questionnaire may ask validly tangential questions that do not tip off program participants about which aspect of their behavior is of concern. Alternatively, if workers in an agency learn that they are continually being evaluated using the forms they complete daily, their form completion behavior may drastically change to protect themselves. Obtrusive and unobtrusive are, therefore, general categories of methods. Evaluators must be constantly concerned about the obtrusiveness of all measures and what effect that may have on the results.

Self-Completion Questionnaires

A self-completion (or self-report) questionnaire is an instrument that the respondent can complete by reading the questions and providing answers, without an interviewer or other person taking part. Such a questionnaire can be used with a single individual or with groups at a time.

Strengths. The self-completion questionnaire is the most convenient and frequently used method of data collection for program evaluation. It allows data to be collected from many people in a very short period of time; almost all types of measures can be assessed by questionnaire; the costs are minimal (interviewers are not needed, printing costs are low); and all people are exposed to the same instrument. Good references on self-completion questionnaires include Berdie and Anderson (1974), Bradburn and Sudman (1979), and Barker and Blankenship (1975).

Since no interviewer is involved in asking the questions, a well-designed questionnaire can control for interviewer effects, i.e., differences in responses because of differences in the way in which interviewers asked the question. Moreover, the proportion of unusable data in a self-report questionnaire is quite low. In contrast, an interviewer may have to listen to irrelevant comments, and an observer may waste time on unproductive observations. In a questionnaire, all the questions are directed at the phenomenon of concern. Similarly, the replicability of a questionnaire is quite high. The same questionnaire can be used in multiple studies.

The questionnaire is particularly useful when the phenomenon being studied is amenable to self-observation and well-defined, data about it can be elicited in simple straightforward questions, and respondents can read and write.

Phenomenon Amenable to Self-Observation. For some phenomena, e.g., attitudes, values, and beliefs, self-report may be the only method of data collection. For others, e.g., cognitive processing of information, self-report may be appropriate but not exclusive. And for some, e.g., skill at performing particular tasks, self-report instruments are suspect. When the phenomenon of concern is amenable to self-reflection and self-report, a self-completion questionnaire can be a very useful instrument.

Phenomenon Well-Defined. When the phenomenon of concern has been studied extensively and much is known about it, a self-report questionnaire can be used. For example, there are extensive data on the many facets of smoking, so an interviewer may not be needed to probe and interrogate subjects to elicit the possible responses. The response possibilities are known from other research, and the purpose of the questionnaire is to document which is most appropriate for this particular respondent.

Some phenomena are poorly defined, e.g., the reasons why healthy people do not engage in aerobic activity or the factors promoting and inhibiting breast-feeding. Much of the basic research has not been done about these subjects, so the possible responses are not clearly outlined. Data collection about them would benefit from the active questioning of a trained interviewer to identify and document the response possibilities.

Simple, Straightforward Questions. The longer and more complex a question, or the more subtle the distinctions a question requires, the more likely it is that a respondent will misinterpret it or have difficulty understanding and answering it. An interviewer may be necessary to explain a long, complex, or subtle question or ask further questions to be sure the respondent understood it. A self-report questionnaire assumes that the respondent is motivated to read the questions completely, whereas an interviewer can encourage a respondent to attend to longer questions. Self-report questionnaires, therefore, are most valid and reliable with short, simple, and straightforward questions.

Cognitive Ability of Respondents. Although it may seem obvious, it is worth noting that self-report questionnaires assume that respondents can read and write. By inference, a self-report questionnaire is inappropriate for the blind, the retarded, nonreaders, and people not familiar with the language. To ensure the greatest applicability, a questionnaire is often developed to be readable at a fifth or sixth grade reading level.

Weaknesses. The self-completion questionnaire is susceptible to several biases. Respondents can easily fall into role selection when answering questionnaires, since no one is present to observe their role taking, clarify it, and challenge it. The phenomenon of response sets was originally identified using self-completion questionnaires. Other problems are: (1) the questionnaire itself may promote change, (2) changes may occur in the respondents' understanding of the questionnaire; or (3) limits may exist on the phenomena to which a questionnaire can be applied.

Although a questionnaire theoretically controls for interviewer effects, the person who distributes the questionnaire often answers questions about it and may give subtle or overt cues to how it should be answered. Another disadvantage is that, although a variety of validating questions can be asked, a questionnaire is limited in the use of descriptive cues. For example, a dietary interviewer may use portion size pictures to obtain data on a respondent's quantity of consumption. It would be very costly to build portion size pictures into every question of a dietary self-completion questionnaire.

Steps in Questionnaire Development. A questionnaire obtains information from a respondent through self-reported answers to a series of questions, usually using paper and pencil, although computers can be used to do this as well. Good references on questionnaire development include Berdie and Anderson (1974), Bradburn and Sudman (1979), Schuman and Presser (1977), Kalton et al. (1978), Barker and Blankenship (1975), and Noelle-Neumann (1970). Four general areas in questionnaire development are discussed next: instrument selection, questionnaire development, field testing, and quality control.

Instrument Selection. You do not need to reinvent the wheel. When an instrument has already been shown to be valid and reliable, and it directly measures the variables of interest to you, it makes sense to use that instrument. Many investigators have developed and applied a broad variety of instruments for a broad variety of purposes. Using already developed instruments is valuable for several reasons. First, you can capitalize on the thoughts of other investigators in the design of an instrument. Other investigators often have spent time reviewing the literature and considering various alternatives for developing an instrument. Using a developed instrument will therefore save you this time. Second, other investigators may have spent time assessing and refining the instrument to maximize its validity and reliability. For example, some investigators go through several generations of a questionnaire to increase its reliability. Using their instrument will, therefore, ensure some level of reliability and validity of measurement in your evaluation. Third, using an existing instrument enables you to make comparisons across studies. In most cases the need for, or effectiveness of, a program is assessed in comparison to other areas, populations, or programs. Assuming similar populations, using measures developed for another study will allow you to make comparisons between evaluations that might not otherwise be possible.

Using already developed measures has been encouraged in theoretical as well as applied research. To facilitate this use, several authors have compiled compendia of measures used in a variety of areas: health behaviors (Reeder et al., 1976), family (Strauss and Brown, 1978), attitudes (Shaw and Wright, 1967; Robinson and Shaver, 1973; Bonjean et al., 1967), and psychodiagnostic testing (Buros, 1972). The Center for Disease Control has published seven volumes that document instruments in seven areas of health and behavior research, which should be extremely useful for health promotion program evaluation. (Contact the Center for Health Promotion and Education.)

Developed instruments should not, however, be used blindly. In a recent study on the effect of a family intervention to promote behaviors that reduce cardiovascular risk, a knowledge test was used that had been developed for another study. This test had been developed in a population of primarily white, middle-class adults, and item-to-total correlations had been used to assess its internal consistency. The knowledge test was then applied to a population of primarily lower-class, black and Mexican-American adults and children in a different area of the country. Furthermore, the knowledge test dealt with several risk factors not of concern in the second study, and the intervention in the second study did not attempt to cover the knowledge domain as comprehensively as the knowledge test did. The results in the second study showed statistically significant, but educationally insignificant, differences between experimental and control adults, and no significant differences between children. Selecting that knowledge test was an exercise in poor judgment, because of the many differences in purposes between the study for which the instrument had been developed and the second study in which it was used. At the least, the evaluators in the second study should have intensively reviewed the content for face validity and field tested the instrument with the local population, before using it in their program evaluation.

Instrument Development and Field Testing. In some cases, instruments have not been developed for a particular topic, or existing instruments are not appropriate. Even when instruments are available, you usually have to develop some questions specific to your study. You should refer to one or more texts (Berdie and Anderson, 1974; Bradburn and Sudman, 1979) and articles (e.g., Barker and Blankenship, 1975) on questionnaire development, to consider and address the essential development issues.

Windsor, Roseman, et al. (1981) have proposed the following ten steps in instrument questionnaire development:

1. *Formulate objectives*: The first consideration in generating a questionnaire is to ensure that it measures what it was intended to measure. If you have consensually agreed on a model of the structures and processes underlying your service, this often facilitates developing a questionnaire. With the model in hand, you can clearly state specific objectives for the questionnaire.

2. *State objectives in behavioral terms*: The objectives of your evaluation should be stated in behavioral terms, that is, in terms of what the program participant should be expected to do. Behavioral objectives enhance the likelihood that people will agree on what the objectives are and that appropriate measures can be created.

3. *Review instruments*: If an instrument measuring the phenomenon of concern exists, seriously consider using it. At a minimum, you should review existing instruments for ideas to be included in a new instrument.

4. *Review necessary skills*: To achieve the desired outcome behaviors, a person must have certain prerequisite knowledge and skills (Parcel and Baranowski, 1981). You must make a complete list of these knowledge and skill items in order to create the questionnaire.

5. *Construct a preliminary version*: Prepare a questionnaire that covers each knowledge, skill, and behavior outcome you wish to measure. Write items so that they can be clearly understood. Clarity is often achieved by basing a questionnaire on a fifth grade reading level. This means use of simple sentences (single subjects, verbs, and objects) and the simplest possible words. Although clear time limits for questionnaire completion have not been established, the longer the questionnaire (beyond four pages or so), the more likely it is that a person will refuse to enter the study, provide quick but erroneous answers, or not complete the questionnaire. Careful attention must be paid to question wording and question sequencing (Kalton et al., 1978; Schuman and Presser, 1977; Noelle-Neumann, 1970). Distributing early drafts of a questionnaire to colleagues for review and comment will often identify obvious problems. The coordination

committee for the evaluation (see chapter 2) may also be of value in reviewing early drafts.

In general, use closed-ended as opposed to open-ended questions. A program participant may not accurately understand an open-ended question; may not want to provide a full answer, because it will take too much time; or may give a full and complete answer in the respondent's view but one that the program staff finds misleading or uninterpretable. For example, if you are interested in specific foods a person has eaten, an open-ended question might read: "What did you eat yesterday?" or "Please list below all the foods you ate yesterday." For some respondents the answer may take a full page and may not cover all the foods of interest to you. If you are interested in a limited number of foods (e.g., foods high in sodium), a reasonable closed-ended alternative would be to list all these foods and ask whether the respondent had eaten any of the foods on that list. This approach is less likely to miss foods of concern, because the foods are listed and the list acts as a memory prompt for the program participant. Developing closed-ended questions, however, requires more time and attention to detail than open-ended questions. You must review the literature to make sure that the response categories are mutually exclusive and exhaustive, i.e., that they include all the logically or frequently identified alternatives. You must also test the questionnaire to ensure that the alternatives are understandable to the intended program participants.

There is one occasion when open-ended questions are useful in a questionnaire: when you want to learn about the motivations of respondents. In this case, a closed-ended question is posed (usually in a yes–no format), followed by an open-ended question asking for an explanation. For example, the following question provided fascinating results: "Have you decided to breast-feed your baby?   ☐ Yes ☐ No   Why? _____ ." It elicited a broad variety of reasons that maintained a high level of internal consistency (Baranowski et al., 1982).

The questionnaire should be appealing to the respondents. Berdie and Anderson (1974) have identified many facets of an appealing questionnaire. Keeping the pages free of clutter and using a lot of empty space make the form visually appealing. Asking several questions that are stimulating or pleasing early in the questionnaire increases the likelihood that respondents will maintain the motivation and attention to complete the instrument. Developing and using clear and simple instructions increase the accuracy of responses to the questionnaire.

Multi-item instruments should be constructed to avoid response sets that can bias the results. This problem can be overcome by keeping the number of questions in which yes is the appropriate response equal to those in which no is appropriate and including equal numbers of positively and negatively worded items. The response biases may then be detected and corrected.

Finally, you should develop the questionnaire with the method of data processing in mind. Since computers are most frequently used to process data, the following guidelines are often helpful: Questions that employ a similar response format (e.g., yes–no versus a five-point scale versus an open-ended response) should be grouped together so that the keypuncher can enter the data right from the form; or the form should have a column on the right side of the page in which responses from the main body of the questionnaire are coded for keypunching. Answer spaces should be kept to the right-hand side of the page for easy coding or keypunching. The questionnaire should be precoded for keypunching, i.e., each response alternative should be assigned a response value, and each question should have an identified and numbered set of columns for coding or keypunching. Figure 7.1 illustrates a questionnaire with these characteristics.

6. *Develop data collection training protocols*: Once the instrument has been developed, protocols for collecting and coding the data must be written. Writing them at this time will help the staff answer many questions that will arise. These protocols in turn provide materials for training the people who will collect the data. Protocols are often revised during and soon after training.

7. *Pilot testing the questionnaire*: Whether the questionnaire is an existing instrument or was developed for this particular evaluation, it should be field-tested. At a minimum, the purpose of the field test is to see whether the intended respondents can complete the set of questions under the specified circumstances.

In the most basic field test, a draft of the questionnaire is given to a sample of people (maybe 10 to 15) who are representative of the target group of the larger evaluation, under the same circumstances. After these people have completed the questionnaire, the person distributing the questionnaire intensively interviews the respondents to find out whether any questions were unclear, produced anger or anxiety (e.g., used terms considered racist or sexist), or were too complex. The interviewer also asks detailed questions about the most important aspects of

HEALTH QUESTIONNAIRE	For Computer Use Only

HEALTH QUESTIONNAIRE
ID #

For Computer Use Only

Are you married? (check only one) Yes ☐ 1

No ☐ 2   (1,06) V2

Do you have any children? (check only one) Yes ☐ 1

No ☐ 2   (1,07) V3

About how often do you go to a fast food restaurant? (check only one)

Never ☐ 1

Rarely ☐ 2

About once a week ☐ 3

Several times a week ☐ 4   (1,08) V4

About once a day ☐ 5

Several times a day ☐ 6

Do you like to go to fast food restaurants? (check only one) Yes ☐ 1

No ☐ 2   (1,09) V5

Why? (please explain) _____

_____

_____

SKIP
(1,10-1,79)
Card 1

(1,80)

Figure 7.1 Example of a Precoded Questionnaire

the questionnaire to be sure that the respondents understood what the program staff intended. A more complex field test might include several wordings of the same items at different points in the same questionnaire and might compare responses of separate groups of respondents or compare questionnaires completed under various circumstances. In such field-testing, the program staff might look at differences both in responses to the same questions (reliability) and in relationships between questions (validity).

Although it is often valuable to test a questionnaire early in its development with friends and colleagues, the actual field test should be done with respondents representative of the population to be included in the major evaluation.

8. *Redesign the questionnaire and protocol*: As a result of the pilot test, the questionnaire and protocol are redesigned and rewritten to capitalize on what was learned.

9. *Retesting the questionnaire*: The program staff repeats step 7 with the revised instrument.

10. *Make a final redesign*: The staff repeats step 8.

Although a lot of work has been done, the questionnaire is not yet ready for use in the program evaluation.

Quality Control. Selecting, developing, and field-testing a questionnaire are necessary but not sufficient to collect valid and reliable data. Error can creep into data collected by a questionnaire in many ways. The health promotion program staff should assume that Murphy's law is the law of the land. Therefore, a questionnaire quality control check should be made.

Estimates of reliability should be obtained for the most important items or instruments. They can be made in several ways—test–retest, internal consistency, or multiple-form reliability (see chapter 6). At a minimum, an investigator should calculate Cronbach's alpha (or the KR–20, as appropriate) on all multi-item instruments, to obtain an estimate of internal consistency.

Questionnaires are often returned incomplete (e.g., a person turned two pages, instead of one, and missed a whole page of questions) or with obvious inconsistencies (e.g., a person answered a set of questions when an earlier response indicated that this person should not have completed those questions). To control for these sources of error, a staff person should be available at the return of a questionnaire to review it for completeness and obvious inconsistencies. This staff person can approach the respondent immediately (while the information is still fresh in memory) for item completion or clarification.

A more intensive review of responses must be conducted fairly soon to recheck incomplete responses, to detect illegal codes to a question, and to detect more detailed inconsistencies. This review is important so that respondents can be contacted while answers are still relatively fresh in their memory.

Other data editing and cleaning procedures can be conducted after the data have been entered into the computer. This set of checks also detects keypunching errors.

Although this appears to be a lot of work, following these steps will avoid a lot of problems in making inferences from questionnaire data.

Agency or Organizational Forms

In many agencies, the best approach to evaluating a particular service is to collect data every time a unit of service is provided. The instrument for collecting such data is most often a *form*. Two articles have discussed the specifics of form creation: Carey (1972) and Staggs (1972).

Carey's comments on the value of a form in business also apply to the health agency setting:

> The form, or document, or report is a management instrument that ties the several parts of the business system, or sub-system, together. It is the cement or adhesive, of any business. A well designed form confirms, instructs, directs and informs. A quality form insures that business policies, regulations and directives are accommodated. Just as it is axiomatic that a home run has no value unless the hitter touches all bases, so it is with a form. Its utility is in direct relationship to the effort made to ensure it will be used effectively. Checks and balances, standards and measures all contribute to quality and to effective use.

This is a tall order for any form to fill, but forms can be useful in evaluating an agency's services. The strengths and weaknesses discussed under the section on self-completed questionnaires apply to forms and need not be repeated here (see pp. 99–111).

Steps in Form Development. All the guidelines for creating a questionnaire apply to creating a form, and there are additional considerations in designing an evaluation form. The primary restriction on a form in comparison to a questionnaire is brevity. While a questionnaire should be kept brief (four to ten pages), a form should rarely be more than a single page. This is often a challenge for the form developer. The single page must include the instructions as well as the questions; questions must therefore be self-evident, keeping instructions to the absolute minimum.

To be accepted by the program staff members who will be filling it out, the form should pose few barriers or hurdles to completion. Besides being simple and uncluttered, it should request information in the manner that is easiest for the staff to complete. The easiest manner is often the sequence in which the information is obtained by the staff person from the task being recorded. If a form follows a client through a health program with multiple staff members completing parts of the form, it is important to keep the information provided by one staff member together on a portion of the form, perhaps separated from other portions by boxes or lines. The sequence of the boxes or lined sections should reflect the sequence in which they are completed in the service delivery process.

Developing incentives for the staff to complete the form is also important. Sometimes it is valuable to use or modify existing forms to collect the desired evaluative information. In this way, you capitalize on whatever incentives exist for completion of the existing form and avoid the natural resistance to newly developed forms. At times each person in a form completion chain wants a copy of the form completed to that point. A form can be created using NCR paper (the paper that reproduces impressions on lower sheets without the use of carbon paper) and appropriately pyramided—that is, each person in the chain can detach a color-coded copy from the form as it goes from staff member to staff member, with each successive copy showing and collecting additional information. Showing the staff members that the data are used, and how, creates an important incentive. Form data should be reviewed on a frequent periodic basis (every day is best) by a clerk, who can call the form completer to clarify any incomplete, confusing, or otherwise unclear information. Providing periodic reports that summarize these form completion behaviors will promote quality form completion and may even be useful in improving or maintaining a high quality of service (Andrasik and McNamara, 1977; Andrasik et al., 1978).

To be most useful, a form should be reviewed in several drafts by the people who will complete it and the people who will use the collected information. In one case, evaluators of an emergency medical services system (Bernstine and Baranowski, 1976) had to develop a single-sheet form to serve many purposes: (1) recording clinical information for the use and legal protection of the emergency medical technicians (EMTs) and paramedics providing emergency care, (2) transmitting clinical information for use at the next stage in the patient care delivery process, e.g., the hospital emergency room, (3) tracking (for the state) the flow of emergency patients' care from preambulance to ambulance care to life support care at a local emergency room to sophisticated regional emergency care, and (4) evaluating the quality of medical care at each stage in delivery. The form had to be flexible enough to record the many types of emergency problems

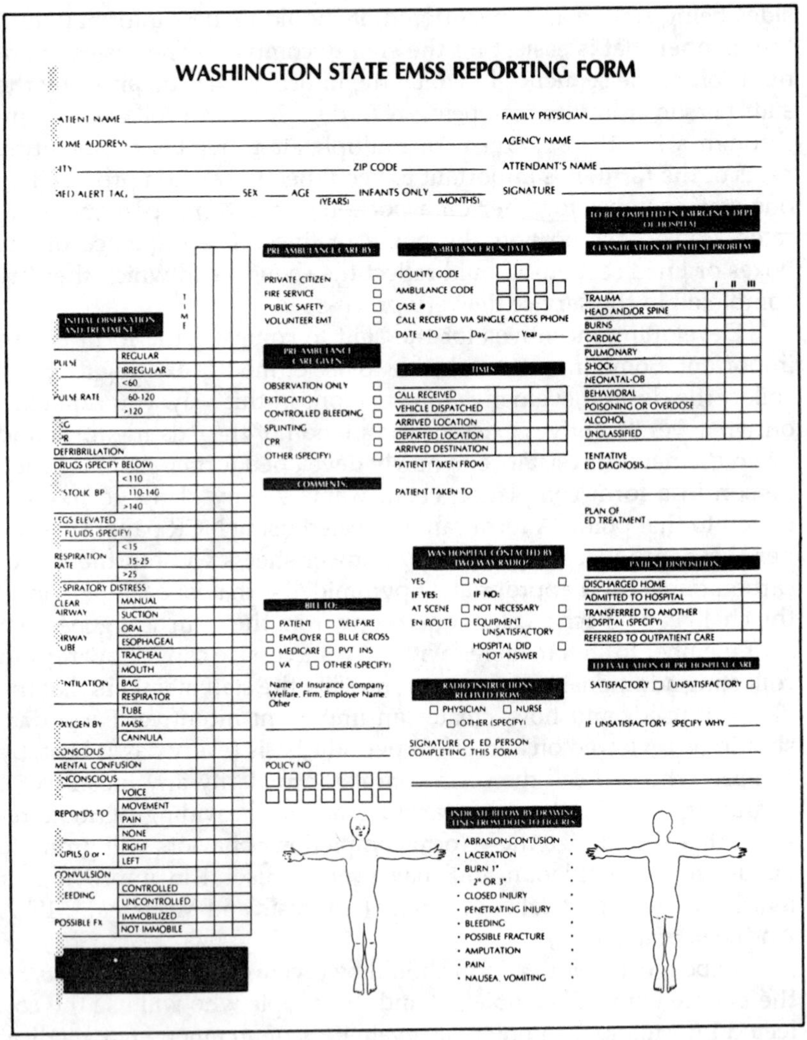

WASHINGTON STATE EMSS REPORTING FORM

PATIENT NAME _____ FAMILY PHYSICIAN _____

HOME ADDRESS _____ AGENCY NAME _____

CITY _____ ZIP CODE _____ ATTENDANT'S NAME _____

MED ALERT TAG _____ SEX ___ AGE ___ (YEARS) INFANTS ONLY ___ (MONTHS) SIGNATURE _____

Figure 7.2 Example of Agency Reporting Form

from snakebites in remote rural areas to automobile accidents to cardiovascular or cerebrovascular accidents.

A draft of this form is found in figure 7.2. It has many of the desirable characteristics discussed. The clinical data are prominent and grouped on the left and bottom of the form. The data on tracking of care appear in the order in which they occur. It is brief and well defined, with all data appearing on a single page. Each section is clearly introduced by a blocked title. The form was developed and refined over a number of meetings with EMTs, various hospital staffs, and state health department employees. At each stage the various groups demanded data in a different format. The state required data in a form that was thorough yet easily computerized, because the state had to process hundreds of thousands of these forms each year. This most often meant closed-ended responses to a series of strategic questions. The EMTs and paramedics demanded that major portions of the form be blank lines to record text about the patient. They wanted this open-ended format because they did not want to hunt through checklists on a form to define the patient's status, and they believed they could easily, quickly, and accurately interpret clinical notes. The hospital staff members wanted nothing to do with the form, because they put no confidence in the procedures, tentative diagnoses, or care provided by EMTs and paramedics (despite their extensive training) and because they did not want the care they themselves provided to be evaluated by the state.

This form was extensively modified in response to the comments of each faction and field-tested in one area of the state. The effort was ultimately a failure because of the conflicts among the various factions using the form. The conflict over open-ended versus closed-ended data was most serious, but the reluctance to be evaluated by the state was a strong undercurrent. This example demonstrates the complexities of form development and the political nature of data collected on forms.

Self-Completion Mail Surveys

When resources are scarce, and the target population for the evaluation is dispersed across a broad geographical area, a mail survey is an attractive method for collecting data. The mail survey uses a self-completion questionnaire with the postal system as the vehicle for delivering and retrieving the instrument. A valuable reference on mail survey research techniques is Dillman (1978).

Strengths and Weaknesses. Comments about the strengths and weaknesses of the self-completion questionnaire also apply to the mail survey. Given the relatively low cost of mail service, these surveys offer an inexpensive method of obtaining data from areas as large as a city, a state, or even a nation.

The strengths of the method under some circumstances can be its weaknesses under others. A mail survey assumes that some sampling frame has a particular respondent's accurate address and that mail can be delivered to that address. Problems may exist with both these assumptions. For example, a mail survey of students in a school district revealed that 30 percent of the addresses were in error. Some were simply out of date; others were nonexistent locations. The latter were probably given by people who wanted their children to attend a preferred school without living in that school district (Nader et al., 1980).

In another study, a mail survey was conducted of all hypertensive patients attending a particular clinic. Roughly 15 percent of the addresses that were obtained from the patients' medical records were in error. The clinic's financial records, kept separately, had more up-to-date information (Baranowski et al., 1982).

Some people want to maintain anonymity and not have mail deliverable to them. Such people may be illegal aliens, people sought by bill collectors, or people afraid of being sought by criminal elements, publicity seekers, or other undesired contacts. Not being able to deliver mail to such people may bias a mail survey in a particular study. People who move frequently (often those wishing to maintain their anonymity or those in constant search of work) have difficulty receiving mail. Although reachable at one point in time, they may be unreachable at others (population stability over time). This mobility of the target population may vary by geographical area (population stability over areas).

The greatest recommendation for the mail survey is its low cost as a method for obtaining data from a large geographical area. The dross rate for unreturned or incomplete questionnaires can be high, depending on the nature of the sampling frame. The dross rate on information on the questionnaire is quite low, however.

Steps in Conducting a Mail Survey. If you are contemplating a mail survey, you need to find a sampling frame that contains names, addresses, and, if possible, phone numbers. You must be concerned about the probable accuracy of that information and whether some people who are of interest to the study may not be included or not accurately represented in the sampling frame.

The following steps should be employed in implementing a mail survey:

1. *Develop a questionnaire*: The ten steps outlined earlier for developing a questionnaire should be followed. In addition the questionnaire should be printed on colorful paper so that respondents can find it later when looking for it in a pile of mail or other papers. The cover letter should be an original typed letter, personally addressed to each respondent, with the message indicating the personal responsibility of the reader to respond immediately. A system should be worked out listing the name, address, and telephone number of each respondent in alphabeti-

cal order, or numerically by identification number, for recording returned questionnaires, updating addresses and phone numbers as new information is obtained, and providing a central data file for conducting follow-ups.

2. *Send a warning postcard*: Investigators have shown that higher initial response rates are achieved if a postcard is sent about a week before the initial mailing of the questionnaire. This postcard informs the respondent of the pending arrival of the questionnaire. It keeps some respondents from initially discarding the questionnaire and entices others to learn more about the questionnaire. With interest piqued, they may look forward to its arrival.

3. *Send out the initial questionnaire*: The questionnaire is initially sent to all potential respondents about a week after the postcard. Including 25 cents in the upper right-hand corner of the cover letter has been shown to increase the response rate significantly over providing no financial reward and as much as providing a $10 reward (Dillman, 1978).

4. *Send a reminder postcard*: Within a couple of days after the initial mailing, there is a high volume of return of questionnaires. After three to five days, the rate of return tapers off. Within two weeks, 95 percent or more of the questionnaires that will be returned from the first mailing alone will have come in. A reminder postcard should be sent at this two-week point.

5. *Send out a second questionnaire*: The pattern of return from the postcard will follow that of the mailing of the first questionnaire, but the rates will not be as high. Within two weeks, 95 percent or more of the questionnaires responding to the postcard reminder will have been returned. Some people will have discarded or otherwise lost the initial questionnaire, however. A second questionnaire should be sent to nonrespondents two weeks after the postcard.

6. *Call nonrespondents by phone*: Reasons for nonresponse to a second questionnaire may be: the questionnaires never got through to the respondent, the respondent refuses to answer, or the respondent wants more personal contact and assurance. A telephone caller can obtain the accurate address of a nonrespondent (to whom a new questionnaire must be sent) and may be able to persuade the respondent of the value of participating in the survey, or can ask the questions immediately over the phone. Phoning, which is an expensive approach to data collection relative to the mail survey, is thus used only as the last resort with the fewest number of potential participants.

Program staff members should expect some percentage of questionnaires to be returned marked "undeliverable." Phone contact should be attempted with these persons immediately to obtain new addresses for a mailing. On the master list of names, addresses, and telephone numbers, the returned questionnaires are monitored, revised addresses and telephone numbers are entered, and attempts to reach the respondents are recorded. Any reasonably organized person can manage the mail and return aspects of a mail survey.

Following this set of procedures, and diligently following up on nonrespondents, has been shown to produce response rates of 70 percent to 95 percent, with a broad variety of respondents (Dillman, 1978). An 80 percent response rate is often considered adequate. Analyses should be conducted with data from the sampling frame (e.g., sex, ethnicity, geographical location), to determine differences between respondents and nonrespondents. Differences may bias interpretation of the results of the survey, and any obtained therefore need to be noted.

Self-Completion Diaries and Logs

Investigators have been concerned about two problems in usual methods of obtaining self-report measures: telescoping and memory loss. *Telescoping* means that respondents tend to remember certain events as having occurred more recently than they actually did. *Memory loss* refers to failure to remember the occurrence of a variety of events. Studying the dietary behaviors of children provides an interesting example. Most dietary assessment methods require intensive recall for the past 24-hour period or for as long as two weeks. Children, however, demonstrate several limitations in reporting the frequency of their consumption of particular foods:

1. They may not easily remember the foods they have eaten for a full 24-hour period.

2. They may have difficulty reporting on frequencies of consumption of particular items across meals and snack times.

3. They are often not aware of the names and nutrient content of food products they consume.

4. They are not aware of the methods of food preparation (e.g., salt shaking habits, use of margarine versus butter) followed by their parents, grandparents, or school cooks.

To compensate for these problems, some investigators have used self-report diaries. One book (Sudman and Lannom, 1980) and three articles (Laurent et al., 1972; Roghmann and Haggerty, 1972; and Verbrugge, 1980) are of particular value on this subject.

Strengths and Weaknesses. Verbrugge (1980) reviewed the available literature on health diaries and came to the following conclusions: (1) diaries produced higher frequencies for most phenomena than other methods and appeared to be particularly better than other self-report methods for reporting low salience phenomena (e.g., transient, low-impact health problems, symptoms, and disability days); (2) telescoping is absent; and (3) memory lapse is minimized. In addition, depending on how the diary data were collected, diaries could provide very rich sources of a wide variety of data for intensive analysis.

Verbrugge further reported that two other methodological concerns of investigators did *not* occur: a very high percentage of people contacted agreed to complete diaries, and very few people who agreed to complete a diary failed to complete one during the full recording period. This high completion rate happened without financial or other incentives to complete the forms.

Verbrugge also reported several problems with diaries. The quality of the data is roughly proportional to the effort expended in collecting it. Frequent (e.g., weekly) attempts must be made to collect the diaries. Recontacts must be made with respondents to clarify missing, inconsistent, or otherwise unclear data, not only to verify the responses but also to demonstrate staff concern about the quality of the data. These collection efforts are obviously made at a high cost in staff time. Verbrugge estimated these costs as higher per respondent than data collected by interviewers, because of the intensive efforts at data collection and because of the need for extensive data coding.

According to Verbrugge, investigators have inferred two other methodological problems (biases) in diaries: sensitization (discussed in chapter 6 as "measurement as a change agent"), and conditioning (discussed in chapter 6 as "changes in the research instrument"). Investigators have inferred that respondents became more aware of the phenomena simply from monitoring their own behavior, at least initially. This increased sensitivity resulted in behavior changes (e.g., the person was more likely to seek medical help when the self-monitored symptoms occurred). These investigators also found that the frequency of events decreased anywhere from 5 percent to 25 percent during the recording period. They inferred that the respondents lost interest in the phenomenon (i.e., became bored) over time, which resulted in the lower reported frequencies. All of the comments about biases in the self-report questionnaire potentially apply to the diary, unless steps are taken to correct them.

The dross rate in diaries varies, depending on how the diary is structured. If the diary calls for open-ended comments, the dross rate may be quite high. If the diary calls for daily checks on a checklist, or frequency counts in a structured format, the dross rate should be quite low.

One recent effort at collecting dietary information from children attempted to capitalize on the virtues of the diary method, while minimizing the dross (Dworkin et al., 1983). The children were asked to record their daily consumption of specific categories of foods that were high in the nutrients of concern to the project: sodium and saturated fats. The categories were food-specific; e.g., the high-salt sauces category included soy, Worcestershire, steak, and related sauces; there were three milk categories—whole milk (4 percent milk fat) and two kinds of low-fat milk (2 percent milk fat and ½ percent milk fat). To promote memory of the whole day's intake, the child was asked to remember the frequency of consumption of specific foods within segments of the school day: breakfast, lunch, after school snack, dinner, after dinner snack, and bedtime snack. Pictures of the food items were used to prompt memory and make the instrument visually attractive.

Diaries are an attractive, though expensive, approach to data collection when the program staff has reason to believe that telescoping and memory loss may occur if other instruments are used.

Interviewing—Face to Face

In certain circumstances, there is no substitute for having an interviewer conduct a survey. The literature on survey interviewing methods seems infinite. Several references are useful (Anderson et al., 1979; Bailar and Lanphier, 1978; Bradburn and Sudman, 1979; Cannell et al., 1975; Cannell, Marquis, et al., 1977; Reeder, 1978; Sudman, 1979; Sudman and Lannom, 1980; Survey Research Center, 1976). This literature is too complex to be conveniently summarized in this brief section; only an overview of the method is presented.

Strengths. Conducted face to face, the interpersonal interview is preferable to the self-completion questionnaire when:

1. The content area is not well defined
2. The questions are long, complex, or require subtle distinctions
3. The respondents cannot read or write
4. Personal effort may be needed to contact respondents

The primary strength of the face-to-face interview is the use of a well-trained interviewer to query the respondent intensively and to detect, clarify, and follow up on perplexing answers or questions. A trained person can obtain answers to questions that are not well-defined or for which in-depth answers are needed. Interviewers can be trained to probe interviewees with a variety of questions, attempting to get below surface responses, i.e., flip and simple answers a respondent may provide. For example, if you are interested in why mothers decide to breast-feed or not, no self-report scales are available in the literature for this phenomenon. You could ask a simple question: "Why did you decide to breast-feed or bottle-feed your baby?" and leave several lines for the unstructured response. Alternatively, you might use the power of having an interviewer and ask the following series of questions:

> "What do you see as the benefits to your baby of breast-feeding (or bottle-feeding)?"
>
> "What do you see as the benefits to yourself of breast-feeding (or bottle-feeding)?"
>
> "What do you see as the costs to you of bottle-feeding (or breast-feeding)?"
>
> "What do you see as the costs to your baby of bottle-feeding (or breast-feeding)?"
>
> "How important are the costs of breast-feeding to you?"
>
> "How important are the benefits of breast-feeding to you?"
>
> "How important are the costs of bottle-feeding to you?"
>
> "How important are the benefits of bottle-feeding to you?"
>
> "What is the most important reason why you selected your method of infant feeding?"

A respondent finding these questions in a self-response questionnaire would probably answer them with the quickest easiest responses. For example, she might answer the first question, "Nothing." An interviewer can probe a little deeper looking for things this mother might like about breast- or bottle-feeding. Thus, for certain situations the interview is more appropriate than the self-completed questionnaire.

Interview questions are best framed when the investigator is working from a theoretical framework or a model. For example, the breast-feeding interview was based on a decision-making model that assesses the benefits and costs of two behavioral alternatives (Janis and Mann, 1977). Questions can be designed to assess the key variables in the model, and the interviewer can be instructed how far to probe respondents to ascertain the data of interest to the program staff.

The interview is appropriate for long and complex questions and those requiring subtle distinctions for the same reasons that it is valuable for poorly defined questions. The appropriateness of an interview for respondents who cannot read or write is obvious.

A face-to-face interview is also valuable when extensive effort is necessary to contact a respondent. In some cases a sample of people is selected from a source (e.g., all previous clients in a smoking-cessation program) that does not maintain their current addresses, or the sample group may have addresses not easily reachable by mail (e.g., some people live in inconspicuous lofts, sheds behind other homes, or other quarters not on usual mail routes and without mail-boxes). In rural areas, respondents may live in remote houses down dirt roads or accessible only by hiking up trails. Such people may not have a mailbox or telephone or may come to town only a couple of times a year to pick up their mail. A timely response to a mail questionnaire is highly unlikely in such cases. A more mundane example might be the survey that requires a random sampling of households in a particular geographical area. Maps do not usually list all the dwellings in an area (the maps that do show dwellings always seem to be ten years out of date), nor do they indicate which dwellings are abandoned or otherwise not occupied and which dwellings are multiple household units (e.g., apartments or condominiums). Rules can be generated for taking a random sample in such a situation, but a trained interviewer is needed to identify all the sampling units in an area and implement a set of selection rules.

The interview provides the most flexible method for the use of descriptive cues. A variety of questions can be asked and a variety of judgments can be made by an interviewer about the state of the respondent. With careful attention to detail, an interview can almost always be replicated. Careful attention to detail also promotes reliability in data collection.

Weaknesses. The face-to-face interview is susceptible to a variety of biases. In an interpersonal situation, respondents are likely to anticipate what the interviewer expects of them and act accordingly (role selection). The probing of particular content areas is likely to focus the attention of the respondent on these issues, which may change the way the respondent thinks about the issues and thereby confound future attempts at measuring this content area (measurement as a change agent). All self-report measures are susceptible to yea-saying and social desirability (response set). Interviewer effects, by definition, may occur in interpersonal interviews. Interviewers become more proficient and more subtle at asking questions, so that later interviews may be different from earlier ones (changes in the research instrument). The interview may not obtain accurate information on highly sensitive subjects, e.g., sexual or contraceptive behavior (restrictions on content).

Realizing these biases, the health program staff must take steps to counter or minimize their effects. Interviewers should be trained to ask questions in a warm and nonjudgmental manner and to avoid behaviors that might lead respondents to infer appropriate versus inappropriate responses. Questions should be worded in both positive and negative forms to minimize the effects of response sets. Training should be long enough so that interviewers are no longer learning about the meaning of the questions during the course of the interviews. Periodic retraining may be necessary to be sure that the interviewing remains true to the original intent of the study. If obviously unreliable answers will be obtained using an interview format, the data should be collected in other ways.

The dross rate for an interpersonal interview may be quite high, because there are many events in life (other than the topic of the interview) about which respondents would prefer to talk, and respondents may feel uncomfortable addressing the issues posed.

The interpersonal interview is an expensive method of data collection and should be used judiciously because of its costs. Some combination of self-completed questionnaires and interviews may best achieve an investigator's ends within the available budget. Alternatively, if time permits, a small interview survey may be conducted first to identify all the response alternatives. This complete listing of alternatives can, in turn, be used in a self-completion questionnaire.

Steps in Conducting Face-to-Face Interviews. A good face-to-face interview requires a well-designed interview schedule (list of questions) and a well-trained interviewer. The guidelines and suggestions presented earlier in this chapter for developing questionnaires apply to developing the interview schedule as well. Training interviewers requires an equal attention to detail. A good training program provides:

1. An understanding of the major ideas that underlie the questionnaire

2. A guidebook on probing and on recording responses

3. Materials for clarifying responses

4. Procedures for collecting other data

5. Clear instructions for obtaining and contacting a sample population
6. Experience in conducting the interview, especially probing
7. Common experiences in reporting or coding self-report information
8. Sources of information
9. Testing for reliability

Training should give the interviewers enough knowledge of the subject area to enable them to ask intelligent, probing questions. They should not, however, be informed of the study's specific hypotheses; that knowledge might bias the way in which they ask, interpret, or record responses. An answer to any question may be ambiguous, unless clear guidelines or clear categories of response exist for recording the response. For example, to the question, "Why do you smoke after eating?" a new smoker might answer: "Well, I'm not too sure. Er . . . well, it gives me a boost right after a meal. I feel like tackling a project after a cigarette, but otherwise I'd feel like taking a nap. But I don't like the taste, and all those ashes. I try to puff enough to feel good, but not keep that terrible smoke in my mouth."

This is a complex response to an apparently simple question. Some of the comments are positive; some are negative. The basic response to the question is equivocal. A set of rules is needed to guide the interviewer on the depth to probe for clarification and which parts of this response to record.

For some questions, an interviewer needs materials to show the respondent how to answer. Materials might include categories of income printed on a card, so that the respondent can report which category most accurately reflects the family income; or portion size pictures to enable the respondent to estimate how much food he or she consumed.

The health promotion program staff needs to provide the interviewer with area maps or other unit enumeration materials and give the interviewer clear, precise instructions on what constitutes an interview unit and how to select among these units. Some interview surveys also call for the collection of noninterview data. For example, interviewers can be trained to take blood pressures as part of a survey on the extent of hypertension control in a community. An extensive program may be needed to train such interviewers.

Armed with these materials and instructions, interviewers need experience in conducting interviews on a pilot basis. The pilot interviews test the questionnaire and enable the interviewers to develop confidence at implementing the interview and clarifying issues that did not come up in the initial review of materials and procedures. A valuable procedure is to have each interviewer tape-record a test interview and discuss the interview with the evaluator, program staff, and other interviewers. During the review of the tape recordings, all the interviewers individually record the taped responses to the questions; they then compare their recordings. Such an experience is particularly valuable because the person who conducted the interview gets feedback on interviewing techniques; the other interviewers get feedback from the program staff and each other on the appropriateness of their recordings; program staff members become aware of a variety of unresolved problems in the interview; and the staff has the opportunity to eliminate, or more intensively train, interviewers who do not obtain or record accurate responses. While the interviewers are recording the information from the interviews, the program staff should collect the data and calculate the level of reliability. Such a session should occur weekly thereafter, to ensure that the interviewers are continuing to record in a reliable manner.

If a health program staff is conducting a community survey, the interviewers must be given a phone number to call when they need information or clarification on interview techniques, sample locations, or the many other problems that occur. The program staff must take many steps to promote the reliability of all facets of the interviewing process. Interviewers should be encouraged to maintain logs of problems they encounter, and these should be resolved at the weekly meetings. If physiological measures are being collected, the interviewers' basic data collection technique needs to be assessed at weekly intervals, and the machine needs to be assessed to ensure that it maintains its calibration.

Interviewer training may be conducted over a three- to five-day period. A common outline for the sequence of training is presented in table 7.1. Before they are sent into the field, interviewers must be furnished with identification. The program staff should announce the impending interviews to the local authorities and place announcements in the papers so that the populace will expect to be contacted.

Conducting an interview survey is a time-consuming and costly business. This section has overviewed only some of the issues and methods involved. Program staff considering this technique should consult several texts on interviewing methods.

Interviewing—Telephone

Telephone interviewing is considered an attractive alternative to face-to-face interviewing, because the information is cheaper to collect per

Table 7.1   Outline of Training for Face-to-Face Interviewers

Day	Time	Training
1	AM	Presentation of the ideas on which the study is based
	PM	Detailed question-by-question review of the instrument, allowing for extensive questioning by the interviewers
2	AM	Presentation of support materials for obtaining responses
		Conduct of a role-played interview
	PM	Training and testing in obtaining the physiological measures
3	AM/PM	Conduct and taping of two practice interviews (prearranged with people to be interviewed)
4	AM	Review of the problems encountered and questions raised
		Common recording by all interviewers of information from taped interviews and discussion of recordings made
	PM	Continued common recording and discussion of taped interviews
		Testing of physiological measurement ability
5	AM	Training in procedures for selecting samples
	PM	Last questions
		Testing of physiological measurement skills

interview, and greater control can be exerted over the methods of data collection in a central automated center for telephone interviewing. Several telephone survey research centers currently use computerized centers for such interviews (Groves, 1979). A burgeoning literature has developed on methods of telephone interviewing (Dillman, 1978; Groves and Kahn, 1979; Jordan et al., 1979).

All the comments made about face-to-face interviewing apply at some level to telephone interviewing, but telephone interviewing is susceptible to additional biases. A primary concern in use of this technique has been population restrictions. Although recent evidence reveals that over 90 percent of all households have telephones (Thornberry and Massey, 1978), telephone unavailability is more common among people traditionally considered deprived, e.g., those in rural areas, the unemployed, those with lower education and income levels, and the separated and divorced. The telephone company refuses to string telephone cable into many sparsely populated, rural, mountainous areas in Appalachia. Further population restriction problems arise in using the telephone to reach people with unlisted phone numbers, those who have moved, and those who have changed phones for other reasons since the last public listing of telephone numbers. To overcome the latter two problems, some investigators have proposed the method of random digit dialing, which obtains randomly selected phone numbers. The shortcoming of this approach is that it is not usable for contacting some known sampling frame of individuals (e.g., all the former participants in a particular project) or contacting people in specific geographical areas, since the first three digits in the telephone number may not be specific to those areas. Jordan et al. (1979) compared a telephone interview survey with a household interview survey conducted on random samples in the Los Angeles area. They reported that 6.8 percent of the units they attempted to contact in the household interviews were ineligible, while 36.0 percent in the telephone interviews were ineligible. Telephone surveys may therefore be a less efficient approach for contacting particular units. Differences may also exist in the populations that can be reached by telephone over a span of time or a geographic area, but these have not been documented.

There may be greater restrictions on content in the telephone than in the face-to-face interview. It is commonly reported that a telephone interview cannot last more than 30 minutes and is best conducted in 20 minutes or less. In contrast, face-to-face interviews are commonly one hour or longer. The telephone interviewers in the study by Jordan et al. (1979) reported: (1) telephone interviews are faster paced than face-to-face interviews; (2) pauses of routine length in interpersonal interviews were unbearably long in telephone interviews; and (3) no visual cues were available to the interviewers to gauge when and how long they should probe for responses.

The Jordan team also reported comparative analyses of data. In their initial comparison, almost twice as many people refused to answer a question on family income (a highly sensitive question) by telephone than in a face-to-face interview, but few other differences were obtained in demographic variables. This difference in response to family income was lower in comparisons of subsequent telephone and face-to-face interviews, ostensibly because of improved telephone interviewing techniques. What these techniques were, however, was not reported. Jordan et al. found no statistically significant differences in means for attitude items or the numbers of responses to open-ended items, but they did find greater yea-saying, more frequent refusal to answer questions, more frequent extreme responses, and greater acquiescence to the perceived desires of the interviewer among telephone interview respondents. Thus, the same mean responses were obtained using the two methods, but greater error was obtained from telephone interviews. More recent articles (Aneshencel et al., 1982; Siemiatycki, 1979) report few differences in means across the methods for collecting the same data and thereby provide greater hope for use of telephone interviews.

Since greater acquiescence is obtained in telephone interviews, the dross rate is probably lower for telephone interviews than face-to-face interviews; this has not been documented, however. Telephone interviewers can ask for descriptive cues as well as face-to-face interviewers can, so rough parity exists on this issue. The methods are equally replicable. A telephone survey is less expensive than a face-to-face interview, but it cannot be maintained for the same length of time. The relative cost per unit of information remains to be documented.

Direct Observation

Sometimes the accuracy of self-reported behaviors is suspect. In these cases, some investigators turn to direct observation. Three references are particularly useful on direct observation: Weick (1968), Herbert and Attridge (1975), and Johnson and Bolstad (1973). Herbert and Attridge have reviewed a variety of psychometric and practical concerns in the design of observational instruments. Johnson and Bolstad have reviewed a series of methodological studies on observation as the primary method of data collection.

Observational methods are most useful for collecting behavioral and capability data. By definition, behavioral data are amenable to observation. Capability or skill data often require a person's performance of a task in a controlled circumstance to see whether the person can do it. For example, a diabetic may be asked to perform a self-injection in a clinic, to demonstrate effectively doing it. Direct observation includes a broad variety of methods. Observational data can be obtained, for example, directly by observers, by videotapes, by audio tape recorders, and by a variety of other mechanical and electronic means. In some methods the observer attempts to be an objective recorder of phenomena; in others the observer frequently interacts with the subjects and may in fact participate with the subjects in various key social events (Emerson, 1981). Observational studies may be concerned simply with identifying the frequency of certain phenomena or at a more complex level with the relationships between events. There are many other ways to segment the observational research literature. The rest of this section relates primarily to cases in which the observations are done by trained observers, attempting to be objective recorders of the frequency of predefined phenomena.

Direct observation is one of the most expensive approaches to obtaining behavioral data. One or more observers must be present for extended periods of time to document the behavior of concern; extensive observation records must be maintained; multiple coders must search the observation records and code the phenomena of concern. Using the self-report method, a single investigator can use a self-report questionnaire with multiple respondents and in an hour obtain data from each respondent covering an hour, a day, a week, a year, or even a lifetime of experiences. In contrast, a single observer in one hour can obtain data on only an hour in the life of one person or an interacting group of people. Observation, therefore, can be cost-effective when used to validate data obtained on small samples using other methods. These other methods can then be used with larger samples.

Steps in Conducting Direct Observation. Herbert and Attridge (1975) should be consulted on creation of an observational form. They have identified 23 rules for consideration in the design and implementation of the form and a system of data collection.

At a minimum, the method of direct observation of behavior requires:

1. An *observation instrument* that reflects the theory, model, or other purposes of the study
2. A *protocol* that outlines all the rules relating to the issues of observational data collection
3. An *observer* trained in use of the instrument and protocol
4. A system of procedures for assessing the *reliability of the data* collected
5. A *protocol for coding the data* into meaningful units from the observational sheets, with lists of all cases of arbitrary codings
6. *Coders* trained in the use of the coding protocol
7. A system of procedures for assessing the *reliability of the coding*

The observation instrument includes the actual sheet for recording and the definitions of terms. The instrument must display the observational items within categories for easy reference and must include a sufficient number of boxes to check the occurrence of the item at timed intervals. Figure 7.3 is an example of a form for recording observations of a child's physical activities.

Careful attention must be paid to defining the items for observation. The activity categories in figure 7.3 define the major aerobic activities that can lead to cardiovascular benefit. Consensus must exist among the observers and other research staff on the meaning of terms. Distinctions among the proposed items must be amenable to observation, requiring as little judgment on the part of the observer as possible. For example, the distinction between partial activity and full aerobic activity is purely a judgment call. Agreement can be increased by extensive practice and consensus among observers with

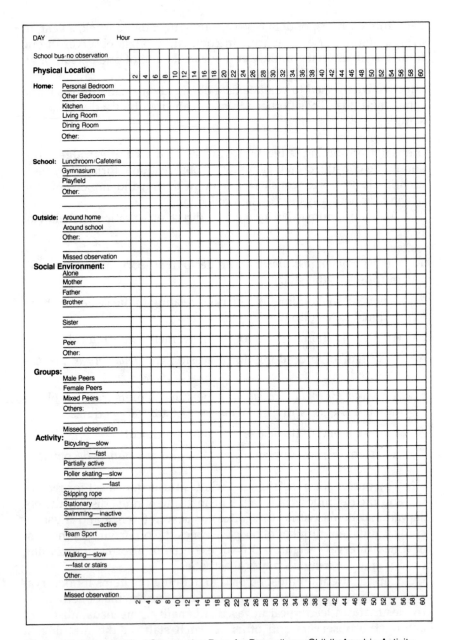

Figure 7.3 Example of an Observation Form for Recording a Child's Aerobic Activity

periodic reliability testing. Observers must also agree on which aspects of the environment correspond to the categories in the instrument. For example, if observations are conducted in homes, which room is the living room and which is the playroom? Where does the kitchen end and the dining room begin? Is the new person who entered the room a cousin, a niece, or an aunt?

The protocol must specify whether the observer should record: (1) the predominant activity during a specific time interval, (2) all activities during a specific time interval, or (3) those activities performed at an instant of observation (the time sampling method). The first method is useful for characterizing predominant activities but may miss important short-duration activities. The second method will obtain short-duration activities but loses any sense of which activities predominate in an interval. The third method is the easiest to implement but misses information on what happened between observations. There are no right and wrong choices of method. The one that obtains the most useful data for the purpose at hand should be selected. In the study in which figure 7.3 was used, the second option, recording all events, was selected, since the investigators were concerned with everything a child did (Baranowski et al., 1983).

The protocol must specify procedures for contacting, training, and/or interviewing the persons to be observed, times at which all activities are to be conducted, sequences of activities within observation sessions, and procedures for ameliorating anticipated problems. The protocol should include the definitions of items and examples of the cases that are difficult to distinguish. It should clarify whether single or multiple checks are disallowed, allowed, encouraged, or required within categories of observational items. Procedures for recording field notes should be stated.

The protocol should also specify periodic times for joint observations to obtain interobserver reliability. The reliability of the observational data can be assessed in a variety of ways depending on the type of data collected and what the program staff want to learn. Several references are useful in discussing these issues: Bartko and Carpenter (1976), Green (1981), House et al. (1981), and Tinsley and Weiss (1975).

Observer training is a primary method for promoting the reliability of direct observational data. Training might proceed according to the outline in table 7.2.

Just as observers may not agree on aspects of how they record what they observe, people coding information from the observational instruments may not agree, due to differences in interpretation or understanding of the coding task, temporary distractions, or errors in memory or perception. A protocol is needed for coding data from the

Table 7.2　Outline of Training for Observers

Day	Time	Training
1	AM	Review of the conceptual framework underlying the research
		Discussion of the observational form and protocol, item by item
	PM	Joint observation of a movie or videotape depicting the expected observation scene
		Assessment of reliability of the joint observation reports
2	AM	Observation of the phenomenon of concern under realistic conditions
	PM	Discussion of the problems encountered
		Revision of the form or protocol, as necessary
3	AM	Simultaneous observations of the phenomenon of concern by two or three observers
	PM	Assessment of interobserver reliability
		Discussion of problems of reliability
		Revision of the form or protocol, as necessary
4 and on	AM/PM	Repeat of day 3 as necessary to achieve the desired reliability

observational instrument into meaningful variables. Many of the same issues covered in the observational protocol must be covered in the coding protocol. People doing the coding need to be trained in performing their task, although the training may not have to be as long, since the task is more clearly defined and the data are not lost once the coding is done. Coding of the same form by two coders must be built into the daily tasks of the coders to obtain periodic estimates of intercoder reliability.

Reliability and validity are significant issues in observational research. Johnson and Bolstad (1973) have identified five key problems in the use of observation methods: (1) reliability estimates may not be made on the same coding and time units; (2) the days on which reliability is assessed may not be representative of other days on which observations are conducted; (3) the instrument may decay due to the passage of time; (4) the observers may respond in some unknown way to having reliability assessed; and (5) the people being observed may respond in some unknown way to being observed. Methods for counteracting these problems have been developed.

First, Johnson and Bolstad were concerned about coding and time units. Constant monitoring of the reliability of observational data is a necessity. Data must be collected in a manner that facilitates comparing the data collected by two people on the same event. Obviously the same event coding system must be used by both observers. In addition, it is important to avoid the possibility that two observers reporting the same frequency of events are each reporting different occurrences. To avoid this, the observational form should use the same time unit for recording events. How long the time unit needs to be will vary with the phenomenon observed. The Johnson and Bolstad study required three- to five-second intervals. Other studies have used one second, one minute, two minutes, and five minutes, depending on the type of behavior observed and the purpose of data collection. The form in figure 7.3 uses two-minute intervals, since this was short enough to obtain relatively discrete information yet long enough not to fatigue the observers during a full day of observation.

Human behavior is variable. Some days may have many occurrences of a particular event; then a long time may transpire before the event of interest occurs again. For example, some people rarely engage in aerobic activity, and an event of aerobic activity may not occur on the day on which observational reliability is estimated. Thus, reliability must be estimated at multiple points in a project. In addition, artificial simulations of infrequent events should be created for observation tests, (e.g., in a movie or videotape), to estimate the interrater reliability.

Johnson and Bolstad reported a study in which the interrater reliability of two observers remained reasonably high during the course of the study, but the correlations of their observations with those of a third party became progressively lower. This phenomenon indicated that the two observers created a mutually approved approach to categorizing events, which progressively diverged from the aim and methods of the original coding scheme followed by the third party. The authors redressed this problem by having more than two observers and conducting interobserver reliability checks on different pairs of observers over the course of the project.

The behavior of observers is as responsive to environmental factors as the behavior of the people being observed. Johnson and Bolstad reported that the reliability of observers significantly declined right after training, but the decline varied depending on which reliability monitoring system was employed. Cases in which reliability was assessed by having a second observer conduct observations on selected and announced days (the spot check method) had the overall largest slide in reliability, except on days when the spot checks occurred. To promote maximum reliability, Johnson and Bolstad recommended the following components of training for a reliability monitoring system:

1. Have all the observers read and study the observation protocol

2. Have the observers complete programmed instruction materials on precoded interactions

3. Conduct daily intensive training programs on precoded scripts enacted on videotape or by actors
4. Provide field training with an experienced observer, followed by reliability testing
5. Randomly assess reliability in the field

Finally, Johnson and Bolstad noted that the people being observed are affected in major and minor ways by the observation process. The literature at this time, however, is not clear about which behaviors are most likely to be affected, in what ways, or for how long. Investigators must be watchful of the reactivity of the observational method. There is reason to believe that the less obtrusive (or obvious) the observer is, the less effect the observer will have on the behavior in question. After some period of time, the effects of the presence of an observer appear to wear off or decrease. Investigators should therefore work to minimize the obtrusiveness of the observer and allow long enough observation periods to reduce the effects of the observer's presence.

UNOBTRUSIVE MEASURES

While interviewing, self-report, and observation methods are marvelously flexible and can tap a broad variety of data, they are also subject to many of the biases identified by Webb et al. (1966). The Webb team argued that, since every method of data collection is subject to one or more (often many) sources of bias, an investigator should use multiple methods. Methods should be selected that are subject to different sources of error. If the same results are obtained despite differing sources of bias, the investigators can be more confident that the sources of bias by themselves do not account for the results. For example, if a health education program promoting dietary change showed that participants reported eating fewer high-calorie foods after completing the program, critics could object that the subjects in the study were only reporting what the investigators wanted to hear. If observational data also showed that the subjects no longer entered a particular candy store, and physiological tests showed a weight loss for these subjects, then skeptics would be harder pressed to question the evaluation conclusions.

There are several methods of collecting unobtrusive data. Under certain circumstances each of these methods is subject to each of the 12 biases identified in chapter 6. For example, if people completing medical records become aware that someone has started using these records to evaluate their performance, they may complete the forms in a self-protective and self-justifying way, thereby making the records a biased source of information. Similarly, hospital accounting records that contain total family income are probably biased downward on this variable, since a lower report of income will often mean a lower, or no, charge for care. The unbiased character of any unobtrusive method is maintained only as long as people are not aware they are being studied and there is no other incentive for them to provide biased information. Several unobtrusive methods used in health research are reviewed next.

Abstraction of Existing Records—Medical/Clinical

Some investigators consider the medical record a readily available and accessible source of rich data at little cost. Imagine the millions of medical records across the country with millions of laboratory and physiological tests on a vast variety of health problems—a veritable gold mine, but filled, perhaps, with fool's gold. There are very limited occasions when a medical record abstraction is appropriate and valuable. These occasions can be identified after listing the biases in record abstraction.

Strengths and Weaknesses. Entries are made in one or more medical records every time a patient receives care from a physician. This is an enormous quantity of data. If the physician or health care institution can be persuaded to share these records, the body of data becomes available for evaluative purposes. The primary cost is incurred by hiring staff to enter and abstract the desired data from all the data available.

There are, however, many limitations. Not every person receives medical care for a particular problem. While some of the major barriers to care have been overcome in the United States and western Europe, study after study has indicated that the poor and ethnic minority groups are less likely to receive care for a health problem than others. Differences in care are lower for painful acute problems (e.g., otitis media) and greater for less painful, more chronic conditions (e.g., hypertension). Thus population restrictions for results of studies made of only those receiving care may be more or less severe depending on the topic of the study.

A more severe problem is restrictions on content. Ferber (1968) abstracted variables primarily related to medical care (information likely to be in the record), and avoided abstracting data related to health education or health promotion (which were much less likely to be in the record). He reported easy access to accurate information on a limited number of demographic variables (e.g., age, sex, hospital accommodation, marital status, employment status, but not occupation), and difficulties in abstracting every other type of information.

Feinstein (1970) has attempted to explain the unreliability of medical record information by examining the three major purposes of maintaining a medical record: patient management, science, and legal concerns. In regard to patient management, Feinstein noted that physicians more frequently relied on their personal memory of a case than on the record. Thus, much clinically useful information is not recorded, and what gets recorded varies with the characteristics of the patient. Physicians also tend to record only "scientific" information, leaving "softer" (but clinically relevant) data out of the record. Physicians typically do not record, or do not consistently record, variables that are pertinent to someone else's study. The same variable may be recorded in several places in the medical record, and, since medical records are not diligently updated, conflicting information on the same variable may appear in different locations in the record.

The way in which scientific facts are clinically obtained in medical practice does not reflect the compulsion and concern for replicability given to data collected for scientific research. In this light, even if the scientific data were systematically recorded, they would be of questionable benefit for research. Few physicians maintain records for scientific reasons, and so replication is not important to them. Medical records do, however, provide evidence in cases of malpractice. If a physician is concerned about malpractice, the information in the medical record may be biased in the direction of protecting the physician from malpractice awards. How this affects any particular variable depends on the variable, the perceived probability that this item is related to malpractice litigation, and the direction of distortions necessary to protect the physician.

The stability of the content of medical records often varies over time and across areas. For example, the International Classification of Diseases (ICD) is a set of codes for major categories of causes of death and disability. Hospitals use several ICD codes in the planning of health services. Different hospitals use different ICD codes, creating variations in data among locations. Moreover, the ICD codes are periodically updated to reflect the latest medical knowledge. Data collected before and after code changes are, therefore, not directly comparable, because the diagnostic criteria for making a particular judgment may have changed. Newly revised ICD codes may be employed earlier in one geographic area and later in others. These differences may preclude comparisons across geographic areas in a particular year or for several years or within an area across time periods. Related issues arise. As medical science advances, new diagnoses are made possible. Diagnoses that were impossible before this research become common. Increasing frequency of a new diagnosis may not reflect an increasing incidence, but simply a new interpretation of a long-term problem. Fads also occur in the popularity of diagnoses. Certain diagnoses that are poorly defined and little used at one point in time become popular at others. Cases that are not clearly defined are more likely to be coded using the more popular disease categories. Any patient may have multiple medical problems; which medical diagnosis gets recorded? For example, was the major cause of this person's death the heart attack, or the 20-year history of diabetes mellitus? Informal conventions on priority in the coding of multiple medical diagnoses will differ by time and geographic area, making comparisons difficult.

Another potentially major bias in using medical records for data abstraction is the guinea pig effect. If medical records are used over an extended period of time, physicians and others become aware of this use of the records and may attempt to change their recording behavior to protect themselves from professional liability. This change in recording may drastically bias the validity of a longitudinal evaluation based on medical record abstraction.

The dross rate in medical record data is quite high. Great quantities of information must be sifted to find the few variables of interest. Familiarity with the record, and training, can assist the abstracter in locating information efficiently. As more information is desired from the medical record, abstracters become less likely to adhere to the abstraction rules, and more inconsistencies become obvious. Only a limited number of variables can be obtained from medical records to describe the selected sample. Effectively done, record abstractions can be replicated.

Steps in Abstracting Medical Records. A medical record abstraction can be useful when demographic data and simple, commonly recorded medical data are desired and attempts to control for reliability are made. One recent study (not yet prepared for publication) that attempted to abstract relevant information on hypertensive patients in a family medicine clinic illustrates the steps required in conducting abstractions of medical records. A page from this study's abstraction form is presented in figure 7.4. Six different drafts of the form were developed. The first three were revised through staff discussion to reflect the purposes of the study more clearly as these purposes became more clearly defined. Reliability analyses were conducted on the next two drafts by having sets of two out of three abstracters jointly abstract 20 records. Reliability indices were calculated on the 20 jointly abstracted records for each variable for each pair of abstracters. All cases in which differing values were obtained were intensively reviewed against the medical record, and rules were generated to refine the search or the recording process. On the second set of reliability

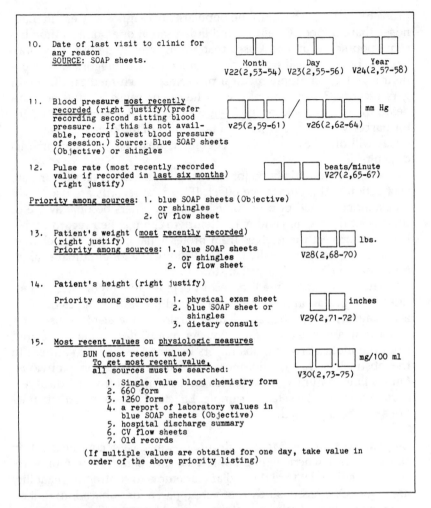

10. Date of last visit to clinic for
    any reason
    <u>SOURCE</u>: SOAP sheets.

    Month   Day   Year
    V22(2,53-54) V23(2,55-56) V24(2,57-58)

11. Blood pressure <u>most recently</u>
    <u>recorded</u> (right justify)(prefer
    recording second sitting blood
    pressure. If this is not avail-
    able, record lowest blood pressure
    of session.) Source: Blue SOAP sheets
    (Objective) or shingles

    /   mm Hg
    v25(2,59-61)   v26(2,62-64)

12. Pulse rate (most recently recorded
    value if recorded in <u>last six months</u>)
    (right justify)

    beats/minute
    V27(2,65-67)

    <u>Priority among sources</u>: 1. blue SOAP sheets (Objective)
                        or shingles
                    2. CV flow sheet

13. Patient's weight (<u>most recently recorded</u>)
    (right justify)
    <u>Priority among sources</u>: 1. blue SOAP sheets
                        or shingles
                    2. CV flow sheet

    lbs.
    V28(2,68-70)

14. Patient's height (right justify)

    Priority among sources: 1. physical exam sheet
                        2. blue SOAP sheet or
                          shingles
                        3. dietary consult

    inches
    V29(2,71-72)

15. <u>Most recent values</u> on <u>physiologic measures</u>
         BUN (most recent value)
         <u>To get most recent value,</u>
         all sources must be searched:

    mg/100 ml
    V30(2,73-75)

            1. Single value blood chemistry form
            2. 660 form
            3. 1260 form
            4. a report of laboratory values in
              blue SOAP sheets (Objective)
            5. hospital discharge summary
            6. CV flow sheets
            7. Old records

         (If multiple values are obtained for one day, take value in
         order of the above priority listing)

Figure 7.4 Sample Page from a Medical Record Abstraction Form

abstractions, rules for abstraction were further refined, and variables for which a reliabilty of abstraction of 0.75 or higher was not achieved were dropped from the study. The sixth draft was used for the final abstractions. Search and coding rules were printed right on the abstraction form to make their use convenient. A limited set of demographic, commonly recorded, and more serious variables was finally obtained from the medical records. Less than half the variables originally desired were included in the final form. Particular attention was given to the development of rules for abstraction, since Boyd et al. (1979) have shown that explicit criteria for abstractions can more than double the interabstracter reliability values.

Abstraction of Existing Records—Financial/Accounting

Financial records are also considered an attractive source of data because of their ready accessibility and availability. Accountants and others have spent many hours developing reliable systems for recording the income and outflow of money to and from organizations. All of the comments made about medical records, however, potentially apply to financial or accounting records as well. There is one major difference. Data in financial or accounting systems tend to be more up to date and more reliable. The primary reason for this is financial incentive. If a company or organization does not maintain accurate, up-to-date financial records, it cannot collect the money necessary to maintain itself. This is especially true for organizations dependent on fees for services, e.g., clinics; it is less true for organizations receiving grants, bequests, or contributions, e.g., voluntary health agencies. Despite the incentives for accurate records in agencies that rely on fees, there is still a wide disparity in the quality of financial records these agencies keep. See Appendix C for data needed in cost studies.

Other limitations exist in abstracting these records. Financial record systems rarely have extensive nonfinancial data. Names and addresses may be systematically recorded, but the rest of the information is often financial. This is a benefit if the primary concern of an evaluation is financial, e.g., it is a cost-benefit or cost-effectiveness study. It is a hindrance otherwise. Even when finances are the data of choice, the abstracters may need special expertise to understand how the financial data are categorized, to locate the desired information, and to check and abstract the most appropriate data. Organizations may be reluctant to permit access to their financial records. Finally, if financial records from more than one organization are of interest, completely different coding systems may be (and often are) used by organizations using differing accounting systems, since the recorded information is defined in a completely different manner. Thus, investigators must be careful in using financial records.

Physiological Measures

Physiological measures are used in a broad variety of health education and promotion studies. In some cases, the physiological measure is the primary outcome measure, e.g., blood pressure determinations as measures of effectiveness of programs to control high blood pressure. In other cases, physiological variables act as checks on the validity of self-reported measures, e.g., serum thiocyanate to validate smoking cessation, urine hydrochlorothiazide to validate diuretic therapy compliance, urine sodium to validate sodium consumption, a sweat patch test to validate alcohol consumption, or hemoglobin A_{lg}

to validate midterm diabetes control. In some studies physiological variables reflect the subject's health status or disease risk, which may be affected by habitual behaviors. Examples include serum cholesterol, which may be affected by diet and exercise and is predictive of atherosclerosis, or a submaximal stress test, which measures physical fitness and should be affected by aerobic activity. The great attraction of physiological measures is that they are not obtrusive in the many senses that behavioral measures are, since it is not obvious to subjects that they are being observed, and the measures are reactive only to the extent that they encourage people to perform the desired behaviors when they are aware of the values.

Despite the aura of complete objectivity that these "hard data" measures have, they are subject to as many sources of error as the "soft data." For example, physiological indicators are often subject to daily, weekly, and other cycles in values. Recent studies of blood pressure, using continuous or frequent monitoring instruments, have shown marked variations between waking and sleeping hours, between mornings and evenings, between conversation times and times alone. Blood pressures taken in an office or clinic are roughly 10 mm Hg higher than those taken in the home. Blood pressures rise and fall in response to the person's emotional or arousal state. Thus, systematic bias may occur in a study from simply taking a blood pressure measurement at different times in the day or in different settings.

Although physiological measures seem simple and straightforward to make, extensive detailed protocols have been developed for obtaining them, including: (1) extended training procedures (for even well-credentialed individuals); (2) specification of the environmental conditions in which the measure is taken (e.g., blood pressures for a research project are typically taken in a well-lit room, with the manometer at eye level, and with low environmental noise); (3) specification of the state of the subject (e.g., an individual who has fasted for 12 hours before a blood sample for serum cholesterol analysis is taken); (4) procedures for handling the specimen (if one was taken); (5) identification of the specific machine and how it should be run, periodically tested, and corrected; and (6) procedures for ongoing quality control of all elements of the data collection process. A primary difference between physiological measures and the behavioral and self-report measures is that the many sources of error in physiological measures are well known and more amenable to control if highly structured procedures are compulsively employed.

Human and other errors can occur at every stage in the measurements, however. Medication compliance provides an interesting example. Biron (1975) has noted that having enough medication flowing in a person's circulatory system to be effective in fighting a disease (a therapeutic plasma concentration) requires prescription of an adequate amount of medication, consumption of all the medication prescribed (patient compliance), and action by the body to make the medication available in the bloodstream as expected (bioavailability). Biron has argued that most physicians do not know enough about pharmacotherapy to prescribe amounts that promote therapeutic bioavailability; there are severe problems in compliance, for many reasons; and there is high variability from person to person in how the body absorbs, metabolizes, and stores the same medication (Alvares et al., 1979). With regard to bioavailability, Biron (1975) also has pointed out that a pharmaceutical company can make the same product within a relatively wide band of variation, some of which promote bioavailability of the product while others retard it. These are all potential sources of error prior to taking a blood sample to test for bioavailability of the drug. Plasma concentrations at less than a therapeutic level, therefore, may be due to factors other than patient compliance.

A variety of other errors can occur. The needle for taking a blood sample from a child may be too narrow, destroying many red blood cells and contaminating the serum sample. The blood sample may not be appropriately chilled, leading to coagulation and destroying the sample for analysis. The centrifuge for separating red blood cells from serum may not be functioning properly. These and a host of other errors should disabuse program staff of blind faith in the value of physiological measures. Furthermore, certain procedures for obtaining a physiological measure (e.g., obtaining a blood sample or making an X-ray film) pose health risks for the individual (e.g., infections from a blood sample, cancer from an X-ray procedure). Does the importance of obtaining the physiological measure override the risk to the individual?

Steps in Using Physiological Methods. The listing of the problems in implementing a physiological measure should not discourage program staff from selecting such a measure when it is appropriate. First, medical and other personnel, e.g., clinical pharmacists, should be consulted on the appropriateness of a particular measure to answer the question at hand. The measure should clearly validate some behavioral measure, be the primary outcome of concern, or be a health or risk indicator of primary concern.

Second, a protocol should be selected (or developed) to monitor *all* phases of physiological data collection and processing. Almost all physiological measures that an evaluator may use have been used in other studies. The protocol that best meets the needs of the evaluative study should be employed.

Third, the evaluator must continually monitor the collection and processing of the data for reliability to ensure that the same high quality data are obtained throughout the project. Most protocols detail a set of quality control procedures. It should be clear from this discussion that collecting physiological variables can be a very expensive proposition, even aside from the substantial laboratory costs for actually conducting the tests.

SUMMARY

The issues in selecting and developing methods are complex. Each method is susceptible to various threats to reliability and validity. Although many of these threats can be overcome, they are overcome at a cost. The job of the evaluator is to select and develop the most reliable and valid methods and instruments appropriate to the issues at hand, within the funding and other resources available.

A common distinction is made between obtrusive and unobtrusive measurement techniques. Unobtrusive measures are often desired, because reactive bias is less likely to appear in these data. Under certain circumstances, however, even the measures that seem most unobtrusive can become obtrusive. Furthermore, unobtrusive measures are not always appropriate for collecting the type of information needed in a particular evaluation. The evaluator must be sensitive to bias issues in every evaluation conducted and must select and employ the most appropriate measurement methods.

Many skills are involved at each stage in selecting and developing methods and instruments. The novice evaluator should not become intimidated or discouraged, however. Despite the collective skills and intelligence of teams of evaluators, anticipated and unanticipated problems occur in the best of evaluative studies. No evaluative (or other) study has been perfect. Budding evaluators should, instead, have a realistic respect for the problems likely to be encountered, build their skills to the maximum possible, and involve consultants knowledgeable in the particular type of evaluation contemplated. The best way to learn these skills is to participate in the selection and development of methods under the supervision of others already skilled in these tasks. Aspiring evaluators should seek professionals conducting program evaluations and volunteer or otherwise participate in these activities.

8

Simple Techniques for Analyzing Program Data

"The results are significant, but how do we explain that?"

"First they ask me for an evaluation; now they tell me to skip the details."

"It has taken me six months to evaluate this project and they simply do what they want!"

"Detailed evaluations often rise in emotional appeal as they decline in intellectual clarity."

Professional Competencies Emphasized in This Chapter:

- specification of types of data

- presentation of data

- description and comprehension of descriptive statistics

- differentiation among selected types of distributions

- selection of analytical methods

- application of analytical methods

One of the world's greatest statisticians, Sir Ronald Alymer Fisher, hated mathematical nitpicking. What made Fisher so great was his intuition and insight into problems. For many health evaluation persons, *statistics* is a word suitable for use only at night with a full moon on Halloween—it's scary! In this chapter we focus on statistics, but as a tool of intuition and insight for persons involved in health education and promotion programs, not for mathematical nitpicking. This is a difficult task. Mathematics is the one area of scholastic performance in which people are comfortable admitting failure. Health workers are not afraid to say, "I haven't had math since algebra, and I failed that." Unfortunately, admission or submission to failure at the outset will prevent the absorption of these valuable tools.

Those who suffer from learned helplessness should not read this chapter. What will follow may surprise you as you read. Learning about statistics is similar to evaluating a nutrition program in rural Mexico—you must understand the language before you can get at the concepts. The notation and jargon get easier and are an insufficient reason to skip this chapter. But do not lose the forest for the trees; the concepts are the meat, the jargon and notation are the mathematical nitpicking. The chapter has been written with the assumption that you have taken an elementary statistics course. This is not a necessity for the earlier portions of the chapter, but it is an asset in the more detailed treatment of statistical methods in the latter portions.

This chapter deals with the use of simple techniques in the analysis of program data. It is not intended to be a statistical text on these topics. Numerous texts already exist, and repeating them would require more than a single chapter. Our basic notion is to give you access to various statistical texts, so that these techniques can be referenced, applied, and understood with the full complement of discussion provided in the array of books available.

The important concepts in evaluation are the *appropriate classification of the design* and the *type of study* that you are using. The use of the statistical tools should be a means rather than an end. The importance of statistics as a tool cannot be overemphasized, but the achievement of statistical significance does not imply, in and of itself, that an intervention has been successful. You must ask a series of additional questions that support the statistical techniques for a full analysis of the data set. Keep in mind that the simple techniques for analyses are (1) understanding of the problem and (2) careful and unbiased assessment of the results obtained.

THE EVALUATOR AS A CONSUMER

The title of this chapter promotes the notion that you as an evaluator can apply simple techniques to program data and obtain sufficient information to shed an objective light on the value of a health education and promotion program. To do this, you must first become a competent consumer of other evaluations. Experience is an excellent teacher. The more you are involved in evaluations and face the difficult decisions, fatal flaws, and critical problems identified in other evaluations, the more efficiently you can perform as a provider of results.

To be a competent consumer, you should become aware of the key issues in presenting information in evaluation reports. Some evaluations consist of nothing more than verbal testimonials on the efficacy of a program. Such statements of faith will not be considered in this chapter. Although potentially meaningful and of some value, they cannot generally be used in an objective manner. The purpose of an evaluation and of statistical techniques for analyzing program data is to assist the decision-making process. Analysis should be done in an unbiased manner, void of the interpersonal issues that come into play after the information is presented. Virtually every tool that is useful in making this kind of objective decision can be summarized in some numerical form. The tool may be nothing more than a simple count of qualitative findings.

TYPES OF DATA

Given the numerical representation of data, several key questions must be asked. The first is: What do these data represent? It is important to recognize which numerical class the data fall into, since analytical techniques are often restricted to one class of information. There are generally three classes of data representation.

Nominal or *naming data* refer to arbitrarily labeled characteristics such as male/female, black/white, infant/child/adolescent/adult, or numbers on a football jersey.

Numerical data consists of two subclasses—discrete and continuous data. *Discrete data* can be placed on an integer scale, such as the numbers 1, 2, 3. Often these data relate to counts or frequencies. *Continuous data* are numerical measures that can be measured to infinitely fine degrees, provided greater measurement capabilities exist. For example, weight is a continuous measure; you can measure it not only in kilograms or grams but also in milligrams or even finer increments if such measurements are deemed appropriate and technically feasible.

The third class is *ordinal data*, a combination of nominal and numerical data. Ordinal data give information that has been arbitrarily labeled, such as low, medium, or high. Corresponding to this labeling is an underlying numerical scale. Thus, if investigators talk about low-risk, medium-risk, and high-risk individuals with regard to serum cholesterol levels, they assume that the low-risk individuals have, by definition, lower cholesterol levels in actual, measured numerical values than medium- or high-risk persons. Nominal and ordinal data are both subsets of a class called *categorical* data.

ACCURACY AND PRECISION

Once you have identified the type of data, you must examine the degree of *accuracy* and *precision* with which the measurements have been made. *Accuracy* is measurement of explicitly what is present, and *precision* is ability to obtain the same results each time the same object is measured. Accurate measurements need not be precise, and precise measurements need not be accurate. Accuracy is analogous to validity, discussed in chapter 6, and precision is the same as reliability. The additional jargon has arisen from the fact that research involving health educators is often multidisciplinary. It is common to have the terms *accuracy* and *precision* used interchangeably with *validity* and *reliability*. However, the latter terms are used almost exclusively when discussing behavioral instruments.

When a measurement is accurate but not precise, the evaluator's confidence in it dwindles. When a measurement is precise but not accurate, the evaluator attempts to identify the extent of inaccuracy and adjust for it. If you were surveying a population and asked people their weight, generally they would underestimate it. Although people are fairly precise, the extent of their consistent underestimate would be the inaccuracy.

The term *bias* is used to describe a measure of inaccuracy. A very precise measurement can be biased. When the bias is known, this presents no problem. One of the major problems in evaluation is unrecognized bias. To detect such bias, it is imperative to have a clear, explicit explanation of how the data were measured. As noted in chapter 6, a danger of bias may exist in the instruments, in their application, or in the recording or transfer of data. It might result from the biases of the interviewers or the biased responses of those being interviewed. Investigators must ask how these individuals were recruited and the data acquired. Questions must be asked perpetually to uncover and assess the underlying information.

Many of the designs used in health education do not lend themselves to random selection of program participants. When your program participants are volunteers, you cannot ignore the population segments you are not measuring. You must think about and anticipate how measurement of the group excluded from your analyses would alter the data and findings you observed.

You must also ask: Are there any logical structures present in the data that bias or limit application of the results? For example, are the responses independent of each other? Are the measurements taken on the same individual before and after an intervention or on two unrelated, independent samples? You must also ask questions about more subtle distinctions. For example, if you are providing a family intervention, the unit of analysis is actually the family, not the individual. You must then be cautious in analyzing data by individuals since the response within a family is likely to be related—that is, a person is more likely to respond the way another family member does than the way a person from a different family does. This violates an important assumption of the statistical procedures used to analyze individual data. In essence, if these questions are neglected, you may end up with statistical analyses that look like textbook examples but are misleading.

READING TABLES

As a consumer of evaluations, you need to know how to get the most out of tables, graphs, and figures.

A table usually consists of rows and columns of numbers or other items. Graphs and charts are pictorial representations of numbers. Graphs usually use lines to connect points on an X-Y axis or bars showing frequencies. Charts usually display data in circles (pie charts) or by

Table 8.1   Number of New Users of Cervical Cancer Screening
Clinics by Year for Five Alabama Counties

	Year of Initial Visit				
County	1977	1978	1979	1980	Total
Hale	63	60	135	94	352
Marengo	250	96	140	96	582
Perry	61	66	41	42	210
Sumter	79	51	90	87	307
Wilcox	*	44	33	54	131
Total	453	317	439	373	1,582

*Clinic not in operation.

size and shape. The distinctions are not universal and usually are un-
important. Developing the ability to extract information from tables,
graphs, and charts is essential to good evaluators. Similarly, they
must be capable of organizing information properly in tables, graphs,
and figures. The key to tabular presentation of data is a properly constructed, adequately labeled table that can be read and understood
without consulting the accompanying text. Table 8.1, for example,
tells a reasonably complete story. The title states that the body of the
table will contain counts—the number of new users of cervical cancer
screening clinics by calendar year for five Alabama counties. The foot-
note explains that in Wilcox County in 1977 the clinic was not in operation; therefore no data could be obtained for that cell of the table. At
the top of the table the column headings under "Year of Initial Visit"
identify the year in which the new users first came to the screening
clinics. The left-hand (or stub) column lists five counties in Alabama.
Knowing these facts, readers can identify any number in the table.
The number 90, for example, represents the number of new users of
the screening program in Sumter County in 1979. The number 96 represents the number of new users in Marengo County in either 1978 or
1980. The total on the row or column is called the *margin*. Margins
provide summaries and are used to give trends.

   All too often, individuals read the text of a document and ignore
the information provided in the tables. Ignoring the tables is a waste
of information. Tables, graphs, and charts are normally provided to
highlight the important points presented. Thus, you should be able to
gain as much from them or more than from the verbiage put forth by
the authors. In addition, your interpretive ability will enable you to

reach a conclusion about the information presented in tables and graphs without the bias of the author's opinion. This does not mean that you should not read the articles, but at least scan the tables and figures first. Then, when the author presents a point, you are armed with the author's own data to decide whether his or her interpretation seems reasonable or is merely a "beauty in the eye of the beholder" statement.

RULES FOR CONSTRUCTING TABLES, GRAPHS, AND CHARTS

There are several general rules to follow in the construction of tables, graphs, and charts:

1. Divide the data into categories
2. Label the axes carefully, and include footnotes if necessary
3. Provide an accurate and descriptive title
4. Include totals of rows and columns
5. Do not clutter the display with too much data
6. Try several displays to see which conveys your best primary message

Regardless of the type of data (nominal, numerical, or ordinal), establishing categories can be a confusing task. Consider the data in table 8.2 on blood pressures of 20 people. Looking at the 20 diastolic blood pressures in this table does not immediately convey a message to you. If 2,000 persons were screened, the display of individual data would be prohibitive.

The majority of categorizing problems come from numerical data. When presenting numerical data in tabular form, you need to group the data into numerical categories called *classes*. A class is a grouping of common characteristics. You want to create neither too many classes nor too few. Having too many classes makes the tabular presentation not very different from looking at the *raw* (uncategorized) data themselves; having too few classes does not provide enough difference to detect the pattern of responses in the raw data. Table 8.3 summarizes the raw data on blood pressures into four classes: 50–64 mm Hg; 65–79 mm Hg; 80–94 mm Hg; and 95–109 mm Hg. From this table, you can better understand a pattern in the data. The greatest number of observations, nine out of twenty, is in the class 65–79 mm Hg. About equal numbers fell in the 50–64 mm Hg and 80–94 mm Hg classes, and two were over 95 mm Hg.

Tables often show what is called the *relative frequency*. This is

Table 8.2 Diastolic Blood Pressure

Person No.	Diastolic Blood Pressure (mm Hg)
1	62
2	93
3	73
4	60
5	70
6	78
7	70
8	94
9	66
10	107
11	97
12	88
13	70
14	64
15	63
16	72
17	61
18	70
19	80
20	76

nothing more than the percentage or proportion of all the observations in the table that fall into the specific class. For example, in table 8.3, 45.0 percent (nine out of twenty) were in the 65–79 mm Hg class. Thus, a general rule of thumb is to use approximately 10 classes. There can be as many as 20 classes for some continuous data and as few as 2 or 3 for certain nominal responses. The actual number of categories depends on the number of observations and the categories used in published literature. Categorical responses generally follow the nomenclature associated with the nominal or ordinal data.

A second criterion useful to follow is that the limits for each class should agree with the precision of measurement of the raw data. Thus, if weight is measured to the nearest tenth of a kilogram, the class limits should not be in terms of the nearest hundredth kilogram.

In general, intervals should be chosen that are of equal width. This facilitates comparison, is not misleading to the reader, and makes other calculations and computations easier. It is important that

Table 8.3 Diastolic Blood Pressure Groups of 20 Subjects Screened

Diastolic Blood Pressure Group (mm Hg)	Frequency	Relative Frequency
50–64	5	25.0
65–79	9	45.0
80–94	4	20.0
95–109	2	10.0
Total	20	100.0

class intervals not overlap, i.e., the classes must be mutually exclusive. Thus, age intervals of 25–35 and 35–45 are not mutually exclusive, for an individual who is 35 years old would not clearly reside in one interval or the other. Open-ended intervals should be avoided, although in many publications they occur very naturally. A common example is the class of persons 65 years of age or older. This creates difficulties in summarizing the data and inhibits maximum use of the results from the table.

Tables should be clearly labeled. The title should describe the body of the table and the various characteristics that appear in the table. Totals should be noted in tables. If proportions or percentages are shown, the denominator should be clearly identified in either the column headings or the title. When there is possible uncertainty about the units of measurement, the units should be clearly identified in the body of the table. Extremely complicated or complex tables should be avoided, even though they tend to save space in an article. Tables should be simple and clear enough so they do not require excessive time to read.

Graphic techniques for displaying data, such as charts, are commonly used and follow many of the same rules of thumb as tables. *Histograms*, commonly called *bar graphs*, are reasonably straightforward and, like nearly all the techniques discussed in this chapter, can be found in any elementary textbook on statistics. Line graphs, frequency polygons, and the like are pictorial ways to present data. Such pictures must be proportional in size to the actual numbers they represent, so that the data are not distorted by appearance and do not cause misinterpretations of the results. In creating graphs and charts, it is exceedingly important to label the scales, space the scales equally, and make the intervals on the axes consistent.

All health educators, at one time or another, need to read or create tables, graphs, and charts. The importance of characterizing

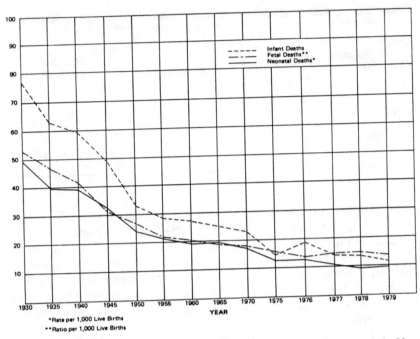

Figure 8.1 Trends in Fetal, Infant, and Neonatal Mortality, Jefferson County, 1930–80

Source: Jefferson County Department of Health, Bureau of Health Statistics and Vital Records, *1979 Annual Report* (Birmingham, Ala. Jefferson County Department of Health, 1980), Figure 5.

them correctly should be clear from this brief discussion. Consider, for example, figure 8.1. This line graph, which shows infant, fetal, and neonatal deaths, suffers several deficiencies, although it is well labeled in terms of a title, a legend, and appropriate footnotes. The unlabeled Y-axis is not clearly delineated; presumably it is the number or rate per 1,000 live births. The X-axis, the year, gives an improper pictorial representation. Looking at it casually, an evaluator might draw the conclusion that little reduction of mortality has come from the efforts put forth by the health department and others in recent years. Administrators might use this graph to argue that additional money should not be spent addressing fetal and infant death, but rather should maintain the status quo, since the pattern has bottomed out. This would be a misinterpretation. Looking closely at the X-axis, an evaluator would see that the spacing of five-year intervals between 1930 and 1975 is the same as the spacing of one-year intervals between 1975 and 1980. An accurately drawn figure would show the 1980 data in the spot where the 1976 data appear. Completing the curve on that scale demonstrates a continued downward trend not inconsistent with the prior data. The mislabeled plot of 1976–80 demonstrates the variability in the yearly rates and gives the appearance of a change in the rate of decline, but this is a visual change rather than a mathematical one.

DESCRIPTIVE STATISTICS

Many of the techniques we describe in this chapter we assume are familiar to you. We will highlight them without elaborate discussion and provide a laundry list of tools that you can use in various circumstances. Our goal is to try to motivate you to use more of the tools in specific circumstances, not to provide a detailed understanding of these statistical tools. For readers lacking an understanding of the tools provided, we recommend any elementary statistics book.

Summary Counts

Program data have attributes that can be summarized in several ways. Frequency data constitute one of the most common summaries found in program analyses. Many interventions are designed to bring people into programs, keep them in the programs, and encourage them to take certain actions. Each of these purposes lends itself to measurement of the number of individuals who take a particular action. This counting, often called *pigeon counting*, is a descriptive statistic that represents the volume in a program. Although numbers of people attending represent achievements, it is important to count nonusers as well as users. Count data frequently appear that attest to the success of a program without giving any notion of the eligible population pool. Lack of descriptive information about the available population gives an inadequate summary for count data. Techniques for count data are described later in the chapter. Analytical techniques to assess differences among various subgroups of count data for certain program decisions are discussed below. However, major issues with count data are whether the counts are adequate and whether they meet the purposes of the evaluation.

Summary Location (Central Tendency) Measures

Continuous data commonly measured as part of community health programs include blood pressure, income, improvement in cognitive score, and baseline score on a behavioral questionnaire. Two useful summary indicators in describing such information are a measure of summary location (central tendency) and a measure of spread or variation. The concept of a summary location measure is the familiar representation of numerous situations by a single experience, a sort of average of what happened. Measures of location, often called *averages*, are the mean, the median, and the mode.

Mean. The mean is the arithmetic average for a series of observations. It is the sum of the observations divided by the sample size:

Important Formula: Mean

$$\bar{x} = \frac{\sum\limits_{i=1}^{n} x_i}{n}$$

This formula uses several important notations. The bar (–) above the x is used almost uniformly to represent a sample mean. The Σ is a standard symbol to represent the addition of a series of numbers. The numbers are represented by the subscripted letters x_i, and the notation $i = 1$ indicates that x_1 corresponds to the first number, x_2 to the second, etc. The letter chosen is arbitrary; it could be y_i, z_i, or any other letter of your choosing. Thus:

$$\sum_{i=1}^{3} x_i = x_1 + x_2 + x_3$$

If we had 200 numbers, then:

$$\sum_{i=1}^{200} x_i = x_1 + x_2 + \ldots + x_{200}$$

The notation $+ \ldots +$ means to continue adding in sequence until x_{200}.

Consider the diastolic blood pressures shown in table 8.2. The mean of these blood pressures is:

$$\bar{x} = \frac{\sum\limits_{i=1}^{20} x_i}{20} = \frac{62 + 93 + 73 + 60 + \ldots + 76}{20} = \frac{1514}{20} = 75.70$$

This implies that the average diastolic blood pressure value is 75.70 mm Hg. This mean value may or may not be equal to the true value; you rarely will measure everyone to determine it exactly. Usually there is only a subset, a sample, from which you estimate the mean. A statistical convention is to use Greek alphabet letters for true values and Latin alphabet letters for estimates, i.e., μ and $\bar{x}$ for the true mean and sample mean, respectively.

The arithmetic mean is the point where, if the data were placed on a number line, you could pick up that number line and have it balance. It is the equivalent of a fulcrum for a teeter-totter. The observations are the weights of the individuals sitting on this teeter-totter, and the fulcrum is the mean. The arithmetic mean has a number of very powerful mathematical properties that make it a very common and important measure of central tendency.

For evaluators to talk about the average blood pressure in a community before and after an intervention is an important, reasonable, commonsense descriptor. The mean, however, can suffer certain deficiencies as measure of central tendency. Its major disadvantage is that it is seriously affected by extreme values. For example, suppose you are describing the average income of the individuals who attended a particular meeting. Five individuals were present whose incomes were $34,000, $25,000, $28,000, $30,000, and $74,000. Using the mean as the measure of central tendency, the average income was $38,000. However, only one of the five individuals had an income greater than $38,000. This mean gives an impression of a wealthier group than on the whole was present. The single aberrant income, $74,000, has distorted the representation of this group by the mean.

Median. A measure that is less sensitive to extreme observations is often used as a competitor or in conjunction with the arithmetic average. It is known as the *median* and is defined as the middlemost observation (the 50th percentile). The median is the observation above which half of the observations occur and below which half of the observations occur. It is not as mathematically powerful as the arithmetic average, although there is increasing interest in it among theoretical statisticians, facilitating increased understanding of the median's properties. As a measure of central tendency, the median is unaffected by extremes. Consider the income example: the mean was $38,000, but the median is $30,000. The median is often used for data such as income, cholesterol levels, and glucose levels, where there is *skewness*—a stretching out of the observed results in one direction compared to the other. The mean and median are the same in certain situations, but when skewness is present they are different. This fact can be useful, since a comparison of arithmetic average to the median can identify skewness, which might be important in interpretation and evaluation.

Mode. The last measure of central tendency is called the *mode*. It is the value that occurs most frequently. Sometimes it is important in evaluation to cite the most commonly occurring point. The mode is rarely encountered as a descriptive measure in the scientific literature and almost never is used in statistical procedures, but it does occur in evaluation research. The mode may be used to point out the peak times at a clinic or the most important day of the week in a program or clinic operation. It is frequently used where ordinal or time-dependent data are found.

Measures of Variation

The mean and the median are by themselves or together not sufficient. They do summarize masses of data into a single number which can be presented as a representative value for an entire group. However, as a single figure they do not provide enough information for all situations. Consider the following sets of numbers: 10, 20, 30, 40, 50 and 28, 29, 30, 31, and 32. Both sets of numbers have the same median, 30, and mean, 30. If these were income figures (in thousands of dollars) for two groups and the evaluation report cited the average income of $30,000 for each group, investigators might erroneously surmise on that basis that the two groups were the same. The five people whose incomes range from $10,000 to $50,000 are likely to be far more diverse in background, education, interests, employment, social standing, etc., than the other group of five, which is economically more homogeneous. Although the means and the medians are the same, the actual data on the two groups clearly convey some sense of difference. To accommodate this apparent failure of the location summary statistics, various measures of spread or variation are often used.

Range. The first and the simplest measure of variation is the range, which is defined as the highest value minus the lowest value. Thus, the range for the two income groups would have been $40,000 for the first and $4,000 for the second. Reporting the descriptive statistic of a mean income of $30,000 with a range of $40,000 and a mean income of $30,000 with a range of $4,000 provides clear summary information. The summary represents the differences that appear in the numbers and does so in the simplified form of two statistics.

Although many individuals think that the range consists of the lowest and highest observations, e.g., the range is from 10 to 50 or 28 to 32, technically this is not correct. The range by definition is a measure of spread, the difference between highest and lowest observations. The main drawback to the range is that it is heavily influenced by the extreme values. It has the further drawback of ignoring all the information in the sample except for two observations, whether there are 1,000 individuals or 10 individuals in the sample. This lack of utilization of the data bothered statisticians, and they searched for a measure that could be used to represent a population and utilize all of the data.

Variance and Standard Deviation. The first choice of a measure to replace the range might seem to be the average deviation from the mean. This represents, on average, how far people were from the central value. Following this logic, you would compute the difference between each observation and the overall mean. Then you would add all these differences together and divide by the number of observations to arrive at an average deviation from the mean. This is a very reasonable measure, but it has one drawback: Since the mean is the point at which all the numerical values of the observations balance, it is also the point at which all positive and negative deviations balance, and adding the deviations together must result in zero.

To get around this problem of the average deviation being zero, statisticians use various approaches. If all the deviations are measured in *positive* units and then averaged, this summary measure describes an average deviation. Such a measure ignores whether the deviation is above or below the mean, and it is called the *mean deviation*. The mean deviation has its limitations, in that it takes the absolute value of the deviation, ignoring the sign of the difference. The mathematical problems associated with that approach are numerous.

Another simple solution has been found. You can take the square of the difference between an observation and the mean, add these squared deviations from the mean, and divide the sum of the squares by the sample size. This quantity is an estimate of what is known as the *variance* of a population. Variance is an esoteric term that really means nothing more than the average square deviation from the mean. Certain mathematical properties are present in this quantity that make it an attractive quantity to mathematicians and statisticians.

What becomes confusing to most individuals when using this as a summary statistic is the denominator, which is a little more complicated than simply sample size. Statisticians found that dividing by the sample size produced a variance slightly smaller than they expected. Discussion of this phenomenon can be found in any statistics book. The solution is quite simple, and the common quantity used to estimate the variance is the sum of the squares divided by the sample size minus one.

Important Formula: Sample Variance

$$S^2 = \frac{\sum_{i=1}^{n}(x_i - \bar{x})^2}{(n-1)}$$

Again, consider the blood pressure example of table 8.2. Following the formula exactly we would obtain:

$$S^2 = \frac{\sum_{i=1}^{20}(x_i - \bar{x})^2}{(20-1)} = \frac{\sum_{i=1}^{20}(x_i - 75.70)^2}{19}$$

Remember that $\bar{x}$ was found to be 75.70. Then, continuing to insert the values from the table into the equation:

$$S^2 = \frac{(62 - 75.70)^2 + (93 - 75.70)^2 + \ldots + (76 - 75.70)^2}{19}$$

$$= \frac{(-13.70)^2 + (17.30)^2 + \ldots + (0.30)^2}{19}$$

$$= \frac{187.69 + 299.29 + \ldots + 0.09}{19} = \frac{3436.20}{19} = 180.85$$

Although this formula is correct, it is rather cumbersome. It requires computing the mean first and then the variance. This is also not efficient. Computers and calculators can generate the mean and variance from a single entry of each data item. Using elementary algebra the formula for S^2 can be rewritten as:

Important Formula: Computing Formula for Sample Variance

$$S^2 = \frac{n\sum x_i^2 - (\sum x_i)^2}{n(n-1)}$$

This requires only adding the numbers and adding the numbers squared, yielding the exact same result as the previous formula but in one pass through the data.

A conceptual problem in utilizing the variance is that, for presentation and interpretation purposes, explaining the variance to an audience is a difficult task. For the income examples above, the variance of the five persons with incomes of $10,000 through $50,000 is $250,000,000. This figure is not only overwhelming but also rather incomprehensible in terms of meaning. For the second group, the variance is $200,500,000. The difficulty arises because variance is computed in units squared, and health educators are not trained to think in terms of squared units. Thus, a simple solution, if the units are squared, is to take the square root of the quantity. This gives a number that is in the same unit as the raw information. Taking the square root provides an estimate of the average deviation from the mean obtained from the average squared deviation from the mean. This measure is known as the *standard deviation*. The standard deviation for the income example is $15,811.39 for the first group and $1,581.14 for the second. This measure of variation is now represented in the units of dollars and is interpretable directly in relation to the raw data.

A common way to present results is to give the mean plus or minus the standard deviation. For example, to report the income example, you might show that the average income of the first group was $30,000 ± $15,811.39 and that of the second was $30,000 ± $1,581.14. A rule of thumb for the number of decimal places is that the mean and standard deviation usually carry one decimal place more than the raw data. This is generally done. If you are reporting on blood pressure, therefore, you would talk about a mean of, say, 80.5 mm Hg, since the measurements of blood pressure are in full integers. Income means and deviations are usually given in customary figures, however. A standard deviation of $1,581.1 is not used; one more decimal place, $1,581.14, would be used to match the customary unit, dollars and cents.

Standard Error of the Mean. The literature often reports another quantity, the standard error of the mean (SEM or SE). This is a statistical measure related to the standard deviation and the sample size:

Important Formula: Standard Error of the Mean

$$SE = \frac{S}{\sqrt{n}} = \frac{\sqrt{\sum_{i=1}^{n}(x_i - \bar{x})^2/(n-1)}}{\sqrt{n}} = \sqrt{\frac{\sum_{i=1}^{n}(x_i - \bar{x})^2}{n(n-1)}}$$

Important Formula: Computing Formula for Standard Error

$$SE = \sqrt{\frac{n\sum_{i=1}^{n}x_i^2 - (\sum_{i=1}^{n}x)^2}{n^2(n-1)}}$$

When reading the literature, you must be careful to note whether the author has presented the mean plus or minus the standard error or the mean plus or minus the standard deviation. Vastly different meanings and conclusions can be drawn depending on which of these quantities was used. Certain rules of thumb apply to the mean plus or minus the standard deviation. It is known for some common situations that the mean ± one standard deviation generally encompasses 66⅔ percent of the observations, the mean ± two standard deviations roughly encompasses 95 percent of the observations, and the mean ± three standard deviations encompasses virtually 100 percent of the observations from most unimodal and symmetrical distributions. This approach provides not only a summary measure of location and the overall variability of the population but also where and how far the sample of values extends.

It is important to emphasize what variation is. You must be clear, in an evaluation, that the sources of variation can be identified. Some sources of variation relate directly to the outcome itself. Any one observation will have some deviation from its mean. This is a natural sampling phenomena. Other sources of variation can be measurement effects, testing effects, and even temporal effects. The various sources of variation provide interesting information and insights into the evaluation process. When you gain experience in perceiving means, variances, and standard deviations, your understanding of the extent and potential sources of variability can give you keen insight into programmatic considerations that can be useful in evaluations.

DISTRIBUTIONS

A distribution is a series of counts or measurements. The numbers in a distribution are called *variates*. Frequently the term *distribution* is used to imply a set of measurements, such as the distribution of weights, blood pressures, cholesterol levels, or educational levels. Often the manner of presenting data as a distribution is in an ordered fashion, such as the frequency of measurements of various blood pressures. At other times, the term *distribution* is used as a theoretical concept, what the data would look like ideally if an underlying mathematical model were true. The mathematical representations permit computations of probabilities, average values, and variances. In any mathematical distribution, the sum of all the probabilities equals 1.

Binomial Distribution

In program evaluations, individuals are commonly characterized as successful or unsuccessful. Persons may attend, comply with their medical regimen, not comply, etc. When evaluators look at the total group, they often are interested in characterizing the number of successes and failures. A simplified mathematical model of this is called the *binomial distribution*.

The binomial distribution characterizes situations in which a number (n) of independent attempts or trials are conducted with only two possible outcomes. The outcomes are arbitrarily called *success* and *failure*. For example, suppose you invite five people at random to a health education training program, and the probability (the relative frequency of occurrence) that a person will attend the meeting is 0.60, the same for all persons. You can compute, in advance, the chance that all five persons will attend the program. Using the assumption that each person is independent (i.e., there is no peer pressure to avoid or come), the chance all of them attend is the product of the individual chances:

$$\text{Probability that all will attend} = (0.60)(0.60)(0.60)(0.60)(0.60)$$
$$= 0.078$$

This means that if you were to invite groups of five over and over again, less than 8 out of 100 times would all five show up.

What is the probability that there will be four attenders and one nonattender? In this situation, you must figure out the probability of four successes and one failure taking into account that any one of the five could be the nonattender. The probability of attending is 0.60. The probability of not attending is the sum of all the probabilities (1.0) minus the probability of attending (0.60), or 0.40. Thus:

$$\text{Probability that four will attend and one will not} = \text{the number of}$$
$$\text{different sets of four attenders and one nonattender} \times$$
$$(0.60)(0.60)(0.60)(0.60)(0.40)$$

That is, there are four successes each with a probability of 0.60 and one failure with a probability of 0.40. You must then figure out the number of different combinations of four attenders and one nonattender that there can be. Since choosing any one person leaves four remaining, you might see that there are five combinations. This logic seems easy, since the counting seems obvious. If the number of attempts or trials gets large, however, it is often easier to use a formula to compute the results. A general formula for figuring out the number of combinations of successes (x) and failures (n − x) from n attempts is:

Important Formula: Number of Combinations

$$_nC_x = \frac{n!}{(n - x)!x!}$$

The symbol ! stands for *factorial*. Factorial simply means continued multiplication of integers descending until the integer 1 is reached:

$$n(n - 1)(n - 2) \ldots 1$$

Mathematicians define 0! to be equal to 1.

Consider, for example, the number of combinations of three successes out of five trials. By formula, this would be:

$$_5C_3 = \frac{5!}{(5 - 3)!3!}$$

$$= \frac{5 \cdot 4 \cdot 3 \cdot 2 \cdot 1}{(2 \cdot 1)(3 \cdot 2 \cdot 1)}$$

$$= 10$$

To see this more clearly, label the five persons A, B, C, D, and E. The combinations of three successes and two failures are:

	Successes	Failures
1	ABC	DE
2	ABD	CE
3	ABE	CD
4	ACD	BE
5	ACE	BD
6	ADE	BC
7	BDE	AC
8	BCD	AE
9	BCE	AD
10	CDE	AB

If each of the five persons has the same probability of success, say 0.60 (probability of attending), then the probability of a single combination of three successes and two failures is:

$$(0.60)(0.60)(0.60)(0.40)(0.40) = (0.60)^3(.40)^2$$

To find the total probability of three successes and two failures, you must count all the correct combinations and add the probabilities together. This is the same as multiplying the probability of a single correct combination by the number of combinations:

$$\text{Probability (3 attenders)} = {}_5C_3(0.60)^3(0.40)^2$$
$$= 10(0.60)^3(0.40)^2$$
$$= 0.346$$

Note that the sum of the exponents (3 and 2) is the same as n (5). Another way of writing this would be:

$$(0.60)^3(0.40)^{5-3}$$

That is, if there are three successes, the rest will be failures. In general, if the probability (the relative frequency of occurrence) of success is p, the same for all persons, you can compute in advance the probability that exactly x of the n persons will be successes, using the following formula:

Important Formula: Binomial Distribution

$$P(x \text{ successes}) = ({}_nC_x)p^x(1-p)^{n-x}$$

If the probability of failure $(1-p)$ is represented instead by the letter q, the formula is:

$$P_x = P(x \text{ successes}) = ({}_nC_x)p^x q^{n-x}$$

Often the problem is not simply to find out the probability of exactly x successes but rather the probability of x or more successes. This is easy with the binomial formula because you simply add the successive probabilities:

$$P_x + P_{x+1} + P_{x+2} \ldots P_n$$

For example, the probability of three or more invited persons attending would be the sum of the probabilities of three or four or five persons attending:

$$\sum_{x=3}^{5} {}_5C_x p^x q^{5-x}$$

$$= [{}_5C_3(0.60)^3(0.40)^2] + [{}_5C_4(0.60)^4(0.40)^1] + [{}_5C_5(0.60)^5(0.40)^0]$$
$$= .3456 + .2592 + .0778 = .6826$$

The chance of observing a particular event (or any event less likely than that one), such as x or more successes out of n trials, is called a *p-value*. The p-value has this meaning regardless of the theoretical model. Sometimes it is stated as a *two-sided* p-value. For example, in a binomial distribution, a two-sided p-value would mean the chance of fewer than some number of successes or greater than some number of successes.

When we discussed descriptive statistics, we said a mean was not sufficient. Often a probability is not sufficient. In evaluating a program, you might want to know the average number of attenders. This figure can be obtained because mathematical distributions have these descriptive statistics. The mean or average number of successes from a binomial distribution is the number of attempts (n) times the probability of obtaining a success (p), or np. This is intuitive to most people. If the average quit rate is 25 percent in a smoking cessation program, and the intervention is applied to 100 persons, how many would probably quit? Most people would answer 25. The other descriptive statistic discussed was the variance. The variance is not as intuitive, but it is easy to compute. The variance of a binomial distribution is the number of attempts times the probability of success times the probability of failure (npq). So, if the probability of cessation were 0.25, the mean would be $n(.25)$ and the variance $n(.25)(.75)$. For an n of 100, the mean would be 25 and the variance 18.75.

Poisson Distribution

When using the binomial distribution, if the number of trials (n) is very large and the probability of success (p) is very small, the binomial distribution becomes difficult to compute. Consider an evaluation of a breast self-examination (BSE) program to detect early cancers. The relatively low incidence of breast cancer may involve tedious computations using the binomial distribution. Suppose the probability of finding a cancer using BSE is 1 in 1,000 or .001. If 2,000 women are screened, what is the probability that three or fewer cases of cancer will be detected? Using the binomial distribution, this would be the sum of the probabilities of detecting 0, 1, 2, and 3 cases:

$$\text{Probability (0 cases)} = 2{,}000^C{}_0 (0.001)^0 (0.999)^{2000} = 0.135$$
$$\text{Probability (1 case)} = 2{,}000^C{}_1 (0.001)^1 (0.999)^{1999} = 0.271$$
$$\text{Probability (2 cases)} = 2{,}000^C{}_2 (0.001)^2 (0.999)^{1998} = 0.271$$
$$\text{Probability (3 cases)} = 2{,}000^C{}_3 (0.001)^3 (0.999)^{1997} = 0.181$$

Computing $(0.999)^{2000}$ etc. can be tedious even with modern calculators. The overall probability of detecting three or fewer cases is 0.858

If we were doing this for the state of Alabama, the number of trials would exceed 3,000,000, but even the exact n is not known.

Mathematicians have found that a formula can be derived that does not depend explicitly on the actual number of trials. This form or distribution assumes that the number is so large that a mathematical constant can be used to summarize the series of multiplications. This distribution is known as the *Poisson*. It is the distribution that results from increasing the number of trials and assuming that the probability of success becomes small. The expression used to calculate the probability of x successes is:

Important Formula: Poisson Distribution

$$P \,(x \text{ successes}) = \frac{e^{-\lambda}\lambda^x}{x!}$$

where $\lambda = np$, the mean number of
successes
e = a mathematical constant, 2.71828
x = the desired number of successes

Consider the BSE screening example. Using this formula, the probability of detecting 0, 1, 2, and 3 cases is a function of λ (or np). In this example:

$$n = 2,000$$
$$p = 0.001$$

Thus:

$$\lambda = 2,000 \,(0.001) \doteq 2$$

In many instances, you do not know n or p exactly. However, you might have tumor registry data that say for a particular time period on average 2 cases or 2.5 cases are detected. These "numerator" data can be used as your estimate of λ. They are very valuable in many community programs where denominator data (the potential target populations) are not explicitly known. Using $\lambda = 2$, you can now find the probabilities:

$$\text{Probability (0 cases)} = \frac{e^{-\lambda}\lambda^x}{x!}$$

$$= \frac{e^{-2}2^0}{0!}$$

$$= \frac{(0.135)(1)}{1}$$

$$= 0.135$$

Probability (1 case) $= \frac{e^{-2}2^1}{1!}$

$$= \frac{(0.135)(2)}{1}$$

$$= 0.271$$

Probability (2 cases) $= \frac{e^{-2}2^2}{2!}$

$$= \frac{(0.135)(4)}{2}$$

$$= 0.271$$

Probability (3 cases) $= \frac{e^{-2}2^3}{3!}$

$$= \frac{(0.135)(8)}{6}$$

$$= 0.180$$

Thus, the probability of three or fewer cases is the sum of these probabilities (0.135 + 0.271 + 0.271 + 0.180) or 0.857. This is quite close to the actual binomial computation of 0.858. The small difference between the two probabilities is from the Poisson assumption of an infinite population; although 2,000 is a large population, it is not infinite.

Consider another example. Suppose that the average number of encephalitis cases in a large community has been two per year. With the cutback in federal funds, spraying for mosquitoes has been substantially reduced. The director of the health department is concerned and wants you to institute a health education program aimed at citizen control and awareness. Six months later she returns to say that your program was obviously not effective, since there were twice as many cases as on average in the past. Using the Poisson distribution, you can compute the probability (p-value) of four or more cases occurring if the mean (λ) were truly two. This would be the sum over all the population of four, five, six, and so on, cases. Mathematically, you would use summation notation and write:

$$P \text{ (4 or more cases)} = \sum_{x=4}^{n} \frac{e^{-2}2^x}{x!}$$

However, remember that n is very large, and this would be quite a bit of computation. If you obtain the probability of fewer than four cases arising, 1 minus that probability must be the probability of four or more cases arising. (This "trick" of finding the complementary event is widely used in statistics.)

$$P \text{ (4 or more)} = 1 - P \text{ (fewer than 4)} = 1 - \left(\sum_{x=0}^{3} \frac{e^{-2}2^x}{x!} \right)$$

$$P \text{ } (x = 0) = \frac{e^{-2}2^0}{0!} = 0.135$$

$$P \text{ } (x = 1) = \frac{e^{-2}2^1}{1!} = 0.271$$

$$P \text{ } (x = 2) = \frac{e^{-2}2^2}{2!} = 0.271$$

$$P \text{ } (x = 3) = \frac{e^{-2}2^3}{3!} = 0.180$$

$$\begin{aligned} P \text{ (fewer than 4)} &= 0.135 + 0.271 + 0.271 + 0.180 \\ &= 0.857 \end{aligned}$$

$$P \text{ (4 or more)} = 1 - 0.857 = 0.143$$

Given this probability or p-value, you can assess the director's statement. After these calculations, you mention to the director that, although you do share some concern about the effectiveness of your program, if the average number of cases had not changed, you would expect four or more cases to arise about 14 times out of 100. Although four cases is a higher incidence than you wish, it can occur somewhat frequently by chance variation alone rather than simply because of a program failure.

The Poisson distribution has further properties that make it very useful in program evaluation. With the binomial distribution, not only the mean but also the variance depended on n and p. The Poisson distribution has the very useful property that the mean and the variance are the same. That is, the mean equals λ and so does the variance. This can be illustrated with an example. As we noted, the Poisson is the result of a binomial when n is very large and p is very small. Suppose n is 1,000,000 and p is .0001, then the binomial mean and variance are:

$$\text{Mean} = np = 1,000,000 \,(.0001) = 100$$
$$\text{Variance} = npq = 1,000,000 \,(.0001)(.9999) = 99.99$$

If n were increased to 10,000,000, the mean would be 1,000 and the binomial variance 999.9. Increasing n would eventually make the mean and variance equal for all practical purposes. This is a very valuable asset, since it gives an estimate of the mean and variance for program planning from numerator data alone.

Normal Distribution

The normal distribution or Gaussian distribution is so commonly used that its complexity (as seen in the formula below) has long been overcome by the utility of the curve. Health educators have encountered this curve in discussions of IQs or grading on a curve or any other instance of the familiar bell-shaped curve. One reason for wide usage of the normal distribution is a remarkable mathematical theorem called the *central limit theorem*, which states that, for most situations in the real world, if you take a random sample of observations, compute the sample mean, and repeat the process over and over, the distribution of the means of the samples will be a normal distribution irrespective of the shape of the distribution of the original observations. The variance would be the standard error of the mean discussed briefly above.

The density function of the normal distribution is:

$$f(x) = [1/(\sigma\sqrt{2\pi})]e^{-(x - \mu)^2/(2\sigma^2)}$$

where e = the exponential constant 2.71828
x = the random variable of interest
σ = the standard deviation
μ = the mean

The way probabilities are generated is by integrating (a calculus concept) the area under particular portions of the curve. This would require tedious computations and a knowledge of calculus except for a simple relationship with what is called a *z-score*. A z-score is nothing more than the number of standard deviation units above or below the mean. Any normal distribution can be transformed into a standard normal distribution, which is the distribution of z-scores. This standardizing is accomplished by subtracting the mean and then dividing by the standard deviation:

Important Formula: z-Score

$$z = \frac{x - \mu}{\sigma}$$

This standard normal deviate z can be compared to a universal table based on standard deviation units from the mean irrespective of the underlying data.

Suppose you know that the mean induration of a TB skin test is 1 cm in a healthy population, with a standard deviation of 0.5 cm. The z-score associated with an induration of 2 cm is:

$$z = \frac{2 - 1}{0.5} = \frac{1}{0.5} = 2$$

The value of z, 2, can be compared to a standard normal table to obtain the probability of any observations two standard deviations or more above the mean. The table shows this probability as 0.02275. Thus, if the critical value of 2 cm induration is used to identify persons for further follow-up, we would expect 2.275 percent to be false positives, given that induration in a healthy population is normally distributed with a mean of 1 cm and a standard deviation of 0.5.

The normal distribution has certain values commonly used.

$z = 0.845 \rightarrow$ corresponds to the 80th percentile

$z = 1.645 \rightarrow$ corresponds to the 95th percentile

$z = 1.96 \rightarrow$ corresponds to the 97.5th percentile

$z = 2.328 \rightarrow$ corresponds to the 99th percentile

90 percent of all observations yield z-scores between -1.645 and 1.645

95 percent of all observations yield z-scores between -1.96 and 1.96

99 percent of all observations yield z-scores between -2.576 and 2.576

These values are frequently used to judge the significance of differences in evaluation research and are found by computing z-scores and comparing them to standard normal tables. Examples of this process are illustrated in the section on Student's t-distribution later in this chapter.

Normal Approximate to the Binomial Distribution

The normal distribution is used as an approximation to other distributions. It is frequently used in evaluation research to approximate a binomial or Poisson distribution to further save on computations. When the sample size or number of successes is large, computation of the factorials needed in the Poisson and binomial distributions becomes rather tedious. To avoid this problem, evaluators use the normal distribution. They are allowed to use it because of the central limit theorem noted above. When computing the probability of x successes out of n trials with a probability of success p, convert this to a z-score, or so-called normal approximation to the binomial, by subtracting the mean, np, and dividing by the standard deviation, $\sqrt{npq}$. Thus, a normal approximation to the number of x or more successes can be found by finding:

$$z = \frac{x - np}{\sqrt{npq}}$$

For example, if you wish to know the probability that 100 or more people will show up at a meeting out of 150 invited, use the probability of their attendance, p, and compute a z-score. If p is 0.40:

$$z \geq \frac{(100) - (150)(0.40)}{\sqrt{(150)(0.40)(0.60)}} = \frac{10}{\sqrt{36}} = \frac{10}{6} = 1.67$$

$$z \geq 1.67$$

Using a standard normal table, you find the corresponding probability of 100 or more successes, which is 0.047.

Similarly, you can approximate a Poisson with a normal distribution. You standardize the variables in the same manner. First, subtract the mean and divide by the appropriate standard deviation. For a Poisson distribution, the mean and variance are λ. Thus:

$$z = \frac{x - \lambda}{\sqrt{\lambda}}$$

Suppose, as the evaluator for a state agency, you find 280 encephalitis cases, when the past data show an average of 250. The question is whether an educational intervention aimed at getting the public to spray for mosquitoes is needed. If there is an indication of an epidemic, such a program would be worthwhile. However, the effort and expense are not trivial. Before you claim that an epidemic exists, you would like to know the probability of 280 or more cases arising when the usual experience is 250. For this you compute a z-score based on a Poisson distribution approximated by a normal distribution. Since λ is 250:

$$z = \frac{(280 - 250)}{\sqrt{250}} = \frac{30}{15.81} = 1.91$$

The probability, using the standard tables, is 0.029 or 29 times out of 1,000. This means that, if the average is really 250, only 29 times out of 1,000 would you expect 280 or more cases to arise. From this, you conclude that a problem exists and begin your education program.

Student's t-Distribution

The normal distribution works well for numerous situations especially when the sample size is large. Many situations in health evaluation involve only small samples, however. It is then unreasonable to assume that σ, the true standard deviation, is known. This is an assumption of the normal distribution above. When n is large, the differences are not great, but for a small n, differences arise when σ is unknown. What is commonly done is to use s, the sample estimate of σ in the computation of the z-score. When this is done, a true z-score is not obtained; rather, a closely related score called *Student's t-score* or simply *t-score* is obtained. The t-score comes from a distribution of scores just as the t-score relates to the normal distribution. The t-distribution is virtually indistinguishable from the normal distribution when the sample size is over 100. The t-distribution has been tabulated, but it requires another parameter (population or fixed constant) besides the mean (μ) and the variance (σ^2), which are all that are necessary for the normal distribution. The t-distribution depends on n, the sample size, whereas the normal does not. This is because the reliability of the estimate of the variance improves as the sample size increases. This dependence is described in terms of $n - 1$, referred to as *degrees of freedom* (d.f.)! The smaller the value of $n - 1$, the greater the variability. The t-distribution probably should be more widely utilized than it is. The use of the t-score is nearly identical to the z-score, the only difference being in the table used to obtain the probabilities after that score is computed.

When you want to know if a mean is different from some hypothesized value, you can use a test based on z-scores or t-scores. The test derived from the t-distribution is the well-known *t-test*, a statistical test used to compare a single value to a hypothesized value.

Important Formula: t-Score for a Sample Mean

$$t = \frac{\bar{x} - \mu}{s/\sqrt{n}}$$

where $\bar{x}$ = the sample mean
  μ = the hypothesized true mean
  s = the estimated standard deviation, $\sum_{i=1}^{n} \frac{(x_i - \bar{x})^2}{(n-1)}$
  n = the sample size
  $s/\sqrt{n}$ = the sample standard error (of the mean)

This t-score is compared to the table value of the theoretical t-distribution with the parameter of $(n - 1)$ degrees of freedom. A value of t less than the lower critical value or above the upper critical value would be an indication that the result obtained occurs so infrequently by chance variation alone that you can reject the supposition that the sample was drawn from a normal distribution with mean μ.

Suppose you are trying to reach young black males with a blood pressure screening program in hopes of reducing the high morbidity and mortality rates that appear to be associated with untreated high blood pressure among black males. As a health educator, you design a multimedia message campaign to increase utilization of the community health clinics. From past data you find that the average age of black males screened has consistently been around 50 years old. The messages are designed to reach the under-40 group, and, after three months of operation, you ask: Is it working? One simple measure is to test whether the average age is lower. Although not a thorough evaluation, this test would provide a simple and quick indicator of success because, if more young men came in to be screened, the average age would have declined. The numbers are collected, and the results are that the mean age of black males screened in the three months of the program was 38.1 years with a standard deviation of 12.5 years. The total number of black males screened was 72. Is this evidence of success or could it have happened by chance?

The average age is lower, indicating the direction you anticipated. However, you do not know how likely the result is from mere chance. If the true average age were 40, 50 percent of the time you would observe a random sample less than 40 years of age and 50 percent of the time a random sample over 40 years of age. Thus, you might say you had a 50/50 chance of supporting your program's effectiveness even if no change occurred. This is due to sampling fluctuations. However, you can assess the *statistical significance* of this result using the t-test. Here, the t-score is:

$$t = \frac{\bar{x} - \mu}{s/\sqrt{n}}$$

$$= \frac{38.1 - 40}{12.5/\sqrt{72}}$$

$$= \frac{-1.9}{1.47} = -1.29$$

Remember, you are seeing if the mean age observed differs from 40 years, which is assumed to be a fixed quantity. The negative sign indicates the observed mean is less than that hypothesized. This result is compared to the lower end of the t-distribution (implicitly, since the actual table values are identical for the positive and negative sides and all tables are given in positive values only). You look at the table value with $n - 1$ degrees of freedom, that is, 71 degrees of freedom, and you find that the probability of observing a sample mean of 38.1 years *if* there had been no change in the true mean of 40 is about 1 out of 10. This gives you some encouragement that the program is working. The result is considered borderline significant. You need more analyses to pinpoint the success. A p-value of 10 percent or less is all right for pilot data.

The t-test can be used for other testing than the sample's mean. Frequently evaluators use this test to compare two means as follows:

Important Formula: t-Test for Two Groups

$$t = \frac{(\bar{x}_1 - \bar{x}_2) - (\mu_1 - \mu_2)}{\sqrt{(s_1^2/n_1) + (s_2^2/n_2)}}$$

where $\bar{x}_1$ and $\bar{x}_2$ = the means of samples 1 and 2, respectively
μ_1 and μ_2 = the respective hypothesized true means (if you
  are testing for equality of these, $\mu_1 - \mu_2 = 0$)
s_1^2 and s_2^2 = the respective sample variances
n_1 and n_2 = the respective sample sizes

This test statistic has approximately $n_1 + n_2 - 2$ degrees of freedom.

Consider a study of the effectiveness of an intervention to improve pill taking among hypertensive patients. Before implementing the intervention in all of the community health centers, you carry out a pilot study. In this pilot, you randomly allocate 25 newly identified hypertensives either to a three-arm intervention including diaries, education, and home blood pressure monitoring or to no intervention beyond medical care. Three months later, you measure compliance through pill counts of each individual. The data in table 8.4 are obtained. If you are attempting to see whether the pilot data support your intervention's effectiveness, the hypothesis you are testing is that there is no difference between the two. Thus, if you can show that the observed difference is unlikely to be a chance occurrence, i.e., if it has a small p-value, the effectiveness is shown and called *significant*. From table 8.4, you learn that the mean compliance index for the intervention group after three months is 83.5 and for the control group it is 80.9. Although the difference is in the direction of your supposition, the t-test is needed to tell you the statistical significance. Only this knowledge tells you the "real world" importance of the numerical difference. The t-test can be computed. Since you are assuming no difference, and testing the likelihood that your observed difference is due to chance alone, $\mu_1 - \mu_2 = 0$. The sample variances 93.6 and 100.1 are computed and shown in table 8.4.

$$t = \frac{(\bar{x}_1 - \bar{x}_2) - (\mu_1 - \mu_2)}{\sqrt{(s_1^2/n_1) + (s_2^2/n_2)}}$$

$$= \frac{(83.5 - 80.9) - (0)}{\sqrt{(93.6/13) + (100.1/12)}}$$

$$= \frac{2.6}{\sqrt{15.5}} = 0.66$$

This quantity, $t = 0.67$, is then compared to tables of student's t-distribution with $n_1 + n_2 - 2$ (in this case, $12 + 13 - 2 = 23$) degrees of freedom. The tables show that the probability of this result occurring by chance alone is greater than one out of four ($p > 0.25$). This suggests that the result is somewhat likely to occur by chance, and, even though it is in the direction of your beliefs, there is not sufficient statistical evidence to say that the intervention group differs from the control.

The t-test for two groups assumes independent samples. Often, pairing of outcomes occurs, such as pretest and post-test outcomes on the same person. This pairing violates the independence assumption; for example, a pulse taken on the same person by two methods is more likely to agree with itself than a pulse taken on one person by

Table 8.4 Compliance Index Based on Pill Counts Related to
Medical Therapy Three Months Postintervention

Intervention Group (n = 13)	Control Group (n = 12)
90	92
88	84
96	99
72	75
71	68
92	76
81	85
63	67
84	85
87	91
91	73
90	76
81	
$\Sigma x_{i1} = 1086$	$\Sigma x_{i2} = 971$
$\Sigma x_{i1}^2 = 91846$	$\Sigma x_{i2}^2 = 79671$
$\bar{x}_1 = 83.5$	$\bar{x}_2 = 80.9$
$s_1^2 = 93.6$	$s_2^2 = 100.1$

one method and on another person by the other method. To get
around this problem, evaluators use a so-called *paired t-test*, which is:

Important Formula: Paired t-Test

$$t = \frac{\bar{d} - \delta}{s_d/\sqrt{n}}$$

where $\bar{d}$ = the average difference of the n pairs of data
  δ = the hypothesized true average difference, often assumed
    to be zero
  s_d = the standard deviation of the differences over the pairs
  n = the number of pairs

This statistic is now the same as a single sample t-test. It makes
inferences about the sample of differences between the n pairs. This
is compared to a theoretical t-distribution with $n - 1$ degrees of
freedom.

Table 8.5   Pretest and Post-test Scores for Knowledge, Attitudes, and Beliefs about Cancer Screening, Diagnosis, and Treatment

Participant	Pretest	Post-test	Change (Difference)
1	53	64	11
2	38	50	12
3	87	94	7
4	72	74	2
5	56	68	12
6	74	78	4
7	62	68	6
8	66	66	0
9	70	70	0
10	48	52	4
11	82	78	−4
12	68	72	4
	$X_{pre} = 64.7$	$X_{post} = 69.5$	$\bar{d} = 4.8$
	$S_{pre} = 14.1$	$S_{post} = 11.7$	$s_d = 5.1$

Suppose you implement a cancer prevention program. The first group attending the program is to be evaluated using a pretest and post-test of knowledge, attitudes, and beliefs about cancer screening, diagnosis, and treatment. You obtain a valid and reliable instrument to use in testing the participants. The scores are those shown in table 8.5. The average pretest score is 64.7, compared to the average post-test score of 69.5. The average difference is 4.8 units higher. Note that the average difference is the difference between the averages. This is always true; what changes is the standard deviation. The standard deviations on the pretest and post-test scores are both larger than the standard deviation of the differences. This is indicative of the benefit of pairing. To test whether your intervention has been successful in raising the scores, you carry out a paired t-test on the 12 pairs (note that δ is assumed to be zero—that is, on average, zero improvement in the scores):

$$t = \frac{\bar{d} - \delta}{s_d/\sqrt{n}}$$

$$= \frac{4.8 - 0}{5.1/\sqrt{12}} = \frac{4.8}{1.47} = 3.26$$

The value, 3.26, is compared with tables of the student's t-distribution with $n - 1$ (or 11) degrees of freedom. The tables show that the result obtained would occur by chance less than one time in one hundred, indicating that it is unlikely to be a chance result. The result is considered statistically significant, demonstrating the effectiveness of the education program in changing knowledge, attitudes, and beliefs.

Chi-Square Distribution

The chi-square distribution is used in testing hypotheses that a sample of data arises from a completely specified distribution. This might test whether a sample could have arisen from a normal distribution. Another use is in testing for associations through specification of probability rules.

Use of the chi-square distribution is relatively straightforward. The following six steps summarize the process:

1. Arbitrarily set intervals covering the range of data for one or more variables
2. Count the number of observations in each interval or class
3. Calculate the probability for each interval based on the hypothesized distribution
4. Calculate the expected number in each interval by multiplying the probability times the total sample size
5. Calculate the chi-square statistic
6. Calculate the significance level or p-value by comparing the results to the upper area of the chi-square distribution

Evaluators are likely to use the chi-square to test whether characteristics could be considered to behave independently of one another in a probability sense. The alternative is that the two characteristics behave dependently, that is, the frequency of one characteristic's occurrence is altered on the basis of the other characteristic's occurrence. More detail of this theory can be found in any statistics book; here it can be summarized as follows: If two characteristics that can occur together behave independently, the probability of both occurring, that is, P(AB), is equal to the probability of one occurring, P(A), times the probability of the other occurring, P(B). For example, the probability of drawing the jack of hearts from a deck of 52 cards is 1/52, since there is only one jack of hearts. However, since suits and numbers can be considered independent characteristics (i.e., there is the same number in each suit) we can apply the basic probability rule. A jack occurs 4 times out of 52 and a heart 13 times out of 52. Thus:

$$P(AB) = P(A) \cdot P(B)$$
$$P \text{ (jack of hearts)} = P \text{ (jack)} \cdot P \text{ (heart)}$$
$$= (4/52)(13/52) = 52/(52 \cdot 52) = 1/52$$

This probability statement is the basis for the chi-square test.

The general formula for a chi-square statistic for a table with r rows and c columns is:

Important Formula: Chi-Square Statistic

$$\chi^2 = \sum_{i=1}^{r} \sum_{j=1}^{c} \frac{(O_{ij} - E_{ij})^2}{E_{ij}}$$

where E_{ij} = the expected frequency in the cell of row i and column j; this expected frequency is usually obtained from the assumption that the element of the cell arises from the independent application of the row probability times the column probability

O_{ij} = the observed frequency in the cell of row i and column j

The statistic has $(r - 1)(c - 1)$ degrees of freedom. The larger the discrepancy between the observed and expected frequencies, the less likely the independence assumption would be. However, if you obtain a frequency of 20 and you expected 10, the difference is 10; if you obtain 200 and you expected 190, the difference is again 10. Intuitively, 200 seems closer to 190 than 20 does to 10. To accommodate this notion, the squared deviation is divided by the number expected. Thus $(20 - 10)^2/10$ yields a contribution to the chi-square statistic of $100/10 = 10$, whereas $(200 - 190)^2/190 = 100/190 = 0.526$.

A computing formula for the chi-square eliminates the need to calculate each expected frequency to yield the overall summary statistic:

Important Formula: Computing Formula for Chi-Square

$$\chi^2 = N \left(\sum_{i=1}^{r} \sum_{j=1}^{c} O_{ij}^2/O_{i.}O_{.j} \right) - N$$

where N = the total number in the table
O_{ij} = the frequency of the cell in row i and column j

$O_{i\cdot} = \sum_{i=1}^{c} O_{ij}$, the row total of row i

$O_{\cdot j} = \sum_{i=1}^{r} O_{ij}$ the column total of column j

r = the number of rows
c = the number of columns

The degree of freedom is the parameter of the chi-square distribution that enables comparison of the computed statistic (also called the *test statistic*) to the percentiles of a theoretical frequency curve. When the chi-square value exceeds the critical value (that percentile above which you would reject the hypothesis of independence), the result is said to demonstrate a significant association.

Suppose the staff of a blood pressure screening program is concerned about the effects of referrals on the kinds of persons utilizing the resource. Since females tend to be seen more frequently than males by physicians, the staff is concerned that differences by sex may occur in whether patients follow referral guidelines. Records are kept of all referrals and, six weeks after the initial referral, patients who have not returned a card documenting a physician's visit are called. The caller elicits information on what happened and then classifies the patient's status as refused, referral pending, or successfully referred. The number of persons completing six weeks of follow-up is 130. The results are categorized by sex as shown in table 8.6. To assess whether males are different from females in following the referrals, a chi-square statistic can be computed. This chi-square would test the independence of sex and referral class, in a probability sense. A significant chi-square would indicate that the row variable, sex, is not independent of the column variable, referral class, implying the sex difference. Applying the computing formula to this example:

$$\chi^2 = N(\sum_i \sum_j O_{ij}^2 / O_{i\cdot} O_{\cdot j}) - N$$
$$= 130[(10^2/76{\cdot}14) + 38^2/76{\cdot}54) + (28^2/76{\cdot}62) + (4^2/54{\cdot}14)$$
$$+ (16^2/54{\cdot}54) + (34^2/54{\cdot}62)] - 130$$
$$= 130(1.06646) - 130$$
$$= 138.64 - 130$$
$$= 8.64$$

This statistic of 8.64 is compared to table values of the chi-square distribution with $(r-1)(c-1)$ degrees of freedom, in this case

Table 8.6 Referral Status of Potential Hypertensives by Sex Six Weeks after Referral

Sex	Refused	Referral Pending	Successfully Referred	Total
Male	10	38	28	76
Female	4	16	34	54
Total	14	54	62	130

$(2 - 1)(3 - 1) = 2$. The probability of observing a chi-square value of 8.54 or greater under the model of statistical independence is less than .013. This low probability indicates the lack of independence between sex and referral. This statistic does not tell which group follows the referral guidelines better; the program staff must return to the actual data to find the direction of the difference. The proportion of males successfully referred is 36.8 percent (28 out of 76) compared to 63.0 percent (34 out of 54) for females. Thus, the staff can conclude that females have a statistically significant difference over males in achieving referral.

F-Distribution

The F-statistic arises from the ratio of two chi-square statistics, usually a variance estimate. Its most common use in evaluation research is in two techniques called *regression analysis* and *analysis of variance*. The F-distribution, a frequency distribution of F-statistics, requires two parameters, the degrees of freedom associated with the estimated variance of the numerator of the statistic and the degrees of freedom associated with the denominator. Commonly, the test or statistic involves the ratio of an estimate of variance between groups (called the *mean square between groups* or *MS between*), and the variance within groups (also called the *MS within* or *mean square error*). Frequently, this statistic takes the form:

$$F = \frac{MS\ between}{MS\ within}$$

with $(k - 1)$ and $(n - k)$ degrees of freedom
where k = the number of groups
n = the sample size

From a regression analysis it takes the form:

$$F = \frac{MS \text{ regression}}{MS \text{ residual}}$$

with k and $(n - k - 1)$ degrees of freedom
where the regression is a linear regression equation

The F-distribution requires more background to motivate the understanding of its use, but such a discussion is beyond the intent of this chapter. Simply, when the variances are equal the ratio should be 1.0. The F-test provides a statement regarding the probability of the observed statistic occurring by chance. How likely is it that the observed ratio is this large compared to 1.0 merely by chance? The value of 1.0 indicates that the variation within groups equals the variation between groups. In other words, there is no difference between the levels of the independent variables. In regression analysis, if the F-statistic is significant, you can conclude that using these independent variables will help you predict or estimate the response or dependent variable. For example, age is important in predicting blood pressure. The variation in blood pressure within a group of 30-year-old persons is smaller than the variation among persons 30 to 60 years old.

Similarly, in analysis of variance, if the F-statistic exceeds 1.0, this indicates that the deviation within a treatment group is less than the deviation between two treatments. For example, if you measure diastolic blood pressure in patients of low, medium, and high socioeconomic status, a significant F-statistic would indicate that average blood pressure differed by socioeconomic status.

ANALYTICAL METHODS AND APPROACHES

When deciding upon appropriate analytical tools for evaluation research, the first major operational decision is choosing a design and, by virtue of that choice, a particular analysis. Will the study involve a single group, two groups, or multiple groups? Although this may seem like an obvious and rather simplistic categorization of studies, it becomes exceedingly critical in the interpretation and understanding provided by the evaluation.

Single-Group Designs

The simplest form of single-group design is a prevalence survey. These studies ascertain the characteristics of a population—attitudes, beliefs, physical characteristics, etc.—at a single point in time. Prevalence surveys may be formally designed cross-sectional surveys, telephone surveys, household interview surveys, convenience samples, clinical samples, etc. The prevalence survey is an important design to evaluators because it can be the basis for a program intervention. Too often information from cross-sectional surveys is not used in understanding a problem. Testimonials and experiences of others are used for the needs assessment of a particular program, especially for nationwide problems. This can lead to the development of under- or overutilized programs, because the planners failed to understand the local setting.

A variety of analyses can be applied in a cross-sectional design. The majority were described above in the sections on display techniques and descriptive statistics. Often, however, it is necessary to go beyond the descriptive statistics in a design and ascertain relationships of various characteristics within the cross-sectional survey. There are two primary methods for doing this.

Chi-Square Test of Association. The first method is use of a chi-square statistic to assess whether two characteristics behave independently of one another or are related. For example, in a smoking-cessation program, the evaluation has focused on identifying the types of individuals who successfully complete the program. Suppose that success is defined as cessation one month following the intervention. Shown in table 8.7 are hypothetical data for 625 individuals enrolled in the program. After one month, 290 were classed as successful and 335 as unsuccessful in their attempts to quit smoking. Of the 625, 158 were single, 226 married, etc. Overall, 46.4 percent stopped smoking. The question arises, is marital status independent of the ability to quit smoking as represented by the population of this smoking-cessation program? In a statistical sense, the program evaluators want to know whether the probability of quitting is different

Table 8.7 Smoking-Cessation Results by Marital Status

Cessation Result	Marital Status					
	Single	Married	Separated	Divorced	Widowed	Total
Successful	68	89	19	101	13	290
Unsuccessful	90	137	16	79	13	335
Total	158	226	352	180	26	625

$\chi^2 = 13.03$ with 4 degrees of freedom
$p = 0.011$

for people who are single, married, separated, widowed, or divorced. Is the program more successful in some marital groups than others?

Although the chi-square test will not tell which category appears to be different, the evaluators can compute the chi-square statistic for an overall test of any association. When this is done for these data, the chi-square value of 13.03 is obtained with $(r - 1)(c - 1)$ degrees of freedom, r being the number of rows (2), and c being the number of columns (5). Thus, this is a chi-square statistic with 4 degrees of freedom. Looking this up in a table, the evaluators find that the p-value is 0.011. That is, 98.9 percent of all computed chi-square statistics with four degrees of freedom would obtain values below 13.03, if the null hypothesis were true. This suggests a lack of independence between marital status and success in quitting smoking.

Although this illustrates the utility of the chi-square test of association in a single-group situation, it does not indicate or imply the existence of a *causative* relationship between these characteristics. Evaluators must then ask themselves: What is this overall test of significance measuring? Since smoking-cessation programs do not obtain a random sample of participants, the meaning of this statistical test must be considered in a dual context. First, what possible selection biases could be operating to bring in people of different marital categories? Which of these might be associated with their motivation to quit? The chi-square statistic could be measuring a lack of independence induced by the selection of people who come into the program, their motivations for coming, and their ability to quit, rather than the effects of the program. Once the concerns of the first question are satisfied, a second question can be asked: Is there something in the message or the program being implemented that works selectively? For example, divorced persons seem to have better success rates than the other categories, and separated individuals might also have better success rates. If the program gives heavy emphasis to family support for quitting smoking, this finding might indicate program deficiencies rather than strengths. Of course, far more analyses are necessary to establish the link between the finding and its importance, but the chi-square statistic provides an initial indicator of areas worthy of subsequent analyses.

Correlation Coefficients. A second common method of analysis for assessing relationships in single-group studies is a correlation coefficient; often, the Pearson Product Moment Correlation Coefficient is used. This coefficient is used only for variables considered to be continuous, such as age, IQ, and other measured responses. Computation of the correlation coefficient is relatively straightforward. It measures the tendency for two variables to deviate from the respective

Table 8.8   Diastolic Blood Pressures by Human Observer and Automated Device

Participant	Pulse by Observer	Pulse by Automated Device
1	80	82
2	65	77
3	51	58
4	67	66
5	72	75
6	68	81
7	64	72
8	91	99
9	71	72
Average	69.9	75.8

$r = 0.905$

sample means in a related way. That is, the correlation coefficient measures the tendency to get similar differences between pairs of scores on two characteristics of interest. Suppose you have the data in table 8.8 on measures of the pulse as taken by an observer and by an automated device at the same time in a blood pressure intervention study. You are confronted with the decision whether to use the automated device. Use of the observer requires personnel time, training, etc. The automated device provides a permanent record and minimizes the use of personnel.

For this particular decision, you are confronted with nine pairs of observations. Each pulse was taken once by a trained observer and simultaneously by the automated device. The correlation, or what may be referred as the *reliability coefficient*, can be computed using the following formula:

Important Formula: Correlation Coefficient

$$r = \sum_{i=1}^{n} \frac{(x_i - \bar{x})(y_i - \bar{y})}{\sqrt{\Sigma(x_i - \bar{x})^2 \Sigma(y_i - \bar{y})^2}}$$

$$= \frac{n\Sigma x_i y_i - (\Sigma x_i)(\Sigma y_i)}{\sqrt{[n\Sigma x_i^2 - (\Sigma x_i)^2][n\Sigma y_i^2 - (\Sigma y_i)^2]}}$$

where x_i = the value of one characteristic or measurement on person i

y_i = the value of the other characteristic on person i

Applying this formula to the data in table 8.8, you obtain a value of $r = 0.905$. What does this value mean? A correlation coefficient can obtain values from -1.0 to 1.0. The negative values indicate that, as one characteristic increases, the other decreases. A value of ± 1 indicates perfect correlation—knowledge of one variable implies the other. However, a more readily interpretable statistic is provided by squaring r, obtaining a quantity known as the *coefficient of determination* (r^2 or R^2). This quantity, derived from a technique known as *regression analysis*, tells how much of the variation in one variable is determined or explained by the other variable. In the pulse example, $R^2 = 0.819$, meaning that over 80 percent of the variability of one observation (pulse by observer) can be explained by the other (pulse by automated device). This correlation coefficient would be found highly significant on standard tests of significance. There is certainly more agreement between these two measures than would be indicated by chance alone. However, the existence of statistical significance between the characteristics should not be overinterpreted without careful scrutiny. Although the correlation is very high, comparison of the data shows that the average mean pulse is nearly six beats lower when taken by observer than when taken by the automated device. A paired t-test on the differences between readings shows that the average difference is 5.89 beats with a standard deviation of 4.91 beats, yielding a statistically significant difference between the observer and the automated device. The basic implication is that the automated device yields higher readings than those obtained by the observer ($t = 3.60$ with 8 degrees of freedom). This information is important for making the decision to use such a device routinely or not. Your responsibility is then to try to ascertain which is the more accurate response. The correlation coefficient can be used to measure the reliability or reproducibility (that is, the precision) of an estimate. The discrepancy between the two responses, if it tends to remain relatively constant, is a measure of bias. In this example, it is not clear which measurement is more accurate. You need to pursue the content area to straighten this out.

Analysis of Pretest, Post-Test Data. Another design often used in a single-group situation is the multiple pretest, post-test design or single time series design. Chapter 5 described the cancer screening study in Hale County, Alabama. Table 8.9 shows the number of new users of cervical cancer screening clinics by quarter for Hale and Marengo counties, a more refined categorization of some of the information in table 8.1. These data might be seen as summarizing program impact in a single time series design. (See Case 1 in chapter 5.)

Consider the data for Hale County in the year 1979. The intervention periods for this study occurred in the second quarter of 1979

Table 8.9 Number of New Users of the Cervical Cancer Screening
Clinics by Quarter for Hale and Marengo Counties, Alabama

Year	1978				1979				1980			
Quarter	1	2	3	4	1	2	3	4	1	2	3	4
Hale	13	20	12	15	14	89	12	20	15	50	18	11
Marengo	22	36	23	15	32	45	34	29	27	29	40	32

and the second quarter of 1980. Substantial and favorable impact during the two intervention quarters is suggested by the array of data. When the data available for analysis are simply frequency data, options are limited, and formal tests of significance are often avoided because of the assumptions. Percentages are used as descriptive statistics, and increases in the percentage of utilization are often used to summarize change. If you can assume that (1) counts arise from a large population, (2) the number of individuals availing themselves of a clinic screening follows a Poisson distribution, and (3) the periods are independent of each other, the Poisson distribution can be used in a simple pretest, post-test design.

Assume that the baseline period or the baseline and postintervention average is the mean value of some Poisson distribution. Given this parameter, you can ask: What is the probability of observing the number of new cases during the intervention period given this mean from a Poisson distribution (as described above in the section on distributions)? This test, although quick, ignores the fact that the pretest period is not a true parameter; a test that takes into account the inherent variability in both the pretest and intervention periods would be more desirable. Although this test requires several assumptions, using a normal approximation to the Poisson, an approximate test can be used. Here you approximate the difference between two Poisson distributions and ask whether the underlying means are the same. To do this, you use as the means of each sample $(x_1$ and $x_2)$ the actual number of new users in quarter 1 and quarter 2. The variances of a Poisson are equal to the mean, so we use the sum of x_1 and x_2 as the denominator representing the variance of the difference:

$$z = \frac{(x_2 - x_1)}{\sqrt{(x_2 + x_1)}} = \frac{89 - 14}{\sqrt{89 + 14}} = 7.39$$

The probability of a z-score greater than or equal to 7.39 is small. Thus, utilizing this pretest, post-test design, you could reject the hypothesis that these two frequencies have arisen from the same under-lying Poisson distribution.

This, of course, is a weak demonstration, but it may improve on the eyeball method. The use of a single time series design with one group has many limitations, as seen in the discussion of threats to validity in chapters 4 and 5. Analogous tests may be conducted using paired t-tests for a pretest, post-test design and testing the hypothesis that the difference is zero, as was done above.

Analysis of Time Series Data. The idea of a time series is neither new nor necessarily complicated. In its simplest form, a time series is a collection of numerical observations arranged in the order in which they occurred. Formal analysis of time series goes back at least as far as the Romans, who made sufficiently accurate observations to construct the cycle of approximately 365¼ days in the Julian calendar. Data that contain only one periodic component are relatively easy to handle. More complicated series are often characterized by methods not appropriate for this chapter; furthermore, those tools are often useful not in the assessment of impact but rather in the search for periodicities, a confounding factor in many intervention programs.

In using time series data to evaluate community programs, four types of issues are of concern (Windsor and Cutter, 1981):

1. The trend in the data (generally increasing or decreasing)
2. Cyclical fluctuations (multiple-year or multiple-month ups and downs)
3. Seasonal variations (annual ups and downs)
4. Intervention effects (increases or decreases after a program)

These issues are critical to the assessment of program impact. Generally, the term *cycle* is used for short or long duration changes or repetitive changes, and *seasonal variation* is used for annual changes. Trend is an important and potentially misleading component. Suppose your program resulted in the utilization results shown in figure 8.2. Average pretreatment use was 70 persons [(80 + 60 + 70)/3] per period. In the intervention period, there were 110 new users, a 57 percent increase in utilization over the pretreatment average. This increase could convince you that the program had a substantive effect. Even the increase in the post-treatment period, an average 110 users [(90 + 100 + 140)/3], might be claimed as a long-term benefit or sustained effect of the intervention. However, you must be honest—even in your wildest dreams did you really think the program could produce such a sustained impact? You must ask whether other forces were at work.

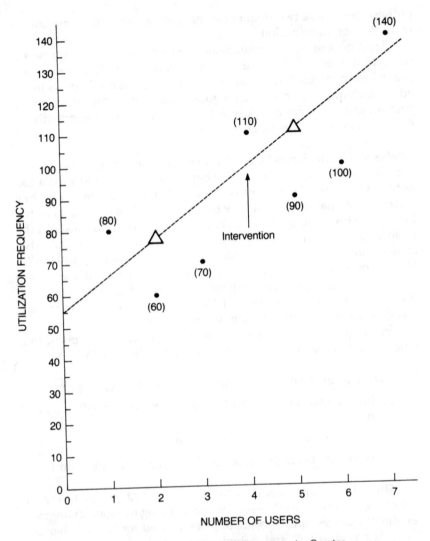

Figure 8.2 Hypothetical Example of New User Frequency by Quarter

Source: R. A. Windsor and G. Cutter, "Methodological Issues in Using Time Series Designs and Analysis: Evaluating the Behavioral Impact of Health Communication Programs," in *Progress in Clinical and Biological Research*, vol. 83. *Issues in Screening and Communications*, ed. C. Mettlin and G. Murphy, 517–535 (New York: Alan R. Liss, 1981)

The simplest assessment of a trend is to plot the data on a properly constructed graph as shown in figure 8.2. Eyeballing this figure gives the impression of an upward trend, represented by the dotted line. The comparison of before, during, and after the intervention periods (averages of 70 versus 110 new users) is called the *method of semi-*

averages. This is because it divides the time series into two parts and a line can be fitted to the two averages. The method of semiaverages is useful in identifying a trend when no intervention effect is present, but it does not clarify a situation where an intervention effect has occurred, because of this method's sensitivity to outliers. A second method, less susceptible to the impact of a single intervention period, is the *method of moving averages.* This computes the mean of a fixed number of successive observations and examines these averages or "smoothed" results. The term *smoothed* is used to indicate that the averaging process reduces some of the random fluctuations expected in real data. The moving averages for three-period increments of the data in figure 8.2 are: $70 = [(80 + 60 + 70)/3]$; $80 = [(60 + 70 + 110)/3]$; $90 = [(70 + 110 + 90)/3]$; etc.

When these three-period moving averages are plotted on a graph, they fall on a straight line, demonstrating the upward trend in utilization, and raising the question of how one intervention could produce this effect. The moving average method is a technique that takes out cyclical variations—regular up and down changes of results (oscillatory movements). Although the series presented in figure 8.2 is too short to determine the cycle explicitly, the pattern of a peak, two lower values and a peak is repeated twice; yet this movement is smoothed by the moving average process. Such cycles are important and may be confused with seasonal variations.

The methods used to isolate seasonal variations are the same as those for identifying oscillatory movements.

Even when the suggestion of trend is graphically present, the significance of it is often an important issue in assessing the program.

Linear Regression. Several methods are useful in assessing a trend, but one of the most common is regression analysis. Simple linear regression is a model that states that the average response or dependent variable y has a straight line relationship to the independent variable x.

Important Formula: Simple Linear Regression Model

$$y = \beta_0 + (\beta_1 x)$$
where β_0 = the intercept of the line
β_1 = the slope of the line

The calculation of the line is usually accomplished by a procedure known as *least squares.* That is, the coefficients β_0 and β_1 are estimated in such a way as to minimize the square of the differences between the actual observations and the expected observations. The equations for β_0 and β_1 are derived from the n pairs of observations (x_i, y_i) by the following formulas:

Important Formula: Coefficients for Simple Linear Regression

$$\hat{\beta}_1 = \frac{n \Sigma x_i y_i - (\Sigma x_i)(\Sigma y_i)}{n \Sigma x_i^2 - (\Sigma x_i)^2}$$

$$\hat{\beta}_0 = \bar{y} - (\beta_1 \bar{x})$$

where $\bar{y}$ and $\bar{x}$ = the respective means of the x's and y's

The slope β_1 is equal to zero when there is no linear relationship between x and y. The slope is equivalent to assessing the correlation coefficient r. The square of the correlation coefficient R^2 tells us the proportion of variance in y explained by x. When there is no relationship $r = 0$, $r^2 = 0$, and no variance is explained. The slope in this situation is zero. The same value is predicted for the dependent variable y no matter what the value of the independent variable is.

Both r and β_1 can be tested, i.e., the probability of the result can be found, using a t-test. Thus, to test the hypothesis that $\beta_1 = 0$, you would compute:

$$t = \frac{\hat{\beta}_1 - \beta_1}{\text{Standard Error } \hat{\beta}_1} = \frac{\hat{\beta}_1 - 0}{\text{Standard Error } \hat{\beta}_1}$$

This is compared to a t-distribution with $n - 2$ degrees of freedom. In analyzing trend data, evaluators often use time (t) as the independent variable x, and y remains the response. Consider the example from figure 8.2. The least squares equation that characterizes these data is:

$$\hat{\beta}_0 = 52.9$$
$$\hat{\beta}_1 = 10.0$$
$$y_i = 52.9 + 10.0t_i$$

That is, average usage is 52.9 persons plus 10 additional persons for each time period of observation.

Applying the regression method to the smoothed data, as discussed above, yields $u = 60.0 + 10.0t$. The R^2 value is 0.64 for the unsmoothed data and 1.00 for the smoothed data. In both situations, the regression is significant, indicating the existence of a trend. You must ask whether the trend is overriding the intervention or whether there is an intervention effect over and above the trend. In this situation, with the strong trend evidence and an apparent seasonal pattern, the success of the intervention could be questioned, especially if the likelihood of a sustained impact is small.

Outliers or Successful Interventions. Given an understanding of the series, the question remains how to measure and assess an impact. When no trend, cycle, or seasonal variation exists, impact can be assessed by comparing the intervention period results to the before and after periods as was done in the earlier example when a trend existed. A statistical appraisal can be made using a method for the detection of outliers in data sets. Although many criteria have been proposed and used, a simple test (Grubbs, 1969) can be used to assess whether the value appears to have arisen by more than chance variation; if so, this indicates a program impact. This statistic, G, is easily computed by the formula:

$$G = \frac{\text{Intervention observation } - \text{ Mean of all observations}}{\text{Standard deviation } \sqrt{n-1}}$$

This parallels a t-test except for the adjustment in the denominator. Where the standard deviation of all observations is used, the resultant value, G, can be compared to available special tables, provided the data can be assumed to be normally distributed. Another test is to compute a z-score by comparing the intervention observation to the mean and dividing by the standard deviation. If this value is larger than 3.2, the result is considered significant.

A similar analysis can be carried out when a significant trend exists, as in the example in figure 8.2. In this situation, the expected value from the trend line is used in the Grubbs formula and compared to the standard error (S) of the regression line:

$$G = \frac{y_i - \hat{y}_i}{S_{\text{regression}} \sqrt{n-2}}$$

Application of this technique to the example in figure 8.2 yields no statistically significant deviation from the trend line.

Example of Applied Analysis. To give a more complete example, we will apply the techniques to the Hale County study of cervical cancer screening described extensively in chapter 5 and briefly above. The data are presented in table 8.10. We will consider only the total users for the moment. The intervention periods occurred at the second quarters of 1979, 1980, and 1981. A brief scanning of the data shows large peaks for those quarters. This is, of course, consistent with the hypothesized effect of the broadcast messages and screening efforts

Table 8.10 Frequency of New and Repeat Cancer Screening Program Users by Quarter, 1978–81

Year	Quarter	New Users	Repeat Users	Total Users
1978	1	13	28	41
	2	20	34	54
	3	12	21	33
	4	14	51	65
1979	1	14	47	61
	2	89	87	176
	3	12	43	55
	4	20	58	78
1980	1	16	54	70
	2	50	96	146
	3	18	51	69
	4	11	62	73
1981	1	19	60	79
	2	40	141	181

and could be taken as a strong indication of success of the cancer screening program (CSP). However, as pointed out, evaluators should not be content with a statement of program impact based merely on observing the data.

These data offer, on closer inspection, additional information that can be used in evaluating the program. For example, in the first five quarters prior to the first intervention period, average utilization was 50.8 total users per quarter. This can be compared to an average in excess of 70 users for the three quarters prior to the last intervention; that is, quarters 3 and 4 of 1980 and quarter 1 of 1981. This suggests an increasing trend and can be evaluated using the techniques described above.

In order to investigate the effect of the trend with attempts to eliminate some of the variability caused by the impact of the intervention, we chose to use a one-year moving average. This one-year moving average in effect dampens the impact of the intervention periods which occurred annually. Shown in table 8.11 are the results of the one-year moving averages from quarter 4 of 1978 through quarter 2 of 1981. In the column under "Total Users," the smooth average shows a striking increasing trend by quarter. Simple linear regression analyses of the total number of users on the sequence number of the 11 quar-

Table 8.11 One-Year Moving Averages by Quarter

Year	Quarter	New Users	Repeat Users	Total Users
1978	4	14.75	33.50	48.25
1979	1	15.00	38.25	53.25
	2	32.25	51.50	83.75
	3	32.25	57.00	89.25
	4	33.75	58.75	92.50
1980	1	34.25	60.50	94.75
	2	24.50	62.75	87.25
	3	26.00	64.75	90.75
	4	23.75	65.75	89.50
1981	1	24.50	67.25	91.75
	2	22.00	78.50	100.50
		$R^2 = 0.01$	$R^2 = 0.88$	$R^2 = 0.59$
		$\beta_0 = 24.25$	$\beta_0 = 36.05$	$\beta_0 = 60.38$
		$\beta_1 = 0.25$	$\beta_1 = 3.67$	$\beta_1 = 3.91$
		Not significant	$p < 0.01$	$p < 0.01$

ters show the rate of increase in total users estimated at 3.9 additional users per quarter, which is significantly different from a zero slope. From this, we see that there is a trend in the data collected. At this juncture, we need to ask how plausible it is that the trend is a result of program intervention.

Because this is a cervical cancer screening program, as a patient enters the system she is encouraged to follow the screening guidelines, which suggest that new users have repeat physicals annually for three years. This implies that the intervention should not only increase the total number of users during the intervention quarter but also cause increases in subsequent years as a by-product of entry into the system. To address the question of impact, the one-year moving averages were computed for new users and repeat users. These averages are shown in table 8.11, and clearly reveal a strong linear increase in the number of repeat users by sequence number. The new users, on the other hand, do not exhibit any trend by quarter; hence, the temporal trend in the total use group is clearly a carryover effect of the screening process and not simply increased utilization across the board over time. This breaking up of the trend enables us to identify findings consistent with the goals of the screening program, both at the utilization level on a cross-sectional basis and in terms of bring-

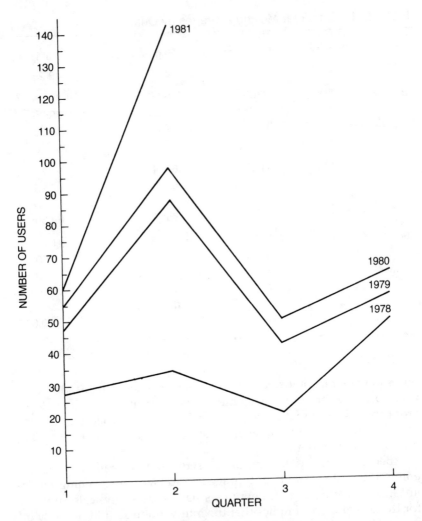

Figure 8.3 Repeat Cancer Screening Program Users by Quarter

ing people into the screening system. *Thus, it provides new evidence that the intervention in fact worked.* With the knowledge of the trends in the data and the trends appropriate to the intervention, the next stage of the analysis is to assess the data on the impact of the intervention effect itself.

Applying the test described above for the existence of an outlier within the data shows that the second quarters of 1979, 1980, and 1981 are all significant, with p-values less than 0.05, even without taking into account the trend. Testing the significance of these values relative to the standard deviation of the regression line shows all values to be significant at the 0.01 level. Similar tests applied to the new and repeat users also show significant increases during each intervention quarter. Further, graphic analysis, as exhibited in figures 8.3 and 8.4, shows both the increase and the seasonal trend. *The increasing peaks during the second quarters and the parallels of the curves for repeat CSP users clearly demonstrate the increased utilization brought about by the communications effort.*

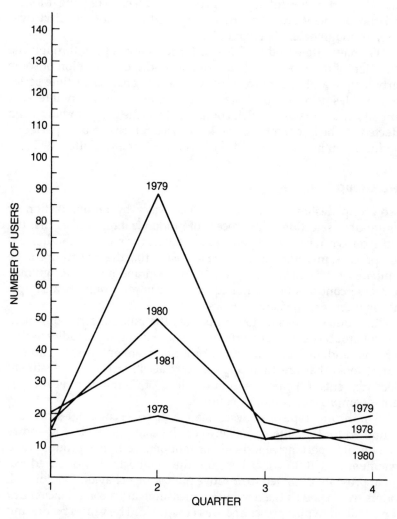

Figure 8.4 New Cancer Screening Program Users by Quarter

The increased number of new users during the second quarters is shown in figure 8.4 decreasing in 1979, 1980, and 1981 This provides exceedingly useful information to the screening program. It illustrates a law of diminishing returns as well as the possibility that the intervention was not applied with as much vigor in later years as in the first year. Thus, the program planners must question how long such an initiative should be continued and for what return. A second issue that is noticeable in the 1978 curve, the baseline period, is a slight increase during the second quarter. This raises the question of whether the effect is seasonal. Upon further investigation, we learned that the second quarter coincided with National Cancer Screening Month, and the publicity attending that effort had a consistent effect over time, although of small magnitude.

We have attempted to show with this analysis that, through the collection of rather simple data elements and the application of some fairly simple and straightforward techniques, analysis of time series data enables us to demonstrate the impact of a community intervention effort, understand which components of the program have been affected by the intervention, and learn what return can be expected in the future on investment of this effort (Windsor and Cutter, 1982).

Two-Group Designs

Two-group designs occur in two basic ways: by randomization or nonrandom selection. The process of randomization implies that the two groups can be considered equal. That is, through the randomization process, investigators attempt to ensure that the two groups to be compared have similar characteristics. A nonrandomized design may be a case control study, a nonequivalent control group, or a sample matched on certain characteristics.

In studies or evaluation proposals, the randomized, equivalent control group is a very powerful tool. These two-group studies assign persons randomly to a treatment or a nontreatment group. The statistical tools that are then applied look at either (1) post-treatment measurements, (2) changes from baseline, or (3) number and/or percentage improved, cured, or controlled.

For the first type of analyses, standardized z-scores or t-scores are computed for the differences between the changes. Table 8.12 shows data on 20 hypertensive individuals randomized to two groups (10 to treatment and 10 to control) before the administration of an educational program designed to improve pill-taking behavior. Random pill counts were used as the dependent measure, and a compliance index of pills taken to pills prescribed was computed. The values before and after treatment are displayed in table 8.12. The changes in the indices

Table 8.12 Compliance Indices Before and After Intervention to Improve Pill-Taking Behavior

	Before		After		Changes	
	Treatment	Control	Treatment	Control	Treatment	Control
Compliance Index	86	85	110	95	24	10
	80	84	102	91	22	7
	86	82	94	101	8	19
	86	83	98	103	12	20
	85	86	100	92	15	6
	84	82	98	94	14	12
	82	82	104	91	22	9
	84	80	102	93	18	13
	88	84	96	89	8	5
	80	78	95	91	15	13
Mean	84.1	82.6	99.9	94.0	15.8	11.4
Standard deviation	2.685	2.366	4.818	4.570	5.67	5.10
t-score	1.33 with 18 degrees of freedom		2.81 with 18 degrees of freedom		0.55 with 18 degrees of freedom	

for each patient are shown in the right-hand set of columns. The evaluators leaving all aspects to randomization may fail to consider the initial before-treatment measurements and simply analyze the after-treatment compliance indices. This yields a mean compliance index of 99.9 in the treatment group and 94.0 in the control group. Using the approach of two independent samples and applying the t-test to the difference between these means, under the hypothesis that there is no difference between treatment and control, yields a t-statistic of 2.81 with 18 degrees of freedom, which is significant at the 1 percent level.

This form of analysis might be used by an evaluator, but actually it is not the desired analysis given the design of this study. Since it is always recommended to take measurements of compliance prior to treatment, those data should be used. The before-treatment data show a tendency for the treatment group to have slightly higher compliance indices than the control group—a mean of 84.1 compared to 82.6. The difference in means, when tested with a t-statistic, yields a t-statistic equal to 1.33 with 18 degrees of freedom, which is not statistically significant. However, in observing the difference between these two treatment groups, even given randomization, an evaluator might be advised to assess the difference in the change scores of the treatment and control groups. (Technically, an approach using what is called *regression gain scores* is preferred, but that will be noted here only in passing. Simply, the technique analyzes the residuals by group of a regression of after-treatment results on before-treatment levels.) Doing this assessment in the third set of columns yields a mean increase in the compliance index of 15.8 for the treatment group compared to an increase of 11.4 for the control group. Applying a t-test to these changes results in a t-statistic of 0.55 with 18 degrees of freedom, which demonstrates no significant difference in increased compliance between the treatment and control groups.

Having applied the statistical tools of t-tests for continuous variables, an evaluator could ask whether the results were not significant because of violations in the assumptions, such as normality, independence between the two groups, or a representative random sample. A second series of questions, however, could be addressed. The initial one is whether there is evidence of a significant program effect. The lack of evidence could be due to the small sample size yielding the expected large variability, which makes it insufficient to detect any changes in the compliance index. The intervention may not have worked, which is a question an evaluator must ask even if it goes against prior beliefs. And finally a series of questions must be asked about sources of bias as described in Chapter 6. For example, one source of unequal performance between the interventions could be interviewer effects. In a health education intervention involving two types of therapists (one administering a dietary protocol and the other a compliance protocol), the skills of the therapists might be substantially different. Such differences may cause differences in results, which are related to the performance of those administering the treatments and not the treatments themselves. This is not apparent from the statistics computed or the tests performed on them. Each of the twelve types of bias given in Chapter 6 and their variations should be considered.

A very special form of bias often occurs when investigators look at only the individuals who had positive results. This bias is known as *stratification by response*. In general, it is a very dangerous form of analysis and harbors many biases not obvious to the evaluator. If evaluators look at only the individuals who had favorable improvements as a result of a treatment, and ignore the rest, they risk showing overpositive results. They also may find correlates of success that are the opposites of the true relationship. For example, in the most extreme case, suppose you are going to mount an intervention designed to reduce stress, based on evidence that all individuals interviewed after having a heart attack (hence all who survived) were individuals who had high stress. You conclude that high stress leads to heart attacks. You could be making a serious mistake, however: Suppose that high stress protects against fatal heart attacks, and individuals who did not have conditioning through high stress died of their heart attacks. You concluded that stress is associated with heart attacks because those individuals interviewed exhibited it. If all the individuals who died did not possess the characteristic, the very characteristic you are setting out to reduce may actually be what allowed the others to survive! Intervening could have the adverse effect of increasing mortality. This is an extreme example of a misinterpretation by evaluation after stratifying by response.

The second type of two-group design is frequently called a *non-equivalent control group design*. In a community-based program, a control group is selected with similar demographic characteristics, a comparable pattern of utilization (if it is a utilization study), and as many of the same characteristics as can reasonably be matched. Frequently such studies are used where the ultimate unit of analysis is an aggregate, such as a county, school, or defined geographical area. The design is selected because the addition of the comparison group improves the chances of attributing observed impacts to program efforts. In the cervical cancer screening program example, a control county, Marengo, was shown in table 8.9. This county was a non-equivalent control group. It was selected on basis of demographic characteristics, a comparable pattern of service use at the baseline, and presence of an ongoing community-based cancer screening and detection program over a comparable time period. Marengo County was chosen as the best county to compare with Hale because of its geographical proximity as well. An increase in new users in Marengo County can be seen in the second quarters of 1978 and 1979 in table 8.9. This parallel increase with the intervention county raises some questions about the demonstrated impact for Hale County. Investigation suggested that the increased utilization may have been due to National Cancer Screening Month, which occurs generally in April or May. Special efforts occur throughout Alabama during that month to promote community awareness of and interest in cancer detection. This probably provided an increase in the utilization in both counties. In the nonequivalent control group design, although t-tests are used to compare continuous results, often studies are evaluated merely in terms of frequency data. The simplest form of analysis is to compare the increases in the magnitude of new users. A 493 percent increase in new users is observed for Hale County, 89 versus 15, while the magnitude of increase in Marengo is 40 percent, 45 versus 32. A gross estimate of the impact of the community intervention can be obtained by subtracting the increase noted in the comparison county, 40 percent, from that noted in the treatment county, 493 percent. A program using this approach might conclude that the "effect size" was approximately 450 percent in the intervention county. *Although this rather extensive difference is likely not to be the true measure, analysis of data from nonequivalent control groups studies allows only cautious interpretation of any statistical techniques.* In general, the percentage increase could be estimated and tested. Assuming a binomial or Poisson distribution for some of these increases, the means and or variances could be tested for equivalence (Windsor and Cutter, 1982).

More complicated methods could be used, such as fitting response curves to both sets of data and testing the equivalence of the two sets of parameters. Although these methods are generally well known, they are oversophisticated and usually do not improve the evaluator's perception of what has taken place. This does not mean that elaborate techniques can never be valuable; however, given available resources and personnel, it is unlikely that such tools will be available to most evaluators. What is useful, though, is not simply an estimate of the percentage increase but also computing a confidence interval for the percentage increase. An approximate method was published by Bross (1954), demonstrating how to assess a percentage increase due to the second quarter intervention. Shown in table 8.13 are new users in Hale and Marengo counties for 1979. The table shows total new users and new users in the intervention quarter alone. The percentage of all new users in 1979 who came in during the second quarter in Hale County was 65.93 compared to 32.14 percent in Marengo. Using this formulation of the data, you can estimate the percentage increase in the second quarter for Hale County compared to Marengo County. The formula is:

$$\hat{\theta} = \frac{100(p_2 - p_1)}{p_1}$$

where $\hat{\theta}$ = estimated percentage increase
p_1 = percentage in group 1, or base percentage
p_2 = percentage in group 2, or increased percentage

Applying the data:

$$\hat{\theta} = \frac{100(0.6593 - 0.3214)}{0.3214} = 105.10$$

The percentage increase in the second quarter in Hale County was 105.10 percent. This shows a substantial increase in the utilization

Table 8.13 New Users of Cervical Cancer Screening Clinics, Hale and Marengo Counties, 1979

County	Total New Users	Number in Quarter 2	Percentage
Hale	135	89	65.93
Marengo	140	45	32.14
Total	275	134	

during the second quarter for this single one-year intervention comparison. *It indicates a substantive effect, and program evaluators can be very comfortable reporting such a percentage increase.* This analytical method takes into account the increase that occurred in Marengo County due to the Cancer Society efforts and shows the additional impact obtained from the educational intervention occurring in Hale County. However, simply a point estimate, such as this percentage increase, may not be sufficient. With small numbers, the estimates vary markedly. Using the methods proposed by Bross, an interval estimate or confidence interval can be obtained, which gives limits for the percentage increase, using the following formula. First we need two interim values:

$$LL = \text{approximate lower limit} = r - [2\sqrt{r(1-r)/n}\,]$$
$$UL = \text{approximate upper limit} = r + [2\sqrt{r(1-r)/n}\,]$$

where r = the ratio of the number of individuals in a specified class of the baseline group (group 1), to the total in the class, n

Applying the data from table 8.13 using new users from Marengo County as the baseline group:

$$r = 45/(45 + 89) = 45/134 = 0.336$$
$$LL = 0.336 - [2\sqrt{(0.336)(0.664)/134}\,] = 0.254$$
$$UL = 0.336 + [2\sqrt{(0.336)(0.664)/134}\,] = 0.418$$

Thus, to obtain an approximate 95 percent confidence interval, we find:

$$L = \text{Lower estimate} = \frac{100[n_1 - (n_1 + n_2)\text{UL}]}{n_2(\text{UL})}$$

$$U = \text{Upper estimate} = \frac{100[n_1 - (n_1 + n_2)\text{LL}]}{n_2(\text{LL})}$$

where n_1 and n_2 = the total number of individuals in each group, respectively

For the above example:

$$L = \frac{100\,[140 - (140 + 135)\,(0.418)]}{135(0.418)} = 44.39\%$$

$$U = \frac{100\,[140 - (140 + 135)\,(0.254)]}{135\,(0.254)} = 204.58\%$$

Although these formulas appear to be rather difficult, reference to Bross's original paper or simply plugging through the formulas can yield the appropriate confidence intervals. Substitution into these formulas shows that the confidence interval for the percentage increase obtained for Hale over Marengo leads to 95 percent confidence intervals of 44.39 percent to 204.58 percent, *a confidence interval that conveys a sense of strong conviction that there was an additional educational impact in Hale County.*

With the nonequivalent control group design (or, in fact, the equivalent control group design) simple time series analysis is often suitable to assess program impact. Referring back to table 8.9 on new user data for 1978–80 for Hale County, analysis of the multiple time series data might be attempted. The literature identifies the multiple time series design as an excellent quasi-experimental method. The data indicate that the baseline year for Hale County, 1978, was stable for the first, third, and fourth quarters, and new users increased during the second quarter, as shown in the table. The baseline data from Marengo County fluctuated more than in Hale, but the observed increase in the second quarter is consistent across counties. The increase in the second quarter in the first intervention year, 1979, was greater for Hale County than for Marengo County. Both intervention and control counties then reverted back to the new user frequencies approximating those in the preintervention quarter. The three quarters between intervention periods of 1979 and 1980 were marked by a relatively stable pattern of use for both intervention and control counties. The data for the second intervention period in 1980 show a marked increase in Hale County, where the intervention was applied, although of a lesser magnitude than the previous year, and do not show a marked increase in the control county. Following the intervention quarter the frequency of new users again reverted to its original level in Hale County. It is possible that the observed increase from 29 to 40 cases in Marengo County in the third quarter may be attributable in part to another factor—this was the last year this screening clinic was to be open in the county. The basic difference between the patterns is not clear. The average numbers of new users per quarter for 1978, 1979, and 1980 in Hale County were 5, 10.4, and 7.2, respectively. In Marengo County, the averages were 4.4, 6.4, and 6.0, respectively. These data suggest that the observed patterns of change in Hale are somewhat larger than in Marengo. They are not, however, as impressive as the data presented in the visual analyses of the intervention quarters.

Analyses of the multiple time series designs are merely an extension of the methods of simple time series. If coefficients are estimated, comparisons of these coefficients can be made. Each coefficient is approximately distributed as a t-distribution when standardized by its standard error. A two-sample t-test can be used to assess the equality of these slopes. A second method is to use analysis of variance with repeated measures or chi-square procedures over both groups. The chi-square test for the quarterly frequency data uses two rows, one for each county, and twelve columns, one for each quarter. *The test answers the question: Are new users per quarter independent of county?* The data shown in table 8.9 yield a chi-square of 63.85 with 11 degrees of freedom or a p-value less than 0.0001. This chi-square test for independence suggests that the quarterly frequency is not independent of county, although this does not in itself demonstrate the success of the intervention. To get some idea of whether the intervention has had the desired effect, an evaluator could eliminate the two intervention periods from the computations and recompute the chi-square test. This yields a chi-square of 7.84 with 9 degrees of freedom, a result consistent with the independence hypothesis. That is, it suggests there is independence between county and quarter when the two intervention quarters, the second quarter of 1979 and the second quarter of 1980, are eliminated. *In combination, these two results suggest an intervention effect* (Windsor and Cutter, 1982).

Multiple-Group Designs

We can merely mention the analyses of multiple groups in this chapter. Generally, these analyses involve some form of regression analysis, analysis of variance, or chi-square procedures. Use of these methods is a straightforward extension of the analyses of two-group designs. The title of this chapter conveys the notion that complex designs are not the subject of this book. Multiple-group designs, by their very nature, tend to be complex. From this perspective, it is our premise that, when you use such designs, you need a complete understanding of the tools required to analyze the program data before you implement the design. There are many times when multiple groups can be used, such as in studies of layered treatment effects (e.g., a dietary program to reduce salt coupled with a weight control program and possibly a control group). Intervention programs might be used alone and in combination with drug treatments, leading to multiple groups. However, analyses of multiple-group comparisons present problems that are not straightforward in the sense of many of the other tools. Explicit designs should be used when more than two groups are envisioned, and the necessity for more than two groups should be carefully weighed. All too often, program planners invest enormous resources in multiple-group studies with small sample sizes, leading to results that are virtually uninterpretable. Because of the high variability in small samples, the results lack power to show differences in treatment effects. From the analytical perspective, the simpler methods often answer the more important questions. It is better to have a reasonable answer to a simple question than no answer to many questions.

Analysis of variance in the simplest form is a mere extension of the t-test. Although the statistics used involve the F-distribution rather than the t-distribution, the basic computations and concepts are the same. The result of an analysis of variance is an analysis of variance table. The single test of the hypothesis answers the question of whether there are significant differences among the means of the populations being considered. This test answers only a single question; the means are equal to each other or they are unequal. The basic procedure followed for the analysis of variance is to ascertain whether the variability that occurs among the various treatment groups is greater than the residual or random error occurring within the treatment groups. An F-test is used to compare the size of the variability among the groups to the variability within groups. If there are substantial treatment effects, then the variability among the groups will be significantly greater than the variability within groups.

A second problem, known as a *multiple comparison problem*, arises when dealing with multiple-group studies. Once the overall significance is found on an F-test, evaluators tend to want to know which treatments are better. To learn this, they tend to make a series of paired comparisons. This ultimately leads to a problem in the overall chance of falsely rejecting a hypothesis of no difference, called a *Type I error*. To compensate for this, various procedures are applied that can be found in any basic statistics book on analysis of variance. Simply, these procedures require the p-values to be smaller before a result is considered significant, so that the overall chance of a Type I error is not increased.

The use of regression analysis in multiple-group studies is generally done in one of several ways, but it yields results equivalent to those found by analysis of variance. Such techniques are described in the numerous texts on regression analyses and are beyond the scope of this book. The overall use of the chi-square statistic is a straightforward extension of what was presented above for two-group designs. Instead of looking at two rows across interventions for frequency data, the evaluator has multiple groups and goes through the same process of identifying independence between, for example, the intervention period of response and the treatment group, yielding a row times column table. More complicated chi-square techniques are available in the literature on categorical data analyses.

SUMMARY

In this chapter we have discussed simple tools to use in the analysis of program data and community health education evaluations. Although inappropriate uses can and do occur, there are no hard and fast rules for exactly when to use each tool. Experience is an artful teacher. Reacting with careful and clearly articulated questions is as much a necessity in the analysis process as choosing the tools to use.

This chapter has dealt with concepts of basic statistics: types of data—nominal, ordinal, and numerical; accuracy and precision; their equivalence to validity and reliability; and the statistical definition of bias. Some basic rules of data presentation in tables, graphs, and charts were discussed, emphasizing the need for clarity, simplicity, and purpose. A major section was devoted to descriptive statistics. These included: summary counts, measures of central tendency (mean, median, mode), measures of spread or dispersion, range, variance, standard deviation, and standard error. The concept of a distribution was introduced, and the binomial, Poisson, normal, t-, chi-square, and F-distributions were discussed. The notions of z-scores, probability, p-values, and computing formulas were presented.

Two basic types of designs, single-group and two-group, formed the context for the remainder of the chapter. The use of chi-square tests and correlation for identifying associations was presented. Examples of pretest, post-test data, time series, and linear regressions were provided. The computation and interpretation of regression coefficients was given, along with testing their significance. The concept of use and identification of outliers in evaluation studies was explored, illustrated with examples of their use. Several examples of two-group designs were provided, along with a method of generating an estimate of a percentage increase and its confidence interval. Finally, the chapter gave an extended example and some mention of multiple-group designs.

The simple tools of this chapter can be used to enhance the efforts of health promotion. The results need not always be positive for a thorough analysis to be useful. These tools can uncover the areas of success, failure, and uncertainty to which future efforts can be directed.

APPENDIX **A**

The Health Education Evaluation Report

As discussed in chapter 3, a good health education program most often results from the application of logical thinking to a health problem and the behavior change that is expected to alleviate or eliminate the problem. The evaluation report is the document that ties together the problem, the program, the intervention impact, and the outcomes of the program. This synthesis is done by presentation of data to illustrate cause-and-effect relationships. When a program fails to yield expected outcomes, the report is a vehicle for exploring the explanations of this fact. The evaluation report is a medium of communication; therefore, while you are preparing it, you must keep in mind the people to whom it is directed. If the audience is quite varied, it is likely that you will prepare different forms of a report emphasizing in each the issues and ideas of greatest interest to a particular group of readers.

The evaluation report is not a massive historical document describing events and results for future generations. Rather it is an immediate, dynamic communication to those with a specific interest in the program. The report discusses program outcomes and serves as a guide to others for making related health education decisions. It is not the length but the quality of the report that makes it acceptable. It may be used to decide if and how to revise the existing program, to expand the program to other sites or settings, or to increase, reduce, or rearrange staff or budget. The major evaluation concern covered in a report is the program's effectiveness: Did it yield what was expected? If not, why not?

In the following pages, we delineate the sections of a comprehensive report. The extent of each section depends on the specific audience to whom the report is directed.

DETERMINING THE AUDIENCE FOR THE REPORT

To what audience must you communicate? In the day-to-day practice of health education, it is quite likely that the unit administrator in the sponsoring organization will be the first to see the report. Next the directors of the agencies or organizations involved in the program may see it. If the program has been funded by outside grants, a report must certainly communicate results of interest to the granting entities. If the program results add to or clarify dimensions of health education practice, your professional colleagues will be interested in the report. When a program complements medical or nursing practice, other health care providers may have an interest in the report. If the program has brought about changes with strong implication for community health and health services, local residents and news media may be interested.

Reports that communicate to each of these audiences differ in range, length, complexity, and language. Each, however, draws from the same data pool or set, and it is likely that much of the material generated in developing the original program plan will be useful in writing each version. It is generally a mistake to try to write one report to address the interests of all the potential audiences. While there may be some standard sections in all reports (that is, chunks of the same material repeated in each), some sections must be specifically directed toward target audiences and provide more complete material about their particular interests. The process of communicating to several audiences is made more efficient by preparing a document with interchangeable parts. The statistical analysis, for example, may be presented in great detail for some audiences and only briefly summarized for others. The administrative pattern for operating the program may be described elaborately for some readers and barely mentioned for others. The first question to ask yourself is: Whom do I want to reach with this document? Then you ask: Which elements and aspects of the evaluation of the program are of greatest importance to that reader?

FORMAT AND PREPARATION OF THE REPORT

If you have followed the evaluation procedures discussed in this book, collected data both at predetermined points in a program and at the end of the program period, then you will have many data in hand when report-writing time arrives. You will also have in hand a logically conceived program plan or blueprint that has enumerated from the outset the expected impact and outcomes of the program. Preparing evaluation reports, therefore, is in large part a matter of reviewing the original plan, the data, and the analysis and interpretation of the data; you then organize this information into a clear, well-documented communication. A suggested outline for the sections of this communication is:

1. Title page
2. Executive summary (abstract)
3. Table of Contents
4. Purpose of the program and evaluation questions
   A. Aims and objectives
   B. Description of participants and setting
   C. Evaluation questions
5. Program description
   A. Nature of the learning
   B. Content
   C. Logistics of the program
   D. Staffing and personnel
6. Evaluation methodology
   A. Outcome evaluation
   B. Process evaluation
7. Data analysis
   A. Quantitative data analysis
   B. Qualitative data analysis
8. Findings and summary of conclusions
9. Costs of the program
10. Recommendations

Each section is discussed in turn next.

The Abstract or Executive Summary

The first section after the title page is the executive summary, or abstract. Because health educators are influenced by their training in academic institutions, some tend to prepare reports that assume the readers have a widespread academic interest and are willing to plod through voluminous material to find the important points. In the day-to-day practice of health education, few people have either the time or the patience to search through many pages to find the pearls. A good evaluation report presents its findings at the very beginning, so the readers know the basic results from the outset. One way to accomplish this is to prepare a one-page abstract or executive summary of the report and to make this the first page of the evaluation document. Of course, the summary may actually be *written* after the full report is completed, but it appears first when the document is compiled. The abstract should concisely describe the program's objectives, methods, processes, and results. You should write the abstract, like the report, without jargon and in the active voice, not the passive (the latter is favored in academic circles but not necessarily by the best scholars). If you need to use scientific or technical words, you should define them for readers.

The abstract should present essential evaluation material in language the intended readers will understand. As you might expect, the quality of the summary often dictates whether the full report will be read. The abstract should be followed by a clearly numbered and accurately referenced table of contents. This is critical. It is quite annoying to busy readers not to find a table of contents to help move easily through a large document. Some people refuse to read reports without a well-labeled table of contents. They may be justified, as the lack demonstrates a significant deficiency in the report writers.

Purpose or Goal of the Program and Key Evaluation Questions

Writing an evaluation report can be a rewarding experience as you review the thinking that led to the program. Readers of the report need to be let in on this thinking, to be told what the program intended to achieve (Baseline editors, 1982). Readers also need to know *why* achieving the goal was important. If the program expected, for example, to assist overweight employees to lose weight, why should the reader accept this as valuable? The reasons may be different for the reader who is the employee's spouse and for the reader who is the chief executive officer of the company.

It is important not to assume that the reader has background information about the program and its potential worth; on the contrary, assume the reader does not. Prepare a clear, direct discourse describing the probram purpose and the value of successful efforts. Describe the characteristics that make the program singular and unique (Morris and Fitz-Gibbon, 1978, Appendix A), and include a profile of the participants or learners. Obviously, a program is valuable because of the particular people it aimed to assist. Who were the learners in the program? Why was it important to reach them?

The major evaluation questions should be spelled out in this section of the report (Fink and Kosecoff, 1979). They are the measuring sticks of whether the program achieved its purpose. This list of the questions that guided your evaluation, whether it is long or short, should be self-explanatory once the reader has gone through your description of purpose.

Program Description

Once readers have grasped the purpose of the program and reviewed the questions that guided evaluation of it, they will want to understand what the program "looked like." To say that the program was "self-management training" is certainly not enough. What constituted the training? Where? When? How did it occur? You need to include five elements in this program description, more or less extensively depending on the audience for your report:

1. The basic nature of the education. What fundamental educational approaches were used? For example, was the program a combination of organized peer group support and rehearsal of specific health skills? Was it counseling from professionals? Was it provision of information through various media? Was it based on group problem solving?

2. The content of the program. What material was presented? How was it presented at each learning session?

3. The logistics of the program. What was the location of the educational sessions, their frequency, and their duration? What number of hours, days, or weeks was assessed?

4. The number and deployment of the health educators or other facilitators of the learning; the kind of training they received before inception of the program; and the average number of learners participating in the learning sessions.

5. The administrative support provided. What number and deployment of program managers, coordinators, secretaries, and other administrative personnel were used?

This description should enable readers to envision a learning session with the health educators and learners doing what they would typically do. A complete narrative would include the behavioral objectives set for learning events, how learners were enabled to reach the objectives, and how achieving the objectives was related to the overall purpose or goal of the program. You may want to include graphs, charts, photos, samples of handouts, and other illustrative materials. These are generally helpful to readers. The trend, however, is to use only one or two particularly clear and concise illustrations within the body of a report and include the rest as appendices. It is unwise to burden your report with interesting but extraneous materials that may distract the readers. Select for the narrative only illustrations that are directly "to the point" and that present ideas or data better than a narrative description would. Do not repeat in the text what is obvious in the illustration. The graphic materials should enhance not reiterate your written word.

The Evaluation Methodology

You must describe for readers the way program assessment was carried out. The methods and design that you selected from the various possibilities presented in chapters 4 through 8 should be presented. You need to discuss two dimensions: the design that enabled you to ascertain the impact and outcomes of the program (for example, whether the employees changed their eating patterns and lost weight); and the process evaluation (chapter 4) that enabled you to make judgments about the quality of the program (for example, whether the staff performed as expected or the anticipated average level of participation in group discussions was reached). These two dimensions are best described separately. The quality assessment measures what actually occurred in the program. The evaluation design measures the results. In health education programs both are exceedingly important and should be reported. Readers will have more or less interest in quality assessment, however. It is likely that, initially, your audience will be more interested in the design to determine the outcome of the program. Once persuaded that this dimension was adequately addressed, many readers will want to know more about process. In this section, like the others, you must determine how much material is appropriate for each set of your readers. When in doubt, mention the material in the body of the report, and include a narrative description as an appendix.

The description of your evaluation design should include use of control groups, sampling procedures, sample size, and the reliability and validity of the data in light of the procedures used. In describing these points you should discuss not only what judgments each element allows you to make about the program but also what judgments cannot be made. In other words, the limitations of the procedures employed should be described. As we discussed in previous chapters, it is frequently difficult to use highly controlled evaluation techniques in natural settings. Almost all quasi-experimental designs and all process assessment methods are flawed. It is your responsibility to recount the ways in which the evaluation procedures are deficient. This is an important part of the report, as it demonstrates to the readers that you have both thought about and tried to account for inherent weaknesses in the evaluation.

Next comes a description of the specific way in which you collected data to answer each evaluation question. If you used several techniques, the limitations of each should be discussed. For example, if some data were collected in face-to-face interviews, how candid and forthcoming were respondents? How did you guard against interviewer bias? If you used hospital records as a source of data, how accurate and consistent were the records completed by health personnel? It is important for you to show that you anticipated, and wherever possible addressed, problems in data collection. Some readers like to see samples of questionnaires or other instruments for collecting data. If yours are of manageable size, you may choose to append them. Readers rarely expect to see questionnaires in the body of a report.

Data Analysis

The way in which you analyzed the data collected should be clearly spelled out for the reader. If a large data set was derived from the study, and you used a computer, you should mention how the data were handled (card? tape?) and what computer program you used. Few health education practitioners have the resources to write special statistical programs. Most use standard packages. It is sufficient, in most cases, to name the program and mention why it was selected. Within each program, several statistical options are generally available. You should report which statistical procedures were used for each kind of evaluation question and describe any adjustments or corrections in the tests that were made. If your audience is comprised of measurement specialists and statisticians, however, you will want to give much more detail on why you selected these tests (the relative benefits they afforded). You will also want to discuss more fully the limitations of the procedures in analyzing the given variables and the evaluation questions considered important.

If you did not use a computer but tabulated and analyzed the data by hand, you must describe the steps you undertook and the statistical tests you applied to the data. Some health educators report only percentages when they have computed data by hand. This is a weak approach; as reported in chapter 8, chi-square and other simple statistical procedures are easy to compute, especially with the ubiquitous pocket calculator. When you have made the effort to design an evaluation and collect quantitative data in the ways suggested in this text, it is a pity not to employ these simple tests. In reporting them, you should make clear the standards for accepting statistical significance. If statistically significant, was it important?

Some of your data will have been analyzed "qualitatively," that is, through content analysis, rating by experts, tabulation of observations over time, or in other ways. The methods used must be described in enough detail so that readers can judge how careful, comprehensive, and consistent the procedures were. If several raters have been used to review data, interrater reliability should be reported. Similarly, your view of the stability of the data should be discussed. If there were major problems in analyzing the data, they should be described and clarified in this part of the report.

The data analysis section should enable readers to see how the data were handled and in what ways they were interpreted by the evaluators. This section should illustrate that the results in the pages to follow are based on reliable data and a careful, generally conservative, analysis.

The Findings from Data Analysis and Conclusions about the Program

Although this section is positioned fairly late in the report, it is frequently the one to which readers flip immediately after the executive summary. It is the focal point of the document; it answers the evaluation questions. There are at least two common errors report writers make here: (1) claiming more than the evidence suggests, and (2) claiming things not suggested in the evidence at all. Both are lethal errors to be avoided at all costs.

In an evaluation report you want to present not only positive findings (significantly more men in the program lost more weight than did men in the control group) but also negative ones (fewer men attended the second half of the program than the first half). The objective of this part of the report is both to present and interpret findings and to explore explanations for results. If fewer men attended as the program continued, what were some possible reasons? Did they tire of the program? Were the later sessions less relevant to their needs? Were there changes in their work schedules? Did every person reach his weight-loss goal early? The world rarely operates just as you expect, and an evaluation report that reads as if all went perfectly is at best inaccurate and at worst dishonest. The report gives you the opportunity to hazard guesses or present additional data to show why the intended results were not achieved as well as why your expectations were reached or exceeded.

It is important to present data for every evaluation question posed and to interpret the meaning of each finding in relation to the overall aims of the program. In other words, you need to say why a particular finding is more or less important, given the impact and outcomes expected. This lends a perspective of the programmatic significance to the result. The statistical significance of a finding is an indication that the changes observed from before to after the program were likely not a random occurrence. Programmatic significance means that the changes had value to the learners and program planners, given all that the program aimed to accomplish.

While tables and graphs are often useful to depict findings, you should not overwhelm readers with them in the body of the report; rather, append them. Only a few, very pertinent and revealing tables or graphs should be included in the findings section. Similarly, the narrative should not repeat what is shown in the tables but should interpret, enhance, or expand on the data presented. You should describe all significant findings in the text in narrative form and refer readers to tables in the appendix for further detail when data are extensive.

The section should end with a summary of the findings and some general conclusions about the program and its accomplishments. The more analytical the review of findings and conclusions the better. This means thoughtful consideration of each result within the context of the learning program designed. It means not drawing conclusions about the program for which there are no empirical data (error 2 mentioned earlier) or making more of a finding than is really there (error 1). According to Isaac and Michael (1971, 159–61), the report writer should explicitly caution readers about conclusions. The soundness of the program can be undermined by sloppy or grandiose "analysis" and presentation of its results. The findings and conclusion section is the most important part of the evaluation report and reflects the evaluator's genuine understanding of the problem, what the program intended to accomplish, and the extent to which aims were met.

The Costs of the Program

With increasing frequency, health educators are being asked to comment in financial terms on the effectiveness and resulting benefits of programs. Indeed, some administrators want a detailed financial picture. As discussed in chapter 3 and appendix C there are several ways to ascertain the benefits and effectiveness of a program given its costs. These formulas are rarely definitive, but where they can be applied they provide some indication of whether the goals attained were financially beneficial and whether the program was the most effective vehicle for reaching the goal. Often it is not possible to illustrate cost effectiveness or benefit, because data needed from other sources are not available. Then, as discussed in chapter 3 and appendix C approximations are used and educated guesses made. Even when data are not available for a sophisticated analysis, you should be able to demonstrate what the program cost the sponsoring organization and estimate or give examples of the kinds of savings the education is likely to yield. These figures, as described previously, are fairly easy to compute.

Recommendations Based on the Evaluation Results

Many readers will expect you to make recommendations based on program outcomes. However, you must determine what kinds of recommendations are suitable based on the characteristics of the audience for the report. It is most appropriate for you to make programmatic rather than policy recommendations unless you were specifically asked to do the latter. A recommendation that a successful program be expanded to a larger audience is well within the prerogative of an evaluator; a recommendation that a hospital change its reimbursement pattern to accomplish this end is not. Recommendations, like conclusions, must grow out of the findings of the evaluation. Adding extraneous recommendations not supported by the data simply weakens the general effectiveness of the report. Some writers even refer to specific evidence in the body of the report when putting forward their suggestions.

Bear in mind that even the most successful program can generally use fine tuning, and the recommendations section is an opportunity to call attention to ways in which a program may be made even stronger. The quality assessment data and findings that describe the processes of program implementation can be particularly useful in recommending change or adustments. The questions usually addressed in a recommendations section are similar to those below:

1. Should the learning approach or content of the program be revised? If so, in what way?

2. Should the program staffing patterns be changed in any way?

3. Should there be changes in the types of personnel implementing the program?

4. Should there be adjustments in the budget allocations to various elements of the program?

5. Is the program generalizable to other groups of learners? If so, in what way might it best be expanded? How might it best be replicated?

GETTING THE REPORT READ BY DECISION MAKERS

One of the biggest complaints of evaluators is the underutilization of data. Findings are rarely used as much as they could be (Alkin, 1980). Getting the report read by the right people does not occur by magic. If you want your evaluation report to influence decisions, you must think through how best to reach the decision makers. One way to do this, as we have discussed, is to ensure that the material in your report is targeted to the interests of a specific audience. But there are other things you can do to generate interest.

According to Zweig and Marvin (1981, 11–22), the educating of any group (in this case, decision makers) by any other group (in this case, evaluators) cannot happen without a process that respects the institutions, culture, and practices of each. In other words, you must carefully consider the individual or groups you hope will use your report. How can you present your case for using the report so that it respects their point of view? Zweig and Marvin also suggest that evaluators need a conception of evaluation that takes into account the secondary place of evaluative information in day-to-day decision making. The decision maker will use your data as only one input into the decision. Your report is *primary* only to you. You must determine how your findings directly and indirectly relate to the priorities of the decision maker you want to reach. Spell out the uses of the data to that person's interests.

Sichel (1982, 82–84) believes that it is critical to give key individuals previews of the report. We agree. Relevant bits of information can be shared with decision makers in advance of open discussion or submission of the report. By reviewing material you can accomplish two things. First, you increase the chances that your material will be accepted by the decision maker. When you speak with him or her on an individual basis, you can better address that person's individual concerns. You will eliminate the element of surprise and can verify that you have been sensitive to the decision maker's position and perspective. Second, you can emphasize the policy implications and usefulness of the report to that particular decision maker. You can seize the opportunity to sell the decision maker on using your findings.

A report that sits on the shelf is of little use. Develop a strategy for reaching key people and assisting them to make data-based decisions.

SOME FINAL THOUGHTS ON THE EVALUATION REPORT

Anonymity

During the data collection period, it is likely that you assured program participants that the actions and opinions they allowed you to document would be anonymous in all evaluation documents. It is crucial that you honor this commitment and in no way write sections of the report so that the identity of individuals is revealed or can be deduced. The institutions, organizations, and services that were part of the health education program may also wish to remain anonymous. Before writing the report, you must determine how specific you can be in your description of people, places, and events while not violating participants' anonymity.

Sensitivity

Few things can unnerve even people with the strongest egos more than the idea of being evaluated. Successful evaluators approach both their subjects and their task in a way that reassures people that they are not being judged or labeled in negative ways. The evaluation report must be written with the same sensitivity. Even in the rare case when only a few people will see the document, a large measure of sensitive wording and phrasing of ideas is the most professional approach. You also want to ensure that the report is in no way offensive to those who have participated in good faith. To accomplish this end, you might ask someone familiar with the program but outside the evaluation team to read the report before it is distributed. The reviewer should be asked to judge its sensitivity to people, places, and events. This reader must, of course, be a trusted person who is pledged to keep confidential all that the document contains.

Confidentiality

Because evaluation reports—even glowingly positive ones—can be sensitive documents, you must accord them a certain confidentiality. It is important to determine at the outset the readership of the report. With members of the program hierarchy, you must then compile lists of those who are to receive the various forms of the document. You should also discuss with the administrators how the report is to be treated after its initial distribution. Will it be made freely available to all who express an interest in the program? Will it be given out only with the permission of someone within the sponsoring organization? Will it be marked "confidential"? Will it be piled at the doorway so that every visitor can pick it up? You need to know the ground rules for distribution and handling of the report.

Objectivity

The chapters of this text have stressed that the primary task of evaluators is to look objectively at a problem and the program designed to address it. Next, they must organize program descriptions and assessment data into clear communications for specific groups of readers. Objectivity must be reflected in every page of every evaluation report. In many ways, developing a health education program is the art of professional health education practice; evaluating it is the science. To develop future programs that will assist people to prevent and manage illness more fully, health educators must learn from the evaluations of current programs. In this sense, every health education program has the opportunity to contribute to the knowledge base of practice in addition to assisting individual learners. It is only by conducting careful, objective program evaluations, and communicating the resulting data to others in the most objective way, that the art and science of health education can be furthered.

APPENDIX **B**

Specification of the Role of the Entry-Level Health Educator

Area of Responsibility V:

The entry-level health educator, working with individuals, groups and organizations, is responsible for:

EVALUATING HEALTH EDUCATION (12%)

The entry-level health educator, working with individuals, groups and organizations, is responsible for:

Function: A.   Participating in developing an evaluation design. (24%)

Skill: 1.   The health educator must be able to assist in specifying indicators of program success.

Knowledge: The health educator must be able to:
              a.   differentiate between what can and cannot be measured (e.g., knowledge gained, changes in morbidity rates due to health education).
              b.   translate objectives into specific indicators (e.g., knowledge gained, values stated, behaviors mastered).
              c.   describe range of methods and techniques

Source: U.S. Department of Health and Human Services, Public Health Service, *Initial Role Delineation for Health Education. Final Report*, prepared for the National Center for Health Education, DHHS Publication no. (HRA) 80–44 (Washington, D.C.. Government Printing Office, 1980), pp. 78–82.

used for educational measurement (e.g., inventories, scales, competency tests).

d. list steps involved in evaluative activities (e.g., setting standards, specifying objectives, developing criteria for achievement of objectives).

Skill:

2. The health educator must be able to help to establish the scope for program evaluation.

Knowledge:

The health educator must be able to:

a. define scope of evaluation efforts (e.g., match standards with goals, explain relationship between activities and outcomes).

b. describe feasibility of evaluative activities (e.g., time availability, resources, setting, nature of the program).

c. explain the beliefs and purposes behind health education activities (e.g., value to consumers, increased control over health matters, informed public).

Skill:

3. The health educator must be able to help develop methods for evaluating programs.

Knowledge:

The health educator must be able to:

a. identify various measures for determining knowledge, attitudes and behavior (e.g., questionnaires, self-assessment inventories, knowledge tests).

b. describe data available for evaluation (e.g., program attendance, reports of behaviors, survey data, letters from consumers and others, test scores).

c. list strengths and weaknesses of various data collection methods (e.g., value of self-report, expense of observing behavior).

Skill:

4. The health educator must be able to participate in the specification of instruments for data collection.

Knowledge:

The health educator must be able to:

a. describe advantages and disadvantages of "home made" and commercial instruments (e.g., utility, cost, timeliness).

b.   identify sources of instruments (e.g., professional organizations, research organizations, consultants, textbook publishers).

Skill: 5.   The health educator must be able to assist in the determination of samples needed for evaluation.

Knowledge: The health educator must be able to:
a.   define sample concepts (e.g., stratified, random, convenience, universe).
b.   identify strengths and weaknesses of sampling techniques (e.g., sampling error, skewed results, normal distributions, precision of estimates).

Skill: 6.   The health educator must be able to assist in the selection of data useful for accountability analysis.

Knowledge: The health educator must be able to:
a.   describe the uses of cost-benefit analysis (e.g., modify programs, select alternative(s) from competing choices).

The entry-level health educator, working with individuals, groups and organizations, is responsible for:

Function: B.   Assembling resources required to carry out evaluation. (22%)

Skill: 1.   The health educator must be able to acquire facilities, materials, personnel and equipment.

Knowledge: The health educator must be able to:
a.   describe facilities, materials and equipment needed (e.g., telephones, typewriters, computers).
b.   identify required expertise and sources for expertise (e.g., survey methodology from universities, physician for clinical study, experts in evaluation).
c.   identify ways of obtaining necessary facilities, materials, expertise and equipment (e.g., personal visitations, formal requests, budgetary requisitions).

Skill: 2.   The health educator must be able to train personnel for evaluation as needed.

Knowledge: The health educator must be able to:

       a. describe the process for assessing training needs (e.g., listing skills needed, reviewing skills of available personnel, comparing skills with program requirements).

       b. describe steps for implementing training programs (e.g., specifying learning objectives, selecting instructional methods, carrying out methods, evaluating).

Skill: 3. The health educator must be able to secure the cooperation of those affecting and affected by the program.

Knowledge: The health educator must be able to:

       a. describe how to involve relevant parties in the evaluation process (e.g., explaining importance, answering questions, asking for cooperation).

       b. identify importance of safeguarding rights of individuals involved (e.g., explanation of purposes and procedures, confidential record-keeping).

       c. explain methods to maintain interest in program evaluation (e.g., importance of the work, reinforcement of effort, communication techniques, presentation of evaluation results).

The entry-level health educator, working with individuals, groups and organizations, is responsible for:

Function: C. Helping to implement the evaluation design. (30%)

Skill: 1. The entry-level health educator must be able to collect data through appropriate techniques.

Knowledge: The health educator must be able to:

       a. identify the applicability of various techniques to a given situation (e.g., observations, interviews, questionnaires, written tests).

       b. describe how to acquire data from existing sources (e.g., scan newspapers, review journal articles, scan morbidity and mortality data, health records).

c. distinguish between quantitative and qualitative data (e.g., counts vs. expressions of satisfaction, changes in physical indices vs. loss of interest).

Skill: 2. The health educator must be able to analyze collected data.

Knowledge: The health educator must be able to:
a. identify basic statistical measures (e.g., counts, means, medians).

b. describe processes of statistical analysis (e.g., selected analysis based on stated concern, collecting data, use of statistical techniques).

c. explain the results of statistical analysis (e.g., report data, make inferences, draw conclusions).

d. identify steps in analyzing qualitative data (e.g., developing categories, ascribing meaning to data, making inferences).

e. explain how data may be kept and used as needed (e.g., record keeping system, computer storage, filing systems, progress reports).

Skill: 3. The health educator must be able to interpret results of program evaluation.

Knowledge: The health educator must be able to:
a. identify relationships between analyzed data and program objectives (e.g., objectives met, reasons for lack of achievement, changes in program reflected in data).

b. recognize importance of looking for unanticipated results (e.g., appearance of seemingly unrelated results, significant deviations from what was expected).

c. identify variables necessary for interpretation of data (e.g., SES, sex, age, medical diagnosis).

d. recognize risks of drawing conclusions not fully justified by the data (e.g., program's value to other fields, program successes, program failures).

The entry-level health educator, working with individuals, groups and organizations, is responsible for:

Function: D.   Communicating results of evaluation. (25%)

Skill: 1.   The health educator must be able to report the processes and results of evaluation to those interested.

Knowledge: The health educator must be able to:
a. describe how to organize, write and report findings (e.g., objectives, activities, results, interpretation, conclusions).

b. translate evaluation findings into terms understandable by others (e.g., professionals, consumers, administrators).

c. explain various ways to depict findings (e.g., graphs, slides, flipcharts).

Skill: 2.   The health educator must be able to recommend strategies for implementing results.

Knowledge: The health educator must be able to:
a. list strategies that can be used for implementation (e.g., involve those affected, explain results to given audiences, propose new or modified programs).

b. identify implications from findings for future programs or other actions (e.g., alert others beyond programs, publish reports on programs and their evaluation).

Skill: 3.   The health educator must be able to incorporate results into planning and implementation processes.

Knowledge: The health educator must be able to:
a. describe how program operations can be modified based on evaluation results (e.g., discussions with personnel, proposed changes in objectives/methods/content).

b. explain how evaluation results are part of the planning process (e.g., formative vs. summative evaluation, self-renewal of programs).

APPENDIX C

First Principles of Cost-Effectiveness Analysis in Health

Donald S. Shepard
Mark S. Thompson

Cost-effectiveness analysis (CEA) is a technique for identifying the most effective use of limited resources. Originally developed in the military realm, CEA has come to be applied to many areas of social policy, including health care. Although the economics and medical literature contain a number of reviews of the technique (1–4), its principles deserve wider understanding as consumers, providers, and regulators increasingly participate in the shaping of health care policy. This paper is a nontechnical discussion of the principles of cost-effectiveness analysis applied to health, in particular, preventive health programs: these principles are illustrated with examples, and the strengths and weaknesses of this approach are discussed.

PRINCIPLES

Cost-effectiveness analysis is a way of summarizing the health benefits and resources used by health programs so that policy makers can choose among them. It summarizes all program costs into one number, all program benefits (the effectiveness) into a second number, and it prescribes rules for making decisions based on the relation between the two. The method is particularly useful in the analysis of preventive health programs, because it provides a mechanism for comparing efforts addressed to different diseases and populations (5). Cost-effectiveness analysis requires fewer troublesome steps than its

Reprinted with permission from *Public Health Reports*, Vol. 94, No. 6 (November–December 1979), pp. 535–543.

close relative, cost-benefit analysis, because CEA does not attempt to assign monetary values to health outcomes or benefits. Rather, CEA expresses health benefits in simpler, more descriptive terms, such as years of life gained. Details of cost-effectiveness analysis vary among practitioners and circumstances, and some problems still have not been resolved satisfactorily. The version we describe is a straightforward one applicable to a broad array of health programs.

An alternative, widely used formulation (2) is that CEA is a method to determine which program accomplishes a given objective at minimum cost. This alternative definition can be derived from the more general formulation for cost-effectiveness analysis: that is, the analysis of tradeoffs between monetary and nonmonetary (in this case health) effects.

The five major steps in our formulation of cost-effectiveness analysis are summarized in the chart.

STEPS IN COST-EFFECTIVENESS ANALYSIS

1. DEFINE THE PROGRAM	2. COMPUTE NET COSTS	3. COMPUTE NET HEALTH EFFECTS (in terms of additional years of healthy life)
• Develop alternative approaches to problem. • Define precisely programs to be analyzed (who, what, where, why, when, and how).	• Compute gross program costs. • Compute monetary savings. • Discount costs and savings to present value. • Compute net costs (gross costs less savings).	• Add —Additional years with full health, —Additional years of disease, —Improvement in health (no extension of life), —Negative effects (inconveniences and morbidity). • Modify by time preference factors.

4. APPLY DECISION RULES	5. PERFORM SENSITIVITY ANALYSIS	
• Identify case based on signs of net costs and net effects. • Apply rule for appropriate case.	• Vary uncertain parameters and recompute costs and health effects. • Examine effects on decision.	

Step 1. Define the program to be analyzed: its focus, processes, and limits. Seemingly minor differences in the definition of the program, such as targeting it to high-risk persons, can have major impacts on costs and effects. For these reasons, a precise definition of the program is critical.

A given problem may be amenable to a variety of approaches. Cost-effectiveness analysis can be used creatively, in conjunction with health expertise, to formulate innovative programs. One might use cost-effectiveness analysis first to compare markedly different programs, such as immunization or treatment, as a means for preventing deaths from influenza. If immunizations are identified as the best general approach, CEA can then be used to refine variants of an immunization campaign and to tailor its design to the specific situation.

Refinements involve such issues as the ages of the vaccinees and the means of delivery. The program to be analyzed can then be described by answering the six questions generally covered in the lead to a newspaper article: who, what, when, where, why, and how.

Step 2. Compute the net monetary cost for prevention and treatment of illness under the proposed program compared with the cost of the status quo. Generally, costs are computed from a societal perspective, that is, the value of all societal resources used in the program are counted as costs, regardless of who pays for them. It is often convenient to compute costs on a per participant basis.

There are four parts to step 2. The first is to compute the gross costs in each year of the program's operation. For example, if the program includes screening, the gross costs are those of screening, followup of positive results, and treatment of persons who might otherwise have gone untreated if their cases had not been found. The timing of each expenditure relative to the beginning of the program is noted.

The second part in computing net costs is to calculate the monetary savings attributable to the program, sometimes called direct benefits. These savings are the costs of avoided treatment that otherwise would have been obtained. Note that this step involves calculating the demand, rather than the need that is obviated. It would be inappropriate to count as monetary savings the avoidance of costs of needed services which are not now provided, so-called unmet need. The effects of services that obviate unmet need will be included as health benefits under step 3.

The third component in computing net costs is discounting to present value. Discounting is a procedure economists use to relate costs and savings occurring at different times to a common basis. The principle is that future costs are less expensive than present costs because (a) most people would accept less money to receive it sooner and (b) a smaller amount of money can be invested by society and allowed to grow at a compound rate of interest (analogous to the growth of a savings account) to yield the amount of money required for future costs. This rate of interest is called the discount rate. For example, suppose that one cost of a program is an expenditure of $1,000, but the expenditure will not be made for 5 years. Suppose the discount rate is 5 percent per year. The $1,000 is then discounted to about $780. In other words, $780 put aside and allowed to grow at 5 percent will become $1,000 in 5 years. The principle of discounting also applies to savings achieved by the health program.

The discount rate, usually in the range of 5 to 15 percent, depends on the cost of obtaining money for the institution for which the analysis is being conducted (for example, society as a whole, an employer, or a health provider). Because there may be uncertainty or disagreement about the rate, the analysis is sometimes repeated using alternative discount rates. The discount rate used should reflect opportunity costs and the rate of time preference for money. Uncertainty and "market imperfections" (especially divergences caused by income taxes between the social productivity of investment and private return) complicate the determination of the appropriate discount rate. Despite a vast economic literature—see for example Meyer (6)—this issue is still not entirely resolved.

Net costs are calculated in the fourth part of this step by subtracting savings from gross costs—both in present-value terms. Net costs can be positive, negative, or zero.

Step 3. Compute the health effects or benefits. Cost-benefit analysis requires that benefits be expressed in monetary terms, but cost-effectiveness analysis permits the use of any commensurate measure of benefits. Lives saved, complications averted, or cases of illness prevented are examples of possible benefit units. A more general and sometimes preferable measure is the additional healthy year of life, also known as the quality-adjusted life year, or QALY (7). Function years and well years are similar concepts (8). Additional years of healthy life are the algebraic differences between the number of healthy years a program recipient expects to live because of the existence of the program being evaluated and the number of healthy years he would have expected had there been no program. Estimation of these numbers must rely heavily on epidemiologic findings, expert opinion, controlled trials and, when available, randomized trials.

Health effects must be calculated from the same perspective (for example, societal or governmental) and basis (total, or per participant) as costs. The change in years of healthy life resulting from a program may be expressed as the sum of four types of health effects.

The first and most valued type of effect is additional years of healthy survival. If, for example, a preventive program postpones death by 1 year during which perfect health is maintained, then the effect is 1 additional healthy year of life.

The second type of effect is also a postponement of death, but during this extension of life, perfect health is not maintained. The proposed program in this instance is said to achieve "additional years of disease." Suppose that, for example, preventive care extends the life of a recipient by 1 year, but during it the recipient is restricted to home. Presumably, the recipient does not value that year as highly as a year of perfect health. The CEA should reflect this valuation. A year restricted to home might, for example, be valued at 80 percent of complete health. Percentages such as these are value judgments that should reflect the preferences of affected persons. Although assessment of these preferences is difficult, progress in determining such values has been made through interviews with patients (9), through forced-choice questionnaires with professionals (7), and through interviews with consumers (8, 10).

The third type of effect is an improvement in health without affecting survival. For example, one's symptoms or the restrictions of being homebound might be relieved. The benefit, in these cases, is the difference between the value of a year at lower life quality and the value of the year at the improved level of health.

The fourth type of effect is negative; the adverse effect arises because some health programs are inconvenient or have some associated morbidity, or restrict activities. Examples of preventive measures with negative effects are requirements that a staunch Bostonian move to Phoenix, Ariz., for asthma relief, that a person visit his physician weekly, or that he discontinue his favorite foods or activities. Presumably, a year with these restrictions is preferred to the alternatives of premature death or sickness, but it may not be valued as highly as a year of full activity without these restrictions. The negative effect is the difference between the value of a year without restrictions and the value of a year with restrictions. The negative effect might, for example, be 5 percent of a year.

Programs with only one type of effect (for example, averting deaths in a narrow age range) are relatively straightforward to evaluate; changes in that effect are compared to costs. More problematic are programs with diverse effects: perhaps extending some lives at perfect health, extending others at impaired health, enhancing the quality of health of other lives without extending them, and having negative effects on still other lives. To measure all these effects by a common metric is a formidable task. While the QALY holds promise of being an appropriate common unit, the practical difficulties of converting various impacts on health into QALY terms should not be underestimated. A more concrete measure of effects, such as cases of cancer prevented, should be used whenever it is common to all programs being compared.

All health effects should be subject to a discount factor, based on the society's time preferences. Generally, people prefer their health benefits sooner rather than later (9). Suppose, for example, that one preventive measure promised 5 additional healthy years and those 5 years were to be the next 5 years. Another preventive program promised 5 additional healthy years that would not start for 20 years. We would probably prefer the program that provided us with the benefits sooner. This observation implies that benefits should be discounted, though not necessarily at the same rate as costs. Many analysts, for example Weinstein and Stason (4, 11), add the further assumption that society's tradeoff between money and marginal health effects remains constant over time. This assumption achieves the convenient result that benefits are discounted at the same rate as costs.

The present values of the four types of effects can be summed to give a measure of present net effects. These net effects will be in units of years of healthy life.

Step 4. Apply a decision rule based on the net costs and net health effects. The rule must be selected from among the four cases, as described in table 1.

In the first case, the net costs and net effects are both positive; that is, there are true benefits but also real costs. In other words, the health of recipients is judged to be better with the proposed program than it would have been without the program, but the program uses resources. In these situations a cost-effectiveness ratio is calculated by dividing the cost by the improvement in years of healthy life. The result is a measure of efficiency, expressed as dollars per year of healthy life. The lower this number, the more efficient is the program, in the sense that it can produce years of healthy life at relatively low cost for a year. If funds are limited, then they should be spent first on the more efficient programs; that is, on those activities that would produce years of healthy life more cheaply.

The second case is that the net costs are negative or zero and the effects are positive. The proposed program improves (or at least does not impair) health, and it reduces costs as well. This kind of program is obviously desirable. Health programs fall into the case 2 situation if they are inexpensive, highly effective, and prevent illness for which expensive treatment would be sought. Provision of sanitary water, immunization against common diseases, fluoridation of community water supplies to reduce dental caries, or antibiotic treatment of streptococcal sore throat are possible illustrations.

Table 1   Decision rules in cost-effectiveness analysis

Net effects	Net costs positive	Net costs zero or negative
Positive	CASE 1. Cost-effectiveness = net costs ÷ net health effects. Select most efficient programs for improving health (lowest ratios).	CASE 2. Program economically valuable. Should generally be implemented.
Zero or negative	CASE 3. Program benefits offset by morbidity and inconvenience. Program generally should not be implemented.	CASE 4. Cost effectiveness = net costs ÷ net health effects. Select most efficient programs for containing costs (highest ratios).

The third case arises when the net effects are negative and the net costs are positive. In other words, the morbidity and inconvenience associated with the preventive program more than offset the health benefits that it produces. Such programs cost money while worsening health. Unless compelling factors excluded from the CEA indicate otherwise, such programs should not be implemented.

In the fourth case, the net effects are negative, but net costs are also negative. A program in this category restrains cost but may sacrifice health. Closing a health facility is a case 4 situation. To measure efficiency in cost containment, a cost-effectiveness ratio like that in the case 1 instances should be calculated. A program that entails no sacrifice in health (an infinite ratio) is best. Otherwise, the decision rule should be to select the program with the largest ratio. The selected program achieves the greatest savings per unit sacrifice in health. Programs that save resources but result in worse health should not be excluded automatically; by shifting those resources to more effective programs, overall improvements in health could be realized for the same total level of expenditure.

Step 5. The final step in a cost-effectiveness analysis is to perform a sensitivity analysis. Many of the procedures required to estimate costs and benefits require estimates of data and preferences that are not known with certainty. For example, it is not possible to predict exactly the future discount rate. Opinions can differ about the value of a year with impaired health relative to a year of perfect health. Finally, medical experts are uncertain about the value of various preventive measures, and their pofessional assessments are constantly updated with new research.

The sensitivity analysis is the process of deliberately varying these uncertain factors to examine their effect on the decision rule. If the final decision is not affected by making different assumptions about these uncertain quantities—by choosing high and low estimates, for example—then one can be relatively confident of the decision. If, on the other hand, the decision would be drastically altered by different estimates, then one should be considerably more cautious in making recommendations. Furthermore, one should, if possible, try to investigate further the precise values of these parameters before proceeding. One should also be alert to ways to gain more information about the uncertain issues.

APPLICATIONS

The hypothetical and two actual applications of cost-effectiveness analysis are presented as illustrations.

Hypothetical Inoculation Program

A hypothetical influenza inoculation program is being contemplated by a department of public health.

Step 1. Define the program. Vaccinations would be administered to 100,000 persons aged 65 and older over the next year by public health nurses in existing clinics and health centers.

Step 2. Compute net costs. On the basis of similar programs elsewhere, it is estimated that vaccinations cost $3 apiece (medications, marginal labor costs, and so forth). The inoculations are expected to prevent 1,000 cases of influenza this year and to result in 50 adverse reactions requiring treatment. The average cost of treatment for influenza is $50, and for the adverse reactions, it is $300. The discount rate for converting money and health effects to present value is 5 percent. Net costs for this program are calculated as follows:

Inoculations (100,000 × $3)	$300,000
Treatment of reactions (50 × $300)	+15,000
Gross program costs	$315,000
Savings due to people not getting influenza (1,000 × $50)	−50,000
Net program costs	$265,000

Because all costs would occur in the first year, discounting is not necessary.

Step 3. Compute net health effects. It is estimated that 10 people will not die of influenza this year as a result of this program. They will live for 8 (all healthy) years. Persons who avoid influenza as a result of the program experience an increase in the quality of their life of .04 of a healthy year. (They would have felt miserable with the illness, but it would not have lasted long.) The 50 persons suffering adverse reactions have their life quality lowered by .09 for the next year. Thus, the three health effects for prolonging 10 lives, enhancing the quality of 1,000 lives by preventing influenza, and impairing 50 lives through adverse reactions. A life prolonged by 8 healthy years is present valued not as 8 years but as 6.79 years, because the worth of all years after the first must be discounted. (The second year is valued as being worth $1 \div 1.05 = .952$ of the first year and so on.) The other effects are first-year effects and need not be discounted. The net health effects are calculated as follows:

Type of effect	Healthy years
Additional healthy years (10 × 6.79)	67.9
Health improvement for those spared the morbidity of influenza (1,000 × .04)	+40.0
Gross health effects	107.9
Negative effects of adverse reactions (50 × .09)	−4.5
Net health effects	103.4

Step 4. Apply decision rules. This is a case 1 situation: definite health gains are achieved, but at net positive costs. Dividing net costs by net health gains, we obtain the cost-effectiveness ratio: $265,000 ÷ 103.4 healthy years = $2,563 per healthy year.

This ratio should help decision makers to determine whether to implement the inoculation program. If alternative programs extend lives at costs of less than $2,563 per life year, they should be given funding preference over the inoculation program. If alternative programs cost more than $2,563 per life year extended, the inoculation program should be preferred.

Step 5. Perform sensitivity analysis. All parameters for the analysis that are subject to doubt may be varied to discover the impacts on the results. Suppose that some experts think that only 800 cases of influenza would be prevented by the inoculations. Such a supposition would reduce net savings by $10,000 (200 × $50), thus increasing net costs by that amount. Net health effects would be reduced by 8 (200 × .04) healthy years. The cost-effectiveness ratio is now: $275,000 ÷ 95.4 healthy years = $2,883 per healthy year.

Would this change affect decisions about the program? The first decision considered—whether or not to implement the inoculation program alone—might be affected. If decision makers conclude that they can afford to save lives and to enhance health at a cost of $2,700 per healthy year and that they cannot afford to pay more than this, then the decision is altered. Under the original analysis, the program would be implemented; under the revised analysis it would not be. The sensitivity analysis indicates to the decision makers how much uncertainty resides in the analysis that guides their actions.

Stool Guaiac Test

Neuhauser and Lewicki (12) analyzed the stool guaiac test in screening for colon cancer. The decisions in this application of CEA are both the basic desirability of the test and the optimal number of retests per patient. The cost-effectiveness approach may be used to address both

Table 2 Incremental cases of cancer detected and marginal cost per year of life saved by successive stool guaiac tests in a population of 10,000

Number of tests	Incremental cases detected	Cost per year of life saved
1	65.9469	$ 294
2	5.4856	1,373
3	0.4580	12,288
4	0.0382	117,384
5	0.0032	1,181,174
6	0.0003	11,776,803

Source: Reference 12.

issues. To reduce the chance of missing a case, the test can be repeated, but there are followup costs for all positive tests, both true and false positives. As shown in table 2, the cost per additional case identified mounts rapidly with test replications. The first screening test is highly cost effective: it gains an additional year of life for only $294. Further tests gain additional life years at progressively increasing costs. The additional benefit from six tests compared to five is so slight that the cost per additional case discovered, and the cost per year of life gained due to the sixth test, are in the millions of dollars. Pursuing such a screening program to the last degree of perfection is inefficient. Cost-effectiveness analysis indicates that resources might better be spent elsewhere, perhaps by more outreach and screening of high-risk persons.

Mobile Coronary Care Units

A mobile coronary care unit is an emergency vehicle with equipment and trained personnel for monitoring the victims and providing emergency treatment for heart attacks. It is intended to reduce mortality prior to hospitalization, the period when half of the heart attack deaths occur. Zeckhauser and Shepard (13) performed a preliminary analysis under the optimistic assumptions that these mobile units cut prehospital deaths in half and that the additional survivors have a prognosis comparable to past heart attack survivors (table 3). Discounting costs at the rate of 5 percent, they estimated the cost per 30-year-old male of having a mobile coronary care unit available for the rest of his life. The present-valued cost over the subject's remaining life-time for the unit and staffing it is $49. The cost of treating heart attacks that the recipient would not otherwise have lived to suffer is

Table 3 Computation of cost effectiveness (per male from age 30 years) of having a mobile coronary care unit in the area

Estimated lifetime cost or effect	Unit
Costs (dollars)[a]	
Unit and staffing	$ 49
Treatment of heart attacks	$ 52
Other medical treatment	$ 29
Total costs	$130
Health effects (QALYs)[b]	
Years before heart attack	0
Years with heart attack (.015 × 80 percent)	.012
Subsequent years (.057 × 95 percent)	.054
Total effects	.066
Cost effectiveness	
Cost effectiveness = $130 ÷ .066 QALY = $1,970 per QALY	

[a]Present value.
[b]QALY = quality adjusted life year.
Source: Reference 13.

$52, and the cost of other medical treatment arising from greater longevity is $29. The total is $130 per person.

As an initial indication of health effects, the authors calculated the impact of the mobile coronary care unit on life expectancy at age 30. They used data from the literature, subjective estimates for some parameters, and computer simulation. The gain in life expectancy estimated by these procedures was a third of a year, or 4 months. This measure was then refined to reflect two facts: (a) that these additional years are likely to be added far in the future, mostly between ages 55 and 80; and (b) that some of these additional years will be ones with impaired health due to heart attack.

In calculating the equivalent number of healthy years added by the mobile coronary care unit, certain assumptions about health quality were necessary. A year of life in which a heart attack occurs was assigned a value of only 80 percent that of a year in full health. The value was reduced to this level because the victim is hospitalized for several weeks, is homebound for several more weeks, and may be unable to work or to carry out normal activities for several months after the infarction. Second and later years after the attack were valued at 95 percent of the value of a year at full health. This value reflects the inability of some survivors, due to anxiety or to some residual disability, to resume full activities. Applying these quality-adjustment factors and a discount factor of 5 percent per year, the authors estimated net benefits to be .066 years—or only 24 days—per person. The final estimate of the cost-effectiveness of the mobile coronary unit is $130 divided by .066 years. This works out to be about $2,000 per perfectly healthy, present-valued year gained. Assuming that this ratio is correct, it indicates that the mobile coronary unit is a relatively efficient way of prolonging life.

Nevertheless, a sensitivity analysis indicates that this estimate should be regarded with caution. Although communities have installed mobile coronary care units, in some areas these units alone (without the backup assistance of citizens trained in cardiopulmonary resuscitation) reduce mortality very little (14). Whereas the analysis assumed that persons saved by these units would have a prognosis similar to that of other heart attack victims who reach the hospital alive, the prognosis may actually be considerably worse. In the latter instance, the benefits will be smaller.

The present value of the costs could be greater than the $130 per person that was estimated. That estimate assumed that the area being served was sufficiently populous to utilize a mobile coronary care unit fully and that the population was sufficiently dense so that the unit could reach the victim quickly. The cost-effectiveness ratio of $2,000 per healthy year cited previously might therefore be regarded as a best-case (or lower-bound) estimate. The cost effectiveness of mobile coronary care units could be 10 times worse, of $20,000 per additional year of healthy life. It would then be of the same order of magnitude as estimates made of the cost effectiveness of the treatment of moderate hypertension (11).

STRENGTH AND LIMITATIONS

Comparisons of Programs

For purposes of illustration, suppose that the hypothetical inoculation program were real and that the differences in discounting among the preceding illustrations could be ignored. Suppose that the health department was willing to invest in health programs only if it could buy years of healthy life at less than $5,000 per year. Then it would fund the cancer detection program with two repetitions (at $1,373 per healthy year), the mobile coronary care unit (at $1,970), and the inoculation program (at $2,563). The third stool guaiac test would not be pursued, and the mobile coronary care unit would be deferred if the unfavorable conditions in the sensitivity analysis prevailed.

Alternatively, suppose that the health department faced a budget ceiling, rather than a maximum amount per year. In these circumstances, we would allocate resources to programs in the order of their cost-effectiveness ratios until the budget was exhausted. That is, it would first fund the cancer detection program with two repetitions. It is the most cost effective of all the possible programs. If budget funds were left over, the department would next fund the mobile coronary care unit, the second most cost-effective program. Next in priority would be the inoculation program. If resources permitted, the third or fourth stool guaiac test could be added. This would not be done, however, until all programs with better cost-effectiveness ratios had already been funded. While cost-effectiveness analysis cannot determine the most appropriate total investment in health, it can indicate the best way to allocate a predetermined budget among health programs.

Data Limitations

The most salient practical problem in performing cost-effectiveness analysis is the lack of adequate data. Definitive data on the likely health effects of preventive programs are rare, and cost data, too, are often insufficient. While this problem complicates and reduces the precision of cost-effectiveness analysis, it may paradoxically increase the attractiveness of performing this analysis. Many important decisions cannot wait until ideal data are obtained. Compared with alternative processes for decision-making—for instance, cost-benefit analysis or intuition—cost-effectiveness analysis is better able to cope with data problems because CEA avoids the difficult problems of money valuation, and it uses a sensitivity analysis to check on the implications of uncertainty in the data. Cost-effectiveness analysis, moreover, provides a framework for using the available objective data and the subjective estimates of experts. Representative experts or consumers can be polled and ranges of values could be considered. A weakness of cost-effectiveness analysis, therefore, is that it rarely yields a single, definitive answer. Its partly compensating advantage is that assumptions are made explicitly and their effect on the analytic results is made clear.

Reflecting the Values of Consumers

A related weakness is the practical difficulty of incorporating consumers' input into an analysis. In theory, the method can incorporate the preferences of any representative consumer in evaluating alternative programs. Valuations of quality of life can be made by past, current, or prospective recipients of a treatment. Because these values are shown explicitly, the resulting analysis can be scrutinized to assure that these preferences, and expert opinions, have been interpreted correctly. With a sensitivity analysis, the opinions of many experts and the values of many consumers can be incorporated. Undoubtedly, however, analysts will need patience and sensitivity to elicit preferences that are expressed in a usable manner, and consumers may require examples and nontechnical explanations before accepting any numerical analysis.

The Unquantifiable Nature of Human Values

Some observers allege that cost-effectiveness analysis may interfere with humanistic values. They assert, as a matter of principle, that health should not be quantified. There is merit in this feeling. A society that based all its decisions on cost-effectiveness analysis might be efficient and healthy, but it could otherwise be cold and sterile. Nevertheless, 1978 health care expenditures amounted to $192 billion, and we cannot rely solely on intuition to choose among competing programs. Some systematic procedures are required. With care, we can obtain the benefits of procedures such as cost-effectiveness analysis while minimizing the dangers of dehumanized decisions. One solution is to use cost-effectiveness analysis primarily to establish general guidelines for the provision of preventive and curative services. Providers and administrators can view these guidelines as general recommendations, not inviolable laws, in making decisions about individual patients.

Determining Most Worthwhile Uses for Limited Resources

Lastly, an important strength of CEA should be mentioned. Many persons feel that preventive health services and educational efforts deserve an enhanced role if national health insurance is enacted. Unfortunately, if every preventive program that has been proposed, or even if every program that has some evidence of effectiveness were undertaken, we would spent much more than the present 9.1 percent of our gross national product on maintaining health. Since society is not prepared to allocate unlimited resources for health, it needs a method for deciding which activities are most worthwhile within ever-present cost restraints. We need to decide how to allocate resources between primary prevention and early detection, or between detection of new cases and followup and more effective treatment of the known ones. Cost-effectiveness analysis can also help us choose between medical approaches to protecting health, such as better emergency medical services versus better highway design. As long as the alternatives under consideration are directed at a common objective, cost-effectiveness analysis can help illuminate the tradeoff.

In summary, cost-effectiveness analysis cannot tell us what health program society should pursue, what preventive programs we should adopt; these answers as Fein wrote, "are up to society" (15). Cost-effectiveness analysis does, however, provide a framework for organizing information about the effectiveness and efficiency of health programs. With these results, consumers and health policy makers can make more enlightened decisions about which programs to adopt.

REFERENCES

1. Dunlop, D. W.: Benefit cost analysis: a review of its applicability in policy analysis for delivering health services. *Soc Sci Med* 9:133–139 (1975).

2. Klarman, H. E.: Application of cost-benefit analysis to health systems technology. In *Technology and health care systems in the 1980s*, edited by M. F. Collen. DHEW Publication No. (HSM) 73–3016. U.S. Government Printing Office, Washington, D.C., 1973.

3. Pliskin, N., and Taylor, A. K.: General principles: cost-benefit and decision analysis. In *Costs, risks, and benefits of surgery*, edited by J. P. Bunker, B. A. Barnes, and F. Mosteller. Oxford University Press, New York, 1977, pp. 5–27.

4. Weinstein, M. C., and Stason, W. B.: Foundations of cost-effectiveness analysis of health and medical practices. *N Engl J Med* 296:716–721, Mar. 31, 1977.

5. Lave, J. R., et al. Economic impact of preventive medicine. In *Preventive medicine USA*. Prodist, New York, 1976, pp. 675–714.

6. Meyer, R. F.: Preferences over time. In *Decisions with multiple objectives: preferences and value tradeoffs*, by H. Raiffa and R. L. Keeney. John Wiley & Sons, Inc., New York, 1977, pp. 473–514.

7. Pliskin, J. S., Shepard, D. S., and Weinstein, M. C.: Utility functions for life years and health status. *Operations Research*. In press.

8. Kaplan, R. M., Bush, J. W., and Berry, C. C.: Health status: types of validity and the index of well-being. *Health Serv Res* 11:478–507 (1976).

9. McNeil, B. J., Weichselbaum, R., and Pauker, S. G.: Fallacy of the five-year survival in lung cancer. *N Engl J Med* 299:1397–1401, Dec. 21, 1978.

10. Sackett, D. S., and Torrance, G. W.: The utility of different health states as perceived by the general public. *J Chronic Dis* 31:697–704 (1978).

11. Stason, W. B., and Weinstein, M. C.: Allocation of resources to manage hypertension. *N Engl J Med* 296:732–739, Mar. 31, 1977.

12. Neuhauser, D., and Lewicki, A. M.: National health insurance and the sixth stool guaiac. *Policy Analysis* 24:175–196 (1976).

13. Zeckhauser, R., and Shepard, D. S.: Where now for saving lives? *Law and Contemporary Problems* 40:5–45, autumn 1976.

14. Guzy, P. M., et al.: Survival of out-of-hospital emergencies requiring cardiopulmonary resuscitation in metropolitan Los Angeles. [Abstract.] *Clin Res* 27:278A (1979).

15. Fein, R.: *The economics of mental illness*. Basic Books, New York, 1958, pp. 137–138.

References

Alkin, M. C. 1980. A user focused approach. In *Conducting evaluations: Three perspectives*. New York: Foundation Center.

Alluisi, E. A. 1975. Optimum uses of psychobiological, sensorimotor, and performance measurement strategies. *Human Factors* 17(4):309–20.

Alvares, A. P.; Kappas, A.; Eiseman, J. L.; Anderson, K. E.; Pantuck, C. B.; Pantuck, E. J.; Hsiao, K. C.; Garland, W. A.; and Conney, A. H. 1979. Intraindividual variation in drug disposition. *Clinical Pharmacology and Therapeutics* 26(4):407–19.

American College of Sports Medicine. 1980. The recommended quantity and quality of exercise for developing and maintaining fitness in healthy adults. *Journal of Physical Education and Recreation* 1:17–18.

American Public Health Association, Committee on Professional Education. 1957. Educational qualifications and functions of public health education. *American Journal of Public Health* 47:1.

Anderson, A. 1976. Policy experiments: Selected analytic issues. In *Validity issues in evaluative research*, ed. I. N. Bernstein, 17–34. Sage Contemporary Social Science Issues, vol. 23. Beverly Hills: Sage Publications.

Anderson, R.; Kasper, J.; Frankel, M. R.; et al. 1979. *Total survey error: Applications to improve health surveys*. San Francisco: Jossey-Bass.

Andrasik, F., and McNamara, J. R. 1977. Optimizing staff performance in an institutional behavior change system: A pilot study. *Behavior Modification* 1(2):235–48.

Andrasik, F.; McNamara, J. R.; and Abbott, D. M. 1978. Policy control: A low resource intervention for improving staff behavior. *Journal of Organizational Behavior Management* 1:125–33.

Aneshencel, C. S.; Frerichs, R. R.; Clark, V. A.; and Yokopenic, P. A. 1982. Telephone versus in-person surveys of community health status. *American Journal of Public Health* 72(9):1017–21.

Argyris, C. 1970. *Intervention theory and method: A behavioral science view.* Reading, Mass.: Addison-Wesley.

● Arnold, M. 1973. Criteria for documentation and evaluation of cancer public education programs. *Health Education Monographs* 36:61–68.

Axelrod, M. 1975. Ten essentials for good qualitative research. *Marketing News* 10 (Mar. 14): 10–11.

Babbie, E. R. 1979. *Practice of social research.* Belmont, Calif.: Wadsworth.

Baggaley, J. 1982a. Electronic analysis of communication technique. *Media in Education and Development* 15(2):70–73.

Baggaley, J. 1982b. TV production research and media development. *Media in Education and Development* 15(1):46–48.

Baggaley, J., and Smith, K. 1982. *Formative research in rural education.* Institute for Research in Human Abilities Research Bulletin no. 82-003. St. John's: Memorial University of Newfoundland.

Bailar, B. A.; and Lanphier, C. M. 1978. *Development of survey methods to assess survey practices.* Washington, D.C.: American Statistical Association.

Baker, F., and McPhee, C. 1979. Approaches to evaluating quality of health care. In *Program Evaluation in the Health Fields*, vol. 2, ed. H. C. Schulberg and F. Baker, 187–204. New York: Human Sciences Press.

Bales, R. 1951. Interaction process analysis. Reading, Mass.: Addison-Wesley.

Bandura, A. 1977. *Social learning theory.* Englewood Cliffs, N.J.: Prentice-Hall.

Baranowski, T. 1978a. Defining a strategy for statewide health education needs assessment. Paper presented to the Second National Conference on Need Assessment in Health and Human Services, Louisville, Ky., March 29.

Baranowski, T. 1978b. Implications of the concepts of need for health education needs assessment strategy. Paper presented to the Second National Conference on Need Assessment in Health and Human Services, Louisville, Ky., March 29.

Baranowski, T.; Bee, D.; Rassin, D.; Richardson, J.; Brown, J.; Guenther, N.; and Nader, P. 1982. Social support, social influence, ethnicity and the breastfeeding decision. (Submitted.)

Baranowski, T.; Dworkin, R. J.; Cieslik, C.; Hooks, P.; Rains, D.; Ray, L.; Dunn, J. K.; and Nader, P. R. 1983. Comparison of observation with children's self-report of aerobic activity: Family Health Project. (Submitted.)

● Baranowski, T.; Evans, M.; Chapin, J.; Wagner, G.; and Warren, S. 1980. Utilization and medication compliance for high blood pressure: An experiment with family involvement and self-blood pressure monitoring in a rural population. *American Journal of Rural Health* 6(1–6):51–67.

Baranowski, T., and Fuller, C. 1981. Third party reimbursement for health education services in rural primary care clinics. *American Journal of Rural Health* 7(2):13–25.

●   Baric, L., ed. 1972. Behavioural sciences in health and disease. *International Journal of Health Education* 15(1):3–32.

●   Baric, L. 1980. Evaluation: Obstacles and potentialities. *International Journal of Health Education* 23(3):142–49.

Barker, R. F., and Blankenship, A. B. 1975. The manager's guide to survey questionnaire evaluation. *Journal of the Market Research Society* 17(4): 233–41.

Bartko, J. J., and Carpenter, W. T. 1976. On the methods and theory of reliability. *Journal of Nervous and Mental Disease* 163(5):307–17.

Baseline editors. 1982. Why evaluate health promotion programs? *Baseline* 1(1):2–4.

Becker, M. H. 1976. Sociobehavioral determinants of compliance. In *Compliance with therapeutic regimens*, ed. D. C. Sackett and R. B. Haynes, 40–50. Baltimore: Johns Hopkins University Press.

Becker, M. H., and Green, L. W. 1975. A family approach to compliance with clinical treatment. *International Journal of Health Education* 18:1–11.

Becker, M., and Maiman, L. 1975. Sociobehavioral determinants of compliance. *Medical Care* 13:10–24.

Berdie, D. F., and Anderson, J. F. 1974. *Questionnaires: Design and use.* Metuchen, N.J.: Scarecrow Press.

Bernstein, I. N., ed. 1976. *Validity issues in evaluative research.* Sage Contemporary Social Science Issues, vol. 23. Beverly Hills: Sage Publications.

Bernstine, R. L., and Baranowski, T. 1976. *Development, testing and evaluation of a Washington State prehospital emergency medical care reporting form.* Report to the Washington State Department of Social and Health Services. Seattle: Battelle Memorial Institute.

Bertrand, J. 1978. *Communications pretesting.* Chicago: University of Chicago, Community and Family Study Center.

Biron, P. 1975. Dosage, compliance and bioavailability in perspective. *Canadian Medical Association Journal*, 115:102–3.

Boatman, R.; Levin, L.; Roberts, B.; and Rugen, M., eds. 1966. Professional preparation in health education in schools of public health: A report prepared for the 1965 annual meeting, Association of Schools of Public Health, Ad Hoc Committee on Health Education. *Health Education Monographs* 21:1–35.

Bonham, G. S., and Corder, L. S. 1981. *NMCES household interview instruments: Instruments and procedures 1.* DHHS Publication no. (PHS) 81–3280. Washington, D.C.: National Center for Health Services Research.

Bonjean, C.; Maclemore, D.; and Hill, R. 1967. *Sociological measurement*. San Francisco: Chandler.

Boruch, R. 1976. Coupling randomized experiments and approximations to experiments in social program evaluation. In *Validity issues in evaluative research*, ed. I. N. Bernstein, 35–57. Sage Contemporary Social Science Issues, vol. 23. Beverly Hills: Sage Publications.

Bosanac, E. M.; Petersen, V. E.; Forren, G. L.; and Baranowski, T. 1982. A resource inventory approach to needs assessment: Examples from a statewide hypertension control program. *Social Science and Medicine* 16:1301–7.

Boyd, N. F.; Pater, J. L.; Ginsburg, A. D.; and Myers, R. E. 1979. Observer variation in the classification of information from medical records. *Journal of Chronic Diseases* 32:327–32.

Bradburn, N. M., and Sudman, S. 1979. *Improving interview method and questionnaire design*. San Francisco: Jossey-Bass.

Broskowski, A. 1979. Management information systems for planning and evaluation in human services. In *Program evaluation in the health fields*, vol. 2, ed. H. C. Schulberg and F. Baker, 147–71. New York: Human Sciences Press.

Bross, I. 1954. A confidence interval for a percentage increase. *Biometrics* 13(2):245–50.

Bruner, J. S. 1973. *Beyond the information given*. New York: Norton.

Buros, O. K. 1972. *Mental measurements yearbook*. 7th ed. Highland Park, N.J.: Gryphon Press.

Cambre, M. 1978. The development of formative evaluation procedures for instructional film and television: The past fifty years. Ph.D. diss., Indiana University, Bloomington.

Cambre, M. 1981. Historical overview of formative evaluation of instructional media products. *Education Communications and Technology Journal* 29(1):3–25.

• Campbell, D. 1969. *Reforms as experiments*. American Psychology 24(4): 409–29.

Campbell, D. 1975. Assessing the impact of planned social change. In *Social research and public policies*, ed. G. M. Lyons. Hanover, N.H.: Dartmouth College, Public Affairs Center.

• Campbell, D., and Stanley, J. 1966. *Experimental and quasi-experimental designs for research*. Chicago: Rand McNally.

Cannell, C. F.; Lawson, S. A.; and Hausser, D. L. 1975. *A technique for evaluating interviewer performance*. Ann Arbor, Mich.: Institute for Social Research.

Cannell, C. F.; Marquis, K. H.; and Laurent, A. 1977. *A summary of studies of interviewing methodology*. Vital and health statistics: Data Evaluation and Methods Research, series 2, no. 69. DHEW Publication no. (HRA) 77–1343. Rockville, Md.: National Center for Health Statistics.

Cannell, C. F.; Oksenberg, L.; and Converse, J. M., eds. 1977. *Experiments in interviewing techniques: Field experiments in health reporting, 1971–1977.* DHEW Publication no. (HRA) 78–3204. Washington, D.C.: National Center for Health Services Research.

Carey, L. C. 1972. The quality form. *Journal of Systems Management* 6(June): 28–30.

Clark, N. M. 1978. Spanning the boundary between agency and community. *American Journal of Health Planning* 3(4):40–46.

Clark, N. M. 1981. Should adult education be competency based? In *Examining controversies in adult education*, ed. B. W. Kreitlow, 126–42. San Francisco: Jossey-Bass.

Clark, N. M.; Feldman, C. H.; Evans, D.; Millman, E. J.; Wasilewski, Y.; and Valle, I. 1981. The effectiveness of education for family management of pediatric asthma: A preliminary report. *Health Education Quarterly* 8(2):166–74.

Clark, N. M.; Feldman, C. H.; Freudenberg, N.; Millman, E. J.; Wasilewski, Y.; and Valle, I. 1980. Developing education for children with asthma through study of self-management behavior. *Health Education Quarterly* 7(4):278–97.

Clark, N. M., and Pinkett-Heller, M. 1977. Developing HSA leadership: An innovation in board education. *American Journal of Health Planning* 2(1):9–13.

Clark, N. M., and Pinkett-Heller, M. 1979. The institution of administrative change in the home health service agency. *Home Health Services Quarterly* 1(1):7–17.

Clark, N. M., and Wolderufael, A. 1977. Community development through integration of services and education. *International Journal of Health Education* 20(3):189–99.

Cochran, D. 1969. Developments in evaluation: Their implications for health education practice. *Health Education Monographs* 29:59–69.

Cohen, J., and Cohen, P. 1975. *Applied multiple regression/correlation for the behavioral sciences.* Hillsdale, N.J.: Lawrence Erlbaum Associates.

Conner, R. F. 1979. The evaluator-manager relationship: An examination of the sources of conflict and a model for a successful union. In *The evaluator and management*, ed. H. C. Schulberg and J. H. Jerrel. Sage Research Progress Series in Evaluation, vol. 4. Beverly Hills: Sage Publications.

Connolly, T., and Porter, A. L. 1980. A user focused model for the utilization of evaluation. *Evaluation and Program Planning* 3:131–40.

Cook, T. D., and Campbell, D. T. 1983. The design and conduct of quasi-experiments and true experiments in field settings. In *Handbook of industrial and organizational psychology*, ed. M. D. Dunnette. New York: Wiley.

Cook, T. D., and Reichardt, C. S., eds. 1979. *Qualitative and quantitative methods in evaluation research.* Beverly Hills: Sage Publications.

Corroll, V. 1980. Employee fitness programs: An expanding concept. *International Journal of Health Education* 23(1):35–41.

Cox, D. R., and Snell, E. J. 1979. The choice of variables in observational studies. *Journal of the Royal Statistical Society,* series C, 23(2):51–59.

Cox, G. B. 1977. Managerial style: Implications for the utilization of program evaluation information. *Evaluation Quarterly* 1(3):499–508.

Creer, T.; Renne, C.; and Christian, W. 1976. Behavioral contributions to rehabilitation and childhood asthma. *Rehabilitation Literature* 37:226–32.

Dale, E., and Chall, J. 1948. A formula for predicting readability. *Educational Research Bulletin* 27(Jan.2):11–20, (Feb. 17):37–54.

Deeds, S.; Chwalow, A.; Green, L.; and Levine, D. 1975. Operational constraints on the design and implementation of health education research in a teaching hospital setting. Paper presented at the annual meeting of the American Public Health Association, Chicago.

Deeds, S.; Hebert, B.; and Wolle, J., eds. 1979. *A model for patient education programming.* Special Project Report. Washington, D.C.: American Public Health Association, Public Health Education Section.

Deeds, S., and Mullen, P., eds. 1981. Managing health education in health maintenance organizations: Part 1. *Health Education Quarterly* 8(4):279–375.

Deeds, S., and Mullen, P., eds. 1982. Managing health education in health maintenance organizations: Part 2. *Health Education Quarterly* 9(1):3–95.

Delbecq, A. L. 1974. Contextual variables affecting decision making in program planning. *Decision Sciences* 5(4):726–42.

Delbecq, A. L. 1978. Relating need assessment to implementation strategies: An organizational perspective. Paper presented to the Second National Conference on Need Assessment in Health and Human Services, University of Louisville, Ky.

Delbecq, A. L.; Van de Ven, A. H.; and Gustafson, D. 1975. *Group techniques for program planning: A guide to Nominal Group and Delphi processes.* Glenview, Ill.: Scott, Foresman.

• Deniston, O., and Rosenstock, I. 1968a. Evaluation of program effectiveness. *Public Health Reports* 83(4):323–35.

• Deniston, O., and Rosenstock, I. 1968b. Evaluation of program efficiency. *Public Health Reports* 83(7):603–10.

• Deniston, O., and Rosenstock, I. 1973. The validity of nonexperimental designs for evaluating health services. *Health Service Reports* 88(2):153–64.

Dickey, B., and Hampton, E. 1981. Effective problem-solving for evaluation utilization. *Knowledge: Creation, Diffusion, Utilization* 2(3):361–74.

Dillman, D. A. 1978. *Mail and telephone surveys: The total design method.* New York: Wiley.

Dinkel, N.; Zinober, J.; and Flaherty, E. 1981. Citizen participation in CMHC program evaluation: A neglected potential. *Community Mental Health Journal* 17(1):54–65.

Donabedian, A. 1966. Evaluating the quality of medical care, Part 2. *Milbank Memorial Fund Quarterly* 44:166–206.

Donabedian, A. 1968. Promoting quality through evaluating the process of patient care. *Medical Care* 6:191–202.

Dunn, W. 1980. The two communities metaphor and models of knowledge use. *Knowledge: Creation, Diffusion, Utilization* 1(4):515–36.

Dworkin, R. J.; Rains, D.; Baranowski, T.; Dunn, J. K.; Ray, L.; Vernon, S.; and Nader, P. R. 1983. Comparisons of dietary self-report methods: Family Health Project. (Submitted.)

Dwyer, F., and Hammel, R. 1978. An experimental study: Patient package inserts and their effects on hypertensive patients. *Urban Health* 7(June):46.

Easton, E.; Easton, M.; and Levy, M. 1977. Medical and educational malpractice issues in patient education. *Journal of Family Practice* 4(2):276.

Emerson, R. M. 1981. Observational field work. *Annual Review of Sociology* 7:351–78.

Employee Health Fitness editors. 1980. Absenteeism drop linked to hospital health promotion. *Employee Health Fitness* 2(11):135.

Ehrenberg, A. C. S. 1982. Writing technical papers and reports. *American Statistician* 36(4):326–29.

Farquhar, J.; Maccoby, N.; et al. 1977. Community education for cardiovascular health. *Lancet* 1(June 4):1192–95.

Feinstein, A. R. 1970. Quality of data in the medical record. *Computers and Biomedical Research* 3:426–35.

Feinstein, A. R. 1977. Clinical biostatistics XLI: Hard science, soft data, and the challenges of choosing clinical variables in research. *Clinical Pharmacology and Therapeutics* 22(4):485–98.

Ferber, B. 1968. Problems in abstracting and using data from hospital medical records. *Inquiry* 5(1):68–73.

Fink, A., and Kosecoff, J., eds. 1979. How to write an evaluation report. *How to Evaluate Health Programs*. Washington, D.C.: Capitol Publications.

Fitz-Gibbon, C., and Morris, L. 1978. *How to design a program evaluation.* Beverly Hills: Sage Publications.

Flanders, N. 1960. Interaction analysis: A technique for quantifying teacher influence. Paper distributed by Far West Laboratory for Educational Research and Development, San Francisco.

Fleiss, J. 1981. *Statistical methods for rates and proportions.* New York: Wiley.

Flesch, R. 1948. A new readability yardstick. *Journal of Applied Psychology* 32:221–33.

French, J. L., and Becker, S. W. 1975. Organizational intervention. In *The diffusion of medical technology*, ed. G. Gordon and G. L. Fisher. Cambridge, Mass.: Ballinger.

Freudenberg, N.; Feldman, C. H.; Clark, N. M.; Millman, E. J.; Valle, I.; and Wasilewski, Y. 1980. The impact of bronchial asthma on school attendance and performance. *Journal of School Health* 50(9):522–26.

Fry, E. 1968. A readability formula that saves time. *Journal of Reading* 11: 513–16. 575–78.

Glanz, K. 1980. Compliance with dietary regimens: Its magnitude, measurement, and determinants. *Preventive Medicine* 9:787–804.

Glaser, E. M., and Taylor, S. H. 1973. Factors influencing the success of applied research. *American Psychologist* 28:140–46.

Glass, G.; Willson, V.; and Gottman, J. 1975. *Design and analysis of time series experiments.* Boulder: University of Colorado, Laboratory of Educational Research.

Gorry, G. A., and Goodrich, T. J. 1978. On the role of values in program evaluation. *Evaluation Quarterly* 2(4):561–72.

Green, L. 1974. Toward cost-benefit evaluations of health education: Some concepts, methods, and examples. *Health Education Monographs* 2(1): 34–64.

● Green, L. 1977. Evaluation and measurement: Some dilemmas for health education. *American Journal of Public Health* 67(2):155–61.

Green, L. 1979. Educational strategies. In *Compliance in health care*, ed. R. B. Haynes et al., 286–94. Baltimore: Johns Hopkins University Press.

Green, L. and Brooks-Bertram, P. 1978. Peer review and quality control in health education. *Health Values: Achieving High Level Wellness* 2(4): 191–97.

Green, L., and Figa-Talamanca, I. 1974. Suggested designs for evaluation of patient education programs. *Health Education Monographs* 2(1):54–71.

Green, L.; Kreuter, M.; Deeds, S.; and Partridge, K. 1980. *Health education planning: A diagnostic approach.* Palo Alto, Calif.: Mayfield.

● Green, L.; Levine, D.; and Deeds, S. 1975. Clinical trials of health education for hypertensive outpatients: Design and baseline data. *Preventive Medicine* 4:417–25.

Green, L.; Werlin, S.; and Schauffler, H. 1976. *Research demonstration issues in self care.* Cambridge, Mass.: Arthur D. Little.

Green, S. B. 1981. A comparison of three indexes of agreement between observers: Proportion of agreement, G-index, and kappa. *Educational and Psychological Measurement* 41:1069–72.

Greene, R. 1976. *Assuring quality in medical care.* Cambridge, Mass.: Ballinger.

Greer, A. L. 1977. Advances in the study of diffusion of innovation in health care organizations. *Milbank Memorial Fund Quarterly, Health and Society* 19:505–32.

Groves, R. M. 1979. A researcher's view of the SRC computer-based interviewing system: Measurement of some sources of error in telephone survey data. In *Health survey research methods, third biennial conference*, ed. S. Sudman. DHHS Publication no. (PHS) 81–3268. Washington, D.C.: National Center for Health Services Research.

Groves, R. M., and Kahn, R. L. 1979. *Surveys by telephone: A national comparison with personal interviews*. New York: Academic Press.

Grubbs, F. E. 1969. "Procedures for detecting outlying observations in samples." *Technometrics* 11:1–21.

Gurel, L. 1975. The human side of evaluating human services programs: Problems and prospects. In *Handbook of evaluation research*, vol. 2, ed. M. Guttentag and E. L. Struening. Beverly Hills: Sage Publications.

Haggerty, R. 1977. Changing life styles to improve health. *Preventive Medicine* 6:276–89.

Hawkins, J.; Rorfman, R.; and Osborne, P. 1978. Decision makers' judgments: The influence of role, evaluative criteria, and information access. *Evaluation Quarterly* 2(3):435–54.

Health Education Monographs editors. 1977. Guidelines for health education preparation and practice. Health Education Monographs 5(1):1–18.

Hecht, R. 1978. Guide to media program development. Stanford, Calif.: Stanford University, School of Medicine, Division of Instructional Media.

Herbert, J., and Attridge, C. 1975. A guide for developers and users of observation systems and manuals. *American Educational Research Journal* 12(1):1–20.

Hladik, W., and White, S. 1976. Evaluation of written reinforcement used in counseling cardiovascular patients. *American Journal of Hospital Pharmacy* 33:155–59.

Hochbaum, G. 1962. *Evaluation: A diagnostic procedure*. Studies and Research in Health Education, vol. 5. Geneva, Switzerland: World Health Organization, International Union for Health Education, International Conference on Health and Health Education.

Hochbaum, G. 1965. Research to improve health education. *International Journal of Health Education* 8(1):141–48.

House, A. E.; House, B. J.; and Campbell, M. B. 1981. Measures of interobserver agreement: Calculation formulas and distribution effects. *Journal of Behavioral Assessment* 3(1):37–57.

Hughes, G.; Hymowitz, N.; Ockene, J.; Simon, N.; and Vogt, T. 1981. The multiple risk factor intervention trial (MRFIT), V: Intervention on smoking. *Preventive Medicine* 10(4):476–500.

Inui, T. 1978. A common bond: Exploring the interface between health education and quality assurance. *Journal of Quality Assurance* 10(Oct.):6–7.

Isaac, S., and Michael, W. 1971. *Handbook in research and evaluation*. San Diego: Robert Knapp Publishing.

Iverson, D., guest ed. 1981. Promoting health through the schools: A challenge for the eighties. *Health Education Quarterly* 8(1):1–117.

Janis, I., and Mann, L. 1977. *Decision making*. New York: Free Press.

Jenkins, C. D.; Rosenman, R. H.; and Zyzanski, S. J. 1974. Prediction of clinical coronary heart disease by a test for the coronary-prone behavior pattern. *New England Journal of Medicine* 290(23): 1271–75.

Johnson, S. M., and Bolstad, O. D. 1973. Methodological issues in naturalistic observation: Some problems and solutions for field research. In *Behavior change: Methodology, concepts, and practice*, ed. L. A. Hamerlynck, L. C. Handy, and E. J. Mash. Champaign, Ill.: Research Press.

Joint Committee on Standards for Education Evaluation. 1981. *Standards for evaluations of educational programs, projects, and materials.* New York: McGraw-Hill.

Jordan, L. A.; Marcus, A. C.; and Reeder, L. G. 1979. Response styles in telephone and household interviewing: A field experiment from the Los Angeles health survey. In *Health survey research methods, third biennial conference*, ed. S. Sudman. DHHS Publication no. (PHS) 81–3268. Washington, D.C.: National Center for Health Services Research.

Kalton, G.; Collins, M.; and Brook, L. 1978. Experiments in wording opinion questions. *Applied Statistics* 27(2): 149–61.

Kaplun-le Meitour, A., ed. 1973. Twenty years of health education: Evaluation and forecast. *Proceedings of the 8th International Conference on Health Education.* Paris: International Conference on Health Education.

Kelly, K. 1979. Evaluation of a group nutrition education approach to effective weight loss and control. *American Journal of Public Health* 69(8): 813–14.

Kenny, D. 1975. A quasi-experimental approach to assessing treatment effects in the nonequivalent control group design. *Psychology Bulletin* 82: 345–62.

Kerlinger, F. 1973. *Foundations of behavioral research.* 2d ed. New York: Holt, Rinehart and Winston.

Klare, G. 1974–75. Assessing readability. *Reading Research Quarterly* 1: 62–102.

Knutson, A. 1952. Application of pretesting in health education. *Public Health Monographs* 42(6): 1–10.

• Knutson, A. 1959. The influence of values on education. *Health Education Monographs* 3: 32–40.

Koskela, K.; Puska, P.; and Tuomilehto, J. 1976. The North Karelia project: A first evaluation. *International Journal of Health Education* 19(1): 59–66.

Kouzes, J. M., and Mico, P. R. 1979. Domain theory: An introduction to organizational behavior in human service organizations. *Journal of Applied Behavioral Science* 15: 449–69.

Kouzes, J. M., and Mico, P. R. 1980. How can we manage divided houses? *New Directions for Mental Health Services* 8: 43–57.

Kurtz, D. L., and Boone, L. E. 1981. *Marketing.* New York: Dryden Press.

• Larry, R., chair. 1973. *Report of the president's committee on health education.* New York: Public Affairs Institute.

Lau, R. R., and Ware, J. F., Jr. 1981. Refinements in the measurement of health-specific locus-of-control beliefs. *Medical Care* 19(12):1147–58.

Laurent, A.; Cannell, C. F.; and Marquis, K. F. 1972. *Reporting health events in household interviews: Effects of an extensive questionnaire and a diary procedure.* National Center for Health Statistics, Data Evaluation and Methods Research, series 2, no. 49. DHEW Publication no. (HSM) 72–1049. Rockville, Md.: Health Services and Mental Health Administration.

Levin, L.; Katz, A.; and Holst, E. 1976. *Self-care: Lay initiatives in health.* New York: Prodist.

Levine, A., and Levine, M. 1977. The social context of evaluation research: A case study. *Evaluation Quarterly* 1(4):515–42.

Ligouri, S. 1978. A quantitative assessment of the readability of PPIs. *Drug Intelligence and Clinical Pharmacy* 12:712–16.

Little, A. 1976. *A survey of consumer health education programs.* Final Report submitted to the Office of the Assistant Secretary for Planning and Evaluation/Health on Contract no. HEW 100–75–0082. Washington, D.C.: Department of Health, Education, and Welfare.

Liu, K.; Cooper, R.; McKeever, J.; Byington, R.; Soltero, I.; Stamler, R.; Gosch, F.; Stevens, E.; and Stamler, J. 1979. Assessment of the association between habitual salt intake and high blood pressure: Methodological problems. *American Journal of Epidemiology* 110(2):219–26.

Lofland, J. 1971. *Analyzing social settings.* Belmont, Calif.: Wadsworth.

Luck, D. J.; Wales, A. G.; Taylor, D. A.; and Rubin, R. S. 1978. *Marketing research.* New York: Prentice-Hall.

McKnight, J. L. 1978. Community health in a Chicago slum. *Development Dialogue* 1:62–68.

McLaughlin, G. 1969. SMOG grading—a new readability formula. *Journal of Reading* 12(May):639–46.

McNutt, K. 1980. Dietary advice to the public: 1957–1980. *Nutrition Reviews* 38(10):353–60.

Manning, D. 1981. Writing readable health messages. *Public Health Reports* 96(5):464–66.

Meals for Millions Foundation. 1981. *Healthy lifestyle for seniors.* Santa Monica, Calif.: Meals for Millions Foundation.

Mezirow, J.; Darkenwald, G.; and Knox, A. 1975. *Last gamble on education.* Washington, D.C.: Adult Education Association.

Michnich, M.; Shortell, S.; and Richardson, W. 1981. Program evaluation: Resource for decision making. *Health Care Management Review* 6:25–35.

Miller, J., and Lewis, F. 1982. Closing the gap in quality assurance: A tool for evaluating group leaders. *Health Education Quarterly* 9(1):55–66.

Mojonnier, M. L.; Hall, Y.; Berkson, D. M.; et al. 1980. Experience in changing food habits of hyperlipidemic men and women. *Journal of the American Dietetic Association* 77:140–48.

Morley, J., and Levine, A. 1982. The role of the endogenous opiates as regulators of appetite. *American Journal of Clinical Nutrition* 35:757–61.

Morris, J. 1980. Vigorous exercise in leisure: Protection against coronary heart disease. *Lancet* 8206:1207–10.

Morris, L. L., and Fitz-Gibbon, C. T. 1978. *Evaluator's handbook*. Beverly Hills: Sage Publications.

◊ Mullen, P., and Iverson, D. 1980. Qualitative evaluation models: Improving the effectiveness of health education programs. Paper presented at the American Public Health Association Annual Meeting, Detroit, October 21.

Mullen, P., and Zapka, J. 1982a. *Guidelines for health education and promotion services: Completing an HMO program*. Washington, D.C.: Department of Health and Human Services, Office of Health Information, Health Promotion, Physical Fitness and Sports Medicine.

Mullen, P., and Zapka, J. 1982b. *Guidelines for health promotion and education services in HMOs*. Washington, D.C.: U.S. Department of Health and Human Services, Public Health Service.

Nader, P. R.; Gilman, S.; and Bee, D. E. 1980. Factors influencing access to primary health care via school health services. *Pediatrics* 65(3):585–91.

National Center for Health Education. 1980. Health education and credentialing: The role delineation project. *Focal Points* 3(July):1–31.

Neaton, J.; Broste, S.; Cohen, L.; Fishman, E.; Kjelsberg, M.; and Schoenberger, M. 1981. The multiple risk factor intervention trial (MRFIT), VII: A comparison of risk factor changes between the two study groups. *Preventive Medicine* 10(4):519–43.

Nickerson, R. 1979a. The formative evaluation of instructional television programming using the program evaluating analysis computer. In *Experimental research in TV instruction*, vol. 2, ed. J. Baggaley. St. John's: Memorial University of Newfoundland.

Nickerson, R. 1979b. Program evaluation using the program evaluation analysis computer (PEAC). Paper presented at the 1979 convention of the Association for Educational Communications and Technology, New Orleans, March.

Noelle-Neumann, E. 1970. Wanted: Rules for wording structured questionnaires. *Public Opinion Quarterly* 34:191–201.

Nunnally, J. C. 1978. *Psychometric theory*. 2d ed. New York: McGraw-Hill.

Ogden, H. 1978. Recent developments in health education policy. *Health Education Monographs* 6(suppl. 1):67–73.

Ogden, H. 1980. Health education as an element of U.S. policy. *International Journal of Health Education* 23(3):150–55.

Ostrom, D. 1978. *Time series analysis: Regression techniques*. Series: Quantitative Applications in the Social Sciences. Beverly Hills: Sage Publications.

Parcel, G., and Baranowski, T. 1981. Social learning theory and health education. *Health Education* 12(3):14–18.

Parkinson, R.; Green, L.; Beck, R.; Pearson, C.; McGill, A.; Collings, G., Jr.; Eriksen, M.; Merwin, D.; and Ware, B. 1982. *Managing health promotion in the workplace: Guidelines for implementation and evaluation.* Palo Alto, Calif.: Mayfield.

Patton, M. 1980. *Qualitative evaluation methods.* Beverly Hills: Sage Publications.

Patton, M.; Grimes, P.; Guthrie, K.; Brennan, N.; French, B.; and Blythe, D. 1977. In search of impact: An analysis of the utilization of federal health evaluation research. In *Using social research in public policy making,* ed. C. H. Weiss, 59–81. Lexington, Mass.: Heath.

Perry, C.; Killen, J.; Telch, M.; Slinkard, L. A.; and Danaher, B. G. 1980. Modifying smoking behavior of teenagers: A school-based intervention. *American Journal of Public Health* 70(7):722–25.

Pilisuk, M., and Minkler, M. 1980. Supportive networks: Life ties for the elderly. *Journal of Social Issues* 36(2):95–116.

Pless, I., and Pinkerton, P. 1975. *Chronic childhood disorder promoting patterns of adjustment.* London: Henry Kempton Publishing.

Polivka, L., and Steg, E. 1978. Program evaluation and policy development: Bridging the gap. *Evaluation Quarterly* 2(4):696–707.

Porter, A., and Chibocos, T. 1975. Common problems of design and analysis in evaluative research. *Sociological Methods and Research* 3:235–57.

Pratt, H. J. 1976. *The gray lobby.* Chicago: University of Chicago Press.

Public Health Reports editors. 1980. Special section: Health promotion at the worksite. *Public Health Reports* 95(2):99–200.

Puska, P.; Koskela, K.; and McAlister, A. 1979. A comprehensive television smoking cessation programme in Finland. *International Journal of Health Education* 22(4, suppl.):1–28.

Reeder, L. G., ed. 1978. *Health survey research methods, second biennial conference.* DHEW Publication no. (PHS) 79–3207. Washington, D.C.: National Center for Health Services Research.

Reeder, L. G.; Ramacher, L.; and Gorelnik, S. 1976. *Handbook of scales and indices of health behavior.* Pacific Palisades, Calif.: Goodyear Publishing.

Reppucci, N. D. 1973. Social psychology of institutional change: General principles for intervention. *American Journal of Community Psychology* 1(4):330–41.

Roberts, B. 1962. Concepts and methods of evaluation in health education. *International Journal of Health Education* 5(2):1–11.

Robinson, J. P., and Shaver, P. R. 1973. *Measures of social psychological attitudes.* Ann Arbor: University of Michigan, Institute for Social Research.

Roghmann, K. J., and Haggerty, R. J. 1972. The diary as a research instrument in the study of health and illness behavior: Experiences with a random sample of young families. *Medical Care* 10(2):143–63.

Roos, N. P. 1974. Influencing the health care system: Policy alternatives. *Public Policy* 22(2):139–67.

Rosenstock, I. 1960. Gaps and potentials in health education research. *Health Education Monographs* 8:21–27.

Rosenstock, I. 1975. General criteria for evaluating health education programs. In *Proceedings of the NHLI working conference on health behavior, May 12–15*, ed. S. M. Weiss. DHEW Publication no. (NIH) 76–868. Washington, D.C.: Government Printing Office.

Ross, H., and Mico, P. 1980. *Theory and practice in health education.* Palo Alto, Calif.: Mayfield.

Rossi, P.; Freeman, H.; and Wright, S. 1979. *Evaluation: A systematic approach.* Beverly Hills: Sage Publications.

Rossi, P., and Williams, W., eds. 1972. *Evaluating social programs: Theory, practice and politics.* New York: Seminar Press.

Roter, D. 1977. Patient participation in the patient-provider interaction: The effects of patient question asking on the quality of interaction, satisfaction, and compliance. *Health Education Monographs* 5(4):281–315.

Rubin, D. 1974. Estimating causal effects of treatments in randomized and nonrandomized studies. *Journal of Educational Psychology* 56(5):688–701.

Saccone, A. J., and Israel, A. C. 1978. Effects of experimental vs. significant other controlled reinforcement and choice of target behavior on weight loss. *Behavior Therapy* 9:271–78.

Schafer, R. B. 1978. Factors affecting food behavior and the quality of husbands' and wives' diets. *Journal of the American Dietetic Association* 72:138–43.

Schulberg, H. C., and Baker, F. 1968. Program evaluation models and the implementation of research findings. *American Journal of Public Health* 58(7):1248:55.

Schulberg, H. C., and Baker, F., eds. 1979. *Program evaluation in the health fields*, vol. 2. New York: Human Sciences Press.

Schulberg, H. C., and Jerrel, J. H., eds. 1979. *The evaluator and management.* Sage Research Progress Series in Evaluation, vol. 4. Beverly Hills: Sage Publications.

Schulberg, H. C.; Sheldon, A.; and Baker, F., eds. 1969. *Program evaluation in the health fields.* New York: Behavioral Publications.

Schuman, H., and Presser, S. 1977. Question wording as an independent variable in survey analysis. *Sociological Methods and Research* 6(2):151–70.

Shaw, M. E., and Wright, J. M. 1967. *Scales for the measurement of attitudes.* New York: McGraw-Hill.

Sherwin, R.; Kaelber, D.; Kezdi, R.; Kjelsberg, M.; and Thomas, H., Jr. 1981. The multiple risk factor intervention trial (MRFIT), II: The development of the protocol. *Preventive Medicine* 10(4):402–25.

Shortell, S., and Richardson, W. 1978. *Health program evaluation.* St. Louis: Mosby.

Sichel, J. 1982. *Program evaluation guidelines.* New York: Human Sciences Press.

Siemiatycki, J. 1979. A comparison of mail, telephone and home interview strategies for household health surveys. *American Journal of Public Health* 69:238–44.

Simmons, J., ed. 1975. Making health education work. *American Journal of Public Health* 65(Oct., suppl.):1–49.

Simon, S.; Howe, L.; and Kirschinbaum, H. 1972. *Values clarification.* New York: Hart.

Society for Public Health Education, Ad Hoc Committee. 1968. *Statement of functions of community health educators and minimum requirements for their professional preparation with recommendations for implementation.* Professional Preparation of Community Health Educators, National Commission on Accrediting. Washington, D.C.: Department of Health, Education, and Welfare, Public Health Service, Center for Disease Control.

Society for Public Health Education, Ad Hoc Task Force on Professional Preparation and Practice of Health Education. 1977a. Guidelines for the preparation and practice of professional health educators. *Health Education Monographs* 5(1):75–89.

Society for Public Health Education, Committee on Professional Preparation and Practice of Community Health Educators at the Baccalaureate Level. 1977b. Criteria and guidelines for baccalaureate programs in community health education. *Health Education Monographs* 5(1):90–98.

Somers, A., ed. 1976. *Promoting health: Consumer education and national policy.* Germantown, Md.: Aspen Systems.

Spector, P. 1981. *Research designs.* Series No. 023: Quantitative Applications in the Social Sciences, ed. J. L. Sullivan. Beverly Hills: Sage Publications.

Spiegel, C., and Lindaman, F. 1977. Children can't fly. *American Journal of Public Health* 67(12):1143–47.

Squyres, W. 1979. Using media in hospitals. In *Handbook of health education,* ed. P. Lazes, 133–62. Germantown, Md.: Aspen Systems.

Staggs, E. W. 1972. Maybe it's your forms. *Journal of Systems Management* 23(Mar.):8–12.

Starfield, B. 1974. Measurement of outcome: A proposed scheme. *Milbank Memorial Fund Quarterly* 5(1):39–50.

Steuart, G. 1965. Health, behavior and planned change: An approach to the professional preparation of the health education specialist. *Health Education Monographs* 20:3–26.

Steuart, G. 1969. Planning and evaluation in health education. In *Behavior change through health education: Problems of methodology,* 193–207. International Seminar on Health Education (Communication, Media, Evaluation). Hamburg, Germany: International Union for Health Education.

Stoner, S., and Fioullo, M. 1976. A program for self-concept improvement and weight reduction for overweight adolescent females. *Psychology* 13:30–35.

Strauss, M. A., and Brown, B. W. 1978. *Family measurement techniques: Abstracts of published instruments, 1935–1974.* Rev. ed. Minneapolis: University of Minnesota Press.

Suchman, E. 1962. *What people know and do about health—more scientific rigor is needed.* Studies and Research in Health Education, vol. 5. Geneva, Switzerland: World Health Organization, International Union for Health Education, International Conference on Health and Health Education.

Suchman, E. 1967. *Evaluative research: Principles and practice in public service and social action programs.* New York: Russell Sage Foundation.

Sudman, S., ed. 1979. *Health survey research methods, third biennial conference.* DHHS Publication no. (PHS) 81–3268. Washington, D.C.: National Center for Health Services Research.

Sudman, S., and Lannom, L. B. 1980. *Health care surveys using diaries.* DHHS Publication no. (PHS) 80–3279. Washington, D.C.: National Center for Health Services Research.

Sukhatme, P., and Margen, S. 1982. Autoregulatory homeostatic nature of energy balance. *American Journal of Clinical Nutrition* 35:355–65.

Sullivan, D., ed. 1977. *Educating the public about health: A planning guide.* Health Planning Methods and Technology Series. DHEW Publication no. (HRA) 78–14004. Washington, D.C.: Department of Health, Education, and Welfare, Public Health Service.

Survey Research Center. 1976. *Interviewer's manual.* Rev. ed. Ann Arbor: University of Michigan, Institute for Social Research.

Thornberry, O. J., Jr., and Massey, J. T. 1978. Correcting for undercoverage bias in random digit dialed national health surveys. In *Proceedings, Survey Research Methods Section, American Statistical Association*, 224–29. Washington, D.C.: American Statistical Association.

Tinsley, H. E. A., and Weiss, D. J. 1975. Interrater reliability and agreement of subjective judgments. *Journal of Counseling Psychology* 22(4):358–76.

Trimby, M. J. 1979. Needs assessment models: A comparison. *Educational Technology* 19:24–28.

U.S. Congress, House. 1975. National Health Planning and Resources Act of 1974, Public Law 93–641, 93d Congress.

U.S. Congress, House. 1976. National Consumer Health Information and Health Promotion Act of 1976, Public Law 94–317, 94th Congress.

U.S. Department of Health, Education, and Welfare. 1978a. *Preparation and practice of community, patient, and school health educators.* DHEW Publication no. (HRA) 78–71. Washington, D.C.: Government Printing Office.

U.S. Department of Health, Education, and Welfare. 1978b. *Pretesting in cancer communications.* DHEW Publication no. (NIH) 78–1493. Washington, D.C.: Government Printing Office.

U.S. Department of Health, Education, and Welfare. 1979. *Healthy people: The surgeon general's report of health promotion and disease prevention.* Washington, D.C.: Government Printing Office.

U.S. Department of Health, Education, and Welfare. 1980. *Smoking and health: Report of the surgeon general.* DHEW Publication no. (PHS) 79–50066. Washington, D.C.: Government Printing Office.

U.S. Department of Health, Education, and Welfare, National Institutes of Health. 1980. Health message testing service. NIH Publication no. 80–2042. Washington, D.C.: Government Printing Office.

U.S. Department of Health, Education, and Welfare, National Institutes of Health, National Institute of Allergy and Infectious Disease Task Force. 1979. *Asthma and other allergic diseases.* NIH Publication no. 79–397. Washington, D.C.: Government Printing Office.

U.S. Department of Health, Education, and Welfare, National Institutes of Health, National Heart, Lung, and Blood Institute. 1977. *Handbook for improving high blood pressure control in the community.* Washington, D.C.: Government Printing Office.

U.S. Department of Health, Education, and Welfare, National Institutes of Health, National Heart, Lung, and Blood Institute. 1981. *Printed aids for high blood pressure education: A guide to evaluated publications.* DHEW Publication no. 81–1244. Washington, D.C.: Government Printing Office.

U.S. Department of Health and Human Services. 1979. *Biennial conference.* DHHS Publication no. (PHS) 81–3268. Washington, D.C.: National Center for Health Services Research.

U.S. Department of Health and Human Services, National Cancer Institute. 1980. *Pretesting in health communications: Methods, examples, and resources for improving health messages and materials.* NIH Publication no. 81–1493, rev. Nov. Washington, D.C.: Government Printing Office.

U.S. Department of Health and Human Services, National Cancer Institute, Office of Cancer Communications. 1979. *Readability testing in cancer communications.* NIH Publication no. 79–1689. Washington, D.C.: Government Printing Office.

U.S. Department of Health and Human Services, Public Health Service. 1980a. *Initial role delineation for health education: Final report,* prepared for the National Center for Health Education. DHHS Publication no. (HRA) 80–44. Washington, D.C.: Government Printing Office.

U.S. Department of Health and Human Services, Public Health Service. 1980b. *Promoting health/preventing disease: Objectives for the nation.* Washington, D.C.: Government Printing Office.

Uzzel, D. 1978. Four roles for the community researcher. *Journal of Voluntary Action Research* 8(pts. 1, 2):62–75.

Van de Ven, A. H. 1980a. Problem solving, planning and innovation, part I: Test of the program planning model. *Human Relations* 33(10):711–40.

Van de Ven, A. H. 1980b. Problem solving, planning and innovation, part II: Speculations for theory and practice. *Human Relations* 33(11):775–79.

Van de Ven, A. H., and Koenig, R., Jr. 1976. A process model for program planning and evaluation. *Journal of Economics and Business* 28(3):161–70.

Verbrugge, L. M. 1980. Health diaries. *Medical Care* 18(1):73–95.

Wang, V. L.; Ephross, P.; and Green, L. 1975. The point of diminishing returns in nutrition education through home visits by aides: An evaluation of EFNEP. *Health Education Monographs* 3(1):70–88.

Webb, E. J.; Campbell, D. T.; Schwartz, R. D.; and Sechrest, L. 1966. *Unobtrusive measures: Nonreactive research in the social sciences.* Chicago: Rand McNally.

Weeks, E. 1979. The material use of evaluation findings. In *The evaluator and management*, ed. H. C. Schulberg and J. H. Jerrel. Sage Research Progress Series in Evaluation, vol. 4. Beverly Hills: Sage Publications.

Weick, K. E. 1968. Systematic observational measures. In *Handbook of social psychology*, ed. G. Lindzey, and E. Aronson. Reading, Mass.: Addison-Wesley.

Weingarten, V.; Goodfriend, S.; and Harris, C. 1976. *Health education demonstration at Roosevelt Hospital.* New York: Institute of Public Affairs.

• Weiss, C. 1972. *Evaluation research: Methods for assessing program effectiveness.* Englewood Cliffs, N.J.: Prentice-Hall.

• Weiss, C. 1973a. Between the cup and the lip. *Evaluation* 1(2):49–55.

• Weiss, C. 1973b. Where politics and evaluation research meet. *Evaluation* 1(3):37–45.

Weller, L.; Arad, T.; and Levit, R. 1977. Self concept, delayed gratification and field dependence of successful and unsuccessful dieters. *Israel Annals of Psychiatry and Related Disciplines* 15:41–46.

Wholey, J.; Scanlon, J.; Duffy, H.; Fukumoto, J.; and Vogt. L. 1970. *Federal evaluation policy: Analyzing the effects of public programs.* Washington, D.C.: Urban Institute.

Wilkie, W. 1974. Analysis of effects of information load. *Journal of Marketing Research* 11:462–66.

Windle, C. 1979. The citizen as part of the management process. In *The evaluator and management*, ed. H. C. Schulberg and J. H. Jerrel. Sage Research Progress Series in Evaluation, vol. 4. Beverly Hills: Sage Publications.

Windle, C., and Cibulka, J. G. 1981. A framework for understanding participation in community mental health services. *Community Mental Health Journal* 17(1):4–18.

Windle, C., and Paschall, N. C. 1981. Client participation in CMHC program evaluation: Increasing incidence, inadequate involvement. *Community Mental Health Journal* 17(1):66–76.

Windsor, R. A. 1973. Mood modifying substances usage among 4H and non-4H youth in Illinois. *Journal of Drug Education* 3(3):261–73.

Windsor, R. A. 1977. Communications and information in international maternal child health (MCH) and family planning programs. Paper presented at the Institute for Reproductive Health, Physicians' Institute for Education in Gynecology and Obstetrics, Johns Hopkins Hospital, Johns Hopkins Medical Institution, Baltimore.

Windsor, R. A. 1978. Evaluation of education and training programs. Report presented to the National Institute for Arthritis, Metabolism, and Digestive Disorders (NIAMDD), Multipurpose Arthritis Centers Planning and Evaluation Workshop, National Institutes of Health, Bethesda, Md., May 22–23.

Windsor, R. A. 1980. *Program description competencies, MPH in community health education.* Birmingham: University of Alabama, School of Public Health, Division of Health Education–Health Behavior.

• Windsor, R. A. 1981. Improving patient education assessment skills of hospital staff: A case study in diabetes. *Patient Counseling and Health Education* 3(1):26–29.

Windsor, R. A. 1984. Planning and evaluating community health education programs in rural areas: Theory into practice. In *Case studies in health education practice,* ed. H. Cleary, J. Kichen, and P. Ensor. Palo Alto, Calif.: Mayfield.

• Windsor, R. A., and Cutter, G. 1981. Methodological issues in using time series designs and analysis: Evaluating the behavioral impact of health communication programs. In *Progress in clinical and biological research,* vol. 83: *Issues in screening and communications,* ed. C. Mettlin and G. Murphy, 517–35. New York: Alan R. Liss.

Windsor, R. A., and Cutter, G. 1982. Quasi-experimental designs for evaluating cancer control programs in rural settings. In *Advances in cancer control research and development,* Proceedings of the Third Conference on Cancer Control, ed. C. Mettlin and G. Murphy, 517–55. New York: Alan R. Liss.

Windsor, R. A.; Cutter, G.; and Kronenfeld, J. 1981. Communication methods and evaluation design for a rural cancer screening program. *American Journal of Rural Health* 7(3):37–45.

Windsor, R. A.; Kronenfeld, J.; Cain, M.; Cutter, G.; Goodson, L.; and Edwards, E. 1981. Increasing utilization of a rural cervical cancer detection program. *American Journal of Public Health* 71(6):641–43.

Windsor, R. A.; Kronenfeld, J.; Crawford, M.; Graves, L.; and Gams, R. 1983, in press. *Using concepts of social marketing to plan a new statewide cancer information service.* Public Education About Cancer, UICC Technical Report Series. Geneva, Switzerland: International Union for Cancer Control.

⦿ Windsor, R. A.; Kronenfeld, J.; Ory, M.; and Kilgo, J. 1980. Method and design issues in evaluation of community health education programs: A case study in breast and cervical cancer. *Health Education Quarterly* 7(3):203–18.

Windsor, R. A.; Roseman, J.; Gartseff, G.; and Kirk, K. A. 1981. Qualitative issues in developing educational diagnostic instruments and assessment procedures for diabetic patients. *Diabetes Care* 4(4):468–75.

Winkler, J.; Kanouse, D.; Berry, S.; Hayes-Roth, B.; and Rogers, W. 1981. *Informing patients about drugs, V: Analysis of alternative designs for erythromycin leaflets.* Santa Monica, Calif.: Rand Corp.

Witschi, J. C.; Singer, M.; Wu-Lee, M.; and Stare, F. J. 1978. Family cooperation and effectiveness in a cholesterol lowering diet. *Journal of the American Dietetic Association* 72:384–88.

World Health Organization, Expert Committee on Health Education of the Public. 1954. *First report.* WHO Technical Report Series no. 89. Geneva, Switzerland: World Health Organization.

World Health Organization, Expert Committee. 1969. *Planning and evaluation of health education services.* WHO Technical Report Series no. 409. Geneva, Switzerland: World Health Organization.

Yalom, I. 1970. *Theory and practice of group psychotherapy.* New York: Basic Books.

• Young, M. 1968. Review of research and studies related to health education practice (1961–66): Program planning and evaluation. *Health Education Monographs* 27:1–112.

Zapka, J., ed. 1982. *Research and evaluation in health education.* SOPHE Heritage Collection of Health Education Monographs, vol. 3. Oakland, Calif.: Third Party Publishing.

Ziegenfuss, J. T., Jr., and Lasky, D. I. 1975a. *Manual of topics for evaluation: A working document.* Harrisburg, Pa.: Dauphin County Executive Commission on Drugs and Alcohol.

Ziegenfuss, J. T., Jr., and Lasky, D. I. 1975b. A rationale for evaluating the quality of services in drug and alcohol programs: Purpose, process, outcome. *Drug Forum* 5(2):171–84.

Ziegenfuss, J. T., Jr., and Lasky, D. I. 1980. Evaluation and organizational development: A management-consulting approach. *Evaluation Review* 4(5):665–76.

Zinober, J. W.; Dinkel, N. R.; Landsberg, G.; and Windle, C. 1980. Another role for citizens: Three variations of citizen evaluation review. *Community Mental Health Journal* 16(4):317–30.

Zweig, F., and Marvin, K., eds. 1981. *Educating policymakers for evaluation.* Sage Research Progress Series in Evaluation, vol. 9. Beverly Hills: Sage Publications.

Index

Please send me _____ copies of EVALUATION OF HEALTH PROMOTION AND EDUCATION PROGRAMS by Richard Windsor, Thomas Baranowski, Noreen Clark, and Gary Cutter at $18.95 each (California state residents add sales tax) plus $1.50 postage and handling.

Enclosed is my check ☐, money order ☐, or credit card number (on reverse) ☐.

_____
Name

_____
Mailing address

_____
City   State   Zip

Please send me _____ copies of EVALUATION OF HEALTH PROMOTION AND EDUCATION PROGRAMS by Richard Windsor, Thomas Baranowski, Noreen Clark, and Gary Cutter at $18.95 each (California state residents add sales tax) plus $1.50 postage and handling.

Enclosed is my check ☐, money order ☐, or credit card number (on reverse) ☐.

_____
Name

_____
Mailing address

_____
City   State   Zip

Please send me _____ copies of EVALUATION OF HEALTH PROMOTION AND EDUCATION PROGRAMS by Richard Windsor, Thomas Baranowski, Noreen Clark, and Gary Cutter at $18.95 each (California state residents add sales tax) plus $1.50 postage and handling.

Enclosed is my check ☐, money order ☐, or credit card number (on reverse) ☐.

_____
Name

_____
Mailing address

_____
City   State   Zip

VISA or
MASTERCARD

Card number

Expiration date   Signature

Mail to: Mayfield Publishing Company
           285 Hamilton Ave.
           Palo Alto, CA 94301

Allow 4 to 6 weeks for delivery.

VISA or
MASTERCARD

Card number

Expiration date   Signature

Mail to: Mayfield Publishing Company
           285 Hamilton Ave.
           Palo Alto, CA 94301

Allow 4 to 6 weeks for delivery.

VISA or
MASTERCARD

Card number

Expiration date   Signature

Mail to: Mayfield Publishing Company
           285 Hamilton Ave.
           Palo Alto, CA 94301

Allow 4 to 6 weeks for delivery.